Risk Management and Litigation in Obstetrics and Gynaecology

Risk Management and Litigation in Obstetrics and Gynaecology

Edited by

Roger V Clements

Foreword by

Lord Daniel Brennan QC

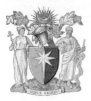

Royal College of
Obstetricians and
Gynaecologists

Setting standards to improve women's health

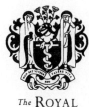

The ROYAL
SOCIETY of
MEDICINE
PRESS Limited

Published by the Royal Society of Medicine Press in association with the Royal College of Obstetricians and Gynaecologists, London

© 2001 Royal Society of Medicine Press Ltd
1 Wimpole Street, London W1G 0AE, UK
207 Westminster Road, Lake Forest, IL, 60045, USA

http://www.rsmpress.co.uk

British Library Cataloguing in Publication Data
A catalogue record for this book is available from the British Library

ISBN 1 85315 480 6

Phototypeset by Phoenix Photosetting, Chatham, Kent
Printed in Great Britain by Bell and Bain Ltd, Glasgow

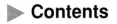 **Contents**

Part I: The Law

Part II: The Principles of Risk Management

Part III: Obstetrics

List of Contributors

David H Barlow Nuffield Professor of Obstetrics and Gynaecology, University of Oxford, Women's Centre, John Radcliffe Hospital, Oxford

Peter Bowen-Simpkins Honorary Treasurer of the Royal College of Obstetricians and Gynaecologists, London

Peter C Buchan Consultant Obstetrician and Gynaecologist

Roger V Clements Consultant Obstetrician and Gynaecologist, Harley Street, London

Peter R F Dear Consultant and Senior Lecturer in Neonatal Medicine, St. James's University Hospital, Leeds

James Owen Drife Vice President, Royal College of Obstetricians and Gynaecologists, London, and Consultant Obstetrician and Gynaecologist, Leeds General Infirmary

Nicholas M Fisk Professor of Obstetrics and Gynaecology, Queen Charlotte's and Chelsea Hospital, Imperial College School of Medicine, London

Robert Francis QC 3 Serjeants' Inn, London

Donald M F Gibb Independent Consultant Obstetrician, Circus Road, London

Elizabeth-Anne Gumbel QC 199 Strand Chambers, London

Gerry Jarvis Consultant Gynaecologist, St James's University Hospital, Leeds

David R Knowles Clinical Co-ordinator, QRM Healthcare Limited, Exeter

Gillian M Lockwood Medical Director, Midland Fertility Services, Aldridge

Simon J Newell Consultant and Senior Clinical Lecturer, St James's University Hospital, Leeds

David Paintin Emeritus Reader in Obstetrics and Gynaecology, Imperial College School of Medicine at St. Mary's, London

Michael J Powers QC Leader: Medical Law Group, 4 Paper Buildings, London

Pat Soutter Reader in Gynaecological Oncology, Hammersmith Hospital, London

Martin Spencer Barrister, 4 Paper Buildings, London

Charles Vincent Professor of Psychology, University College London

Kieran Walshe Health Services Management Centre, School of Public Policy, University of Birmingham

James Watt Retired Solicitor, London

Julian Woolfson Consultant Obstetrician and Gynaecologist, Queen Mary's Sidcup NHS Trust

▶ Foreword

The professions are presently experiencing scrutiny by the media and the public as to their practices and standard of care. Doctors in particular are finding that their approach to medical practice is open to question, and often criticism. This reflects two factors: the concept of patients' rights is now entrenched in public thinking; and the debate on medical issues is now thoroughly exposed by the press and the media in a way that allows no professional secrecy. In many ways, this change is for the better – particularly with respect to calling on the profession, and doctors in particular, to understand fully the medical principles upon which the care of mother and child are practised, and the legal consequences surrounding such medical practice. Lawyers who specialize in clinical negligence are themselves subject to similar scrutiny. The revised system of legal aid public funding now requires that solicitors in the field should meet high standards of competence. If they do not do so, they cannot pursue clinical negligence cases using public funding. Parliament, moreover, and in particular the National Audit Office, carefully analyse the cost of clinical negligence to the National Health Service every year; it is to the nature and cost of legal claims that their analysis is usually directed. All this means that books aimed at educating practitioners as to risk management and litigation are now a necessity. This is such a book. I commend it to the conscientious doctor and lawyer concerned with the practice of, or legal issues arising from obstetrics and gynaecology.

The number of claims against the medical profession – doctors, nurses and ancillary staff – have increased significantly in recent times; and the damages recovered run into hundreds of millions of pounds. Many cases are not pursued after initial enquiries show that there is no evidence of negligence nor any matter that would justify a complaint. But of those that are pursued to trial, many are the result of tragedy arising during the management of pregnancy and birth. The professions, both medical and legal, now deal with negligence claims or public law issues arising from not only the traditional areas of obstetrics, but also gynaecology and fertility treatment.

In obstetrics, claims arising from brain damage occurring during labour or at delivery itself are now commonplace. The circumstances often involve consideration of how those treating mother and baby practised management of known risk. In early pregnancy, prenatal screening is now at an advanced stage. Parents, and in particular mothers, wish to exercise their right to determine whether a pregnancy should continue if it is probable that the child being carried would be born disabled. The House of Lords decided in *McFarlane* (see *McFarlane & Another v Tayside Health Board* [1999] 3 WLR 1301; Clinical Risk 2001; 7[1]: 20–22, and Chapter 6 herein) that there could be no recovery in damages in respect of the birth of a healthy child; however, it is now clear that damages may be claimed for the extra cost referable to bringing up a disabled child (see *Parkinson* (*Parkinson v St. James's and Seacroft University Hospital NHS Trust* [2001] EWCA CIV560, Court of Appeal. Brooke L.J., Hale L.J., Sir Martin Nourse, 11 April 2001).

The law has become more searching in its examination of the standard of care in medicine. The traditional standard of care set out in the *Bolam* test (see *Bolam v Friern*

Hospital Management Committee [1957] 2 All ER 118, and Chapter 6 herein) was that all the law required, and all that the patients were entitled to expect, is that the professional concerned will bring to bear that degree of skill and care which the ordinary skilled man or woman professing that skill can be expected to exercise. In the House of Lords decision in *Bolitho* (see *Bolitho v City and Hackney Health Authority* [1993] 4 Med LR 117, and Chapter 6 herein), it was established that in determining that standard of care, the practice under examination must be shown to withstand logical analysis. In other words, it must be *responsible* and *reasonable*. It is not enough simply to assert that others would have done the same in relation to the act or omission that is being questioned. In addition, the Civil Procedure Rules emphasize that expert evidence in clinical negligence must now involve not only analysis of the issues, but also exposition of contrary views to that expressed by the particular expert. The expert must deal with the contrary view in a logical and reasonable way so as to set out an objective analysis and conclusion.

These medical advances and developments in the law mean that the management of risk is a central issue in medical practice and legal analysis. The authors in this book, whether legal or medical, set out to explain helpfully and convincingly what the law is, and the reasonable standard of care to be expected in risk management by the medical profession.

The publication of the new edition of this book will therefore benefit in great measure not only the medical profession, lawyers and judges, but also the public.

Lord Daniel Brennan QC
June 2001

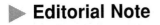 **Editorial Note**

At my request, the authors have adopted a convention in use of the personal pronoun which avoids the repeated use of the alternative gender. Whilst many obstetricians are female and a few midwives are male, for the simplicity of syntax obstetricians are referred to as 'he' and midwives as 'she'.

Part I
The Law

▶1

The Duties of the Obstetrician

Michael J Powers QC

Introduction

This chapter identifies the principal obligations that the obstetrician has to face in the performance of his professional skills. These obligations are defined and delimited by the force of law and by the pressure of social convention.

In every society, duties are recognised and owed under differing circumstances to other individuals of that society. In addition to the duty a doctor owes to his patient,[1] he/she also owes a duty to his/her profession, to his/her employer (if any) and to Society.

A duty may be defined as an act or course of action that is required of an individual by position, social custom, law or religion. Further to the constraints of conventional proscriptive law, under The Human Rights Act 1998 (which came into force on 2 October 2000) patients will be granted legal rights that will impact on NHS obstetric practice.

What then are the obstetrician's legal duties in his/her professional practice? Some are imposed strictly by statute. Others, such as the duties imposed by the common law, are less discrete and, in consequence, susceptible of development through the process of judicial precedent. Confusion often arises between the existence of the duty and the standard to which that duty has to be discharged. Whilst there is a single duty of care towards the patient, it may be breached by an obstetrician's acts or omissions in numerous ways.

The obstetrician is most likely to be confronted with his legal duty when faced with a civil action for damages for alleged negligence. In such circumstances, the claimant not only has to prove that there has been a breach of duty, she also has to prove that the breach resulted in some injury or loss.[2]

Duty to the profession

The basis of the duty owed by a medical practitioner to his/her profession is the public benefit of having the medical profession properly regulated and controlled. Thereby, it should be possible to ensure that acceptable standards of behaviour are followed by those permitted to retain the privilege of being a member of the medical profession. This is recognised in the Hippocratic Oath, which has guided the practice of medicine for over 2000 years. Thus, in addition to the obligations imposed by the civil and criminal law, registered medical practitioners also are subject to disciplinary control by the General Medical Council (GMC) pursuant to statutory powers[3] granted for that purpose. If the Professional Conduct Committee (PCC)[4] find any registered medical practitioner to be guilty of *serious* professional misconduct,[5] it has the power to erase that practitioner's name from the Register. Lesser penalties include suspension for a period not exceeding 12 months or conditional on the doctor's compliance with such requirements as the PCC thinks fit to impose for the protection of the public or in the doctor's own interests. Should an obstetrician be found seriously deficient in his/her performance, after an initial screening the GMC may require a period of rehabilitative training and re-assessment before he/she is allowed to resume practice.

The types of conduct that may lead to disciplinary proceedings include the following:

1. Removing ovaries without consent.[6]
2. Failure to visit a patient or to provide or to arrange treatment for a patient when necessary.
3. Failure to ensure that when clinical work is undertaken for private organizations providing healthcare, there are adequate clinical and therapeutic facilities for the services offered.
4. Failure to ensure that those appointed to deputize are doctors with appropriate qualifications and experience.[7]
5. Failure to take responsibility for delegation of aspects of medical care to a healthcare assistant.
6. Delegation of responsibilities which are imposed upon a registered medical doctor to a person who is not so registered.[8]
7. Prescription or supply of controlled drugs other than in the course of *bona fide* medical treatment.
8. Disclosure of confidential information about a patient.
9. Misuse of drugs or alcohol.
10. Dishonest behaviour.[9]
11. Taking part, in any way, in the trading of human organs or in the transplantation of organs obtained from donors whose consent has been given as a result of any form of undue influence.
12. Indecent or violent behaviour.
13. Any failure to inform the NHS hospital of the private patient status of a patient to enable him/her to be billed for the services provided to them.[10]
14. Any failure to disclose to a private patient any financial interest he/she (or any member of his/her immediate family) has in respect of any course of treatment he/she recommends.

It is an important responsibility of an obstetrician to inform an appropriate person or Body about a colleague whose professional conduct or fitness to practise may be called into question or whose professional performance appears to be in some way deficient. Although it is undoubtedly a difficult matter for any doctor to 'shop' a professional colleague, there is now statutory protection for whistle-blowers.[11] Regard first must be paid to the public interest in maintaining proper standards of medical practice. The culture of secrecy must end.[12] On the other hand, a doctor is under a duty not to undermine trust in a professional colleague's knowledge or skills, and to do so without justification is unethical and may amount to serious professional misconduct in itself.

Control of professional standards is not only in the hands of the GMC. The obstetrician's contract of employment usually includes provisions for the instigation of disciplinary action to be taken in respect of personal and professional misconduct or incompetence.

It is usually a requirement of a contract of employment that a consultant obstetrician should remain not only on the General Medical Register of the GMC but also be a member of the Royal College of Obstetricians and Gynaecologists. Therefore, one might think that the Royal College would have some muscle to effect disciplinary control over its members, with the ultimate sanction of the power to remove a doctor from membership. At the time of writing, the Royal College of Obstetricians and Gynaecologists are considering what can be done about incompetence but the only present event likely to result in such a loss of membership is the failure to pay subscription charges.

Duty to society: compliance with the law

The aspect of the criminal law that most worries any medical practitioner is that circumstances might arise which leave him to face a charge of manslaughter for the death of a patient in his care. Of late, there have been a number of convictions on charges of manslaughter and there does not appear to be any particular diffidence on the part of the Director of Public Prosecutions in bringing charges against doctors where there is sufficient evidence on the elements of the offence. The ingredients of involuntary breach of duty that need to be proved are as follows:[13]

(i)   The existence of the duty;
(ii) a breach of the duty causing death;
(iii) gross negligence which the jury considers justifies a criminal conviction.

The range of possible duties, breaches and surrounding circumstances is so varied that it is not possible to prescribe a standard jury direction appropriate in all cases. The judge should tailor his summing up to the specific circumstances of the particular case. However, . . . without purporting to give an exhaustive definition, we consider proof of any of the following states of mind in the defendant may properly lead a jury to make a finding of gross negligence: (a) indifference to an obvious risk of injury to health; (b) actual foresight of the risk coupled with the determination nevertheless to run it; (c) an appreciation of the risk coupled with an intention to avoid it but also coupled with such a high degree of negligence in the attempted avoidance as the jury consider justifies conviction; (d) inattention or failure to advert to a serious risk which goes beyond 'mere inadvertence' in respect of an obvious and important matter which the defendant's duty demanded he should address.

In particular, (d) is important, and questions directed to this issue first may be addressed to the obstetrician called to give evidence at a coroner's court. As with other courts, as long as the doctor is properly summoned, he/she is under a duty to attend,[14] and, once sworn, he/she is obliged to answer questions put to him/her.[15] Provided the questions are proper and relevant, they must be answered truthfully even though the answer may incriminate a professional colleague. A consultation document, issued in May 2000 by the Home Office, on the government's proposals for the reform of the law of involuntary manslaughter is available (see www.homeoffice.gov.uk/consult/invmans.htm).

Duty to the patient

1. Common law duty of care in tort

There is a general and comprehensive duty owed by the doctor to his/her patient,[16] but it is not so much the existence or extent of that duty which interests practitioners of obstetrics and gynaecology as the knowledge of what is required properly to discharge this duty in order to avoid entanglement with the law. The establishment of standards of medical care[17] carries with it the establishment of a duty of care to comply with those standards. Whether standards of care are set by the profession or by the courts is immaterial, provided there is an effective sanction for their breach. Most, if not all, obstetricians involved in medico-legal work are keen to see advancements in standards of care and, unhappily, many see the judicial process as the principal means of achieving that objective. Whilst some of the following illustrations may appear so obvious as to be laughable, more recent decisions are, if not moulding clinical practice themselves, at least to be seen as a consequence of developments in the standard of care:

1. A pregnant woman should not be placed in the same ward as a patient suspected of having puerperal fever.[18]
2. Having attempted to terminate pregnancy, it is negligent to fail to do so, more particularly in failing to inform the unhappy mother that another attempt could have been made to terminate the pregnancy after the failure of the first.[19]
3. Having attempted to perform a sterilization procedure, it may be negligent to fail to achieve sterilization,[20] but subsequent fertility is not necessarily evidence of negligence[21] and it is not negligent not to offer a hysterosalpingogram where there is no reason to doubt the effectiveness of a sterilization procedure.[22]
4. A doctor should inform a patient of the possible side effects of contraceptive treatment where a reasonable request is made for detailed information.[23]
5. An obstetrician should inform his patient at the earliest practicable moment when an amniocentesis fails to produce a result.[24]
6. Where there is a possibility of pregnancy and the patient has, by her words or actions, made known to the examining doctor that she does not wish to have a baby, it would be negligent of that doctor to dismiss such a possibility without performing a beta-hCG test on the patient's blood or other pregnancy tests on the patient's urine.[25]
7. Unintentional ligation of a ureter during a total abdominal hysterectomy with normal anatomy may be taken to be negligent.[26]
8. A Health Authority has a responsibility to ensure that assistance could be summoned within 10–15 minutes of birth.[27]

9. An anterior colporrhaphy within three months of birth is likely to be found to be negligent.[28]
10. Injury to small bowel during dilatation and curettage is likely to be found to be negligent.[29]
11. The cost of a commercial surrogacy agreement is not recoverable as being contrary to public policy.[30]
12. Cutting an adhesion when there was a risk – albeit a comparatively small risk but with catastrophic consequences – of cutting the small bowel, in circumstances where the surgeon was unable to see what he was cutting, is negligent when there was a reasonable prospect that he could have seen what he was cutting by the apparently simple expedient of opening a third port.[31]

Two particular duties require special attention: the duty to inform (covered in the chapter on consent) and the duty of confidentiality. Patients should be informed when anything has gone wrong with their treatment. Whilst there is no duty in law to inform *relatives* or even tell the truth about the circumstances of a death,[32] the GMC has made telling the truth to relatives (saving where issues of patient confidentiality arise) a matter of professional obligation.

Where there is a breach of duty in negligence, there must be a consequential loss for damages to be recoverable. This duty will be formally established until it can be shown that the failure to provide information to a patient about an adverse consequence of therapy has resulted in recoverable damages.

2. Common law duty of care in contract

The duty of care in private work (where there is a contract between the patient and the obstetrician) is usually no different from that between a NHS hospital doctor and his NHS patient. In looking at a contract in order to ascertain its nature and terms, the court applies an objective test, and what is in the minds of the parties is irrelevant:

> ... I do not think that any intelligent lay bystander (let alone another medical man) ... could reasonably have drawn the inference that the defendant was intending to give any warranty [as to sterility]. ... In my opinion, in the absence of any express warranty, the court should be slow to imply against a medical man an unqualified warranty as to the results of an intended operation, for the very simple reason that, objectively speaking, it is most unlikely that a responsible medical man would intend to give a warranty of this nature.
>
> **Per Slade L.J.[33]**

The common law duty upon a doctor to perform his professional services with reasonable skill and care is in statutory form in section 13 of the Supply of Goods and Services Act 1982. Such a term is statutorily implied into all agreements to provide private medical treatment.

A warranty to produce sterility in a patient about to undergo a sterilization procedure is not to be implied into a contract.[34] Nevertheless, there is nothing to stop a doctor giving an express warranty as to what he will or will not do, nor to subjecting himself to the legal consequences of a binding contract.

In practice, the principal difference to the practising clinician between a contractual duty of care and a duty of care owed in tort is that in the former, the obstetrician will be liable under the terms of the contract for any default of his registrar (or other doctor) to whom he delegates any of the care of his patient.

Duty to the unborn infant

In which circumstances will an obstetrician be liable for the birth of a normal child, and the birth of a defective child? To whom is this duty owed and what is the extent of the liability?

As there can be no contract between an obstetrician and an unborn child, if any duty arises at common law it is in tort. In respect of the mother, it is not necessary for a distinction to be made between tort and contract. The only tort with which we are concerned is the tort of negligence.

In order to succeed for an action in damages, the unborn child has first to be born;[35] and second it must be established that the obstetrician owed the child a duty of care during his/her intra-uterine life.[36]

The duty of care owed by the obstetrician to an unborn child exists at common law even though at the time any breach of the duty occurred no remedy exists for the fetus injured by the breach. The law has long been clear that whatever the interval between the breach of care and the infliction of injury, it is not until the injury is sustained that the matter is actionable and the Limitation Act begins to bite.[37]

Since the Congenital Disabilities (Civil Liability) Act 1976 came into force, there has been a statutory right to bring an action in respect of injuries sustained before birth. This right does not accrue to an unborn child until it is born[38] and the child has to survive birth for a minimum period.[39]

In some circumstances, the claim may only be brought by the child;[40] in other circumstances, the claim is that of the parents.

Wherever damages are recoverable in law for negligence, there is a concomitant and corresponding duty upon the obstetrician to avoid the harm that gives rise thereto.

Claims brought by the mother

Where a child has been born in circumstance where, but for the negligence of the obstetrician, he/she would not have been, the mother usually brings the claim for damages. This is because often she has a claim for personal injuries[41] over and above the claim for the financial consequences of the birth. There are five categories of case. These claims are to be distinguished from those that are brought by the injured infant (see below). Moreover, unlike the latter, where the time period for bringing the action is a minimum of 21 years from the date of birth (and unlimited where there has been significant permanent damage to the infant's intellect), there is a three-year time limit[42] within which the action has to be brought.

Case 1

The pregnancy of the mother may itself be the direct consequence of negligence on the part of the obstetrician (ie he has failed properly to perform a sterilization procedure).[43] The patient, believing that she is sterile, subsequently becomes pregnant. In such circumstances, upon appreciating that she is pregnant, the mother might have an abortion[44] and she would be entitled to the following:

(a) Pain and suffering associated with the termination of her pregnancy.
(b) Consequential financial losses.
(c) Pain and suffering associated with any further sterilization procedure.
(d) Financial losses (eg loss of income) directly lost by mother; this may include a claim for damages for loss of career prospects.[45]

Should the mother decide to continue with the pregnancy, the obstetrician would be liable for the following:[46]

(1) Pain and suffering associated with the unwanted pregnancy and delivery.
(2) Any enduring effects of the pregnancy/delivery which continue to have adverse effects upon her.
(3) Financial losses directly lost by mother associated with the unwanted pregnancy and delivery; this may include a claim for damages for loss of career prospects.[47]
(4) The financial cost of bringing up another child is not recoverable, although in the light of the *McFarlane and Another v Tayside Health Board* case, it remains to be resolved whether, in respect of a child who is disabled[48] and there is a consequential increased financial burden upon its parents, such additional expenses will still be recoverable.[49]

Case 2

Here, the pregnancy itself is not the consequence of any fault of the obstetrician; his negligence was in failing properly to advise his patient undergoing the sterilization procedure of the risks of failure. The mother cannot recover damages for the pregnancy itself. However, if, in consequence of her delayed realization that she was pregnant, she decides against a termination of pregnancy and goes to term, she is entitled to recover the same damages as the mother in Case 1 going to full term *less* a sum for the pain, suffering and any financial loss she would have suffered in any event had she had the pregnancy terminated. It is not considered that the mother has any claim for wear and tear and tiredness in bringing up a healthy child, as this is set off by the benefit of bringing a healthy child into the world.[50]

Case 3

The pregnant mother undergoes antenatal screening, which is performed negligently. She is told that the baby is normal when it is not. Had she been told the nature of the abnormality, the mother would have had a termination. In this case,[51] the mother is entitled to damages for pain and suffering and to the additional costs of raising the disabled child.[52]

Case 4

The pregnant mother undergoes antenatal screening, which is negligently performed. She is told that the baby is abnormal when it is not, and she has a termination of her pregnancy unnecessarily. The mother is entitled to damages for the pain and suffering and any financial loss associated with the termination procedure. It is conceivable that, in the event of the mother not being able to (or, alternatively, being unwilling to) have a further pregnancy, the court, in awarding damages, might discount the damages for the pain and suffering which the patient would have had in the event, had the pregnancy not been wrongly aborted. This would run the risk that the claimant might recover no damages, although I consider this to be an unlikely outcome where the real loss is that of a child which otherwise would have been born.[53]

Case 5

In this case, the mother suffers no direct personal physical injury.[54] She gives birth to a child brain-damaged through obstetric negligence. She is able to recover damages for any 'nervous shock' that she suffers. Insofar as her claim extends beyond that, it may do so successfully only to take into account the prospective costs 'thrown away' in going through a future 'replacement' pregnancy.

Claims brought by the infant

Case 6

Where a child is born with a disability that has been caused by negligence of the obstetrician, a claim may be brought on the child's behalf. The many claims that are now brought for cerebral palsy fall into this category.

Case 7

The child is injured by some force of nature – for example, rubella infection – during the mother's pregnancy. Through the negligence of the obstetrician, the pregnancy progresses without proper steps being taken to investigate and to advise the mother of her right to have a termination of pregnancy. If such a pregnancy goes to term, the child does not have a right to sue for damages on the basis that the child should never have been born ('wrongful life'). As such, a claim is considered to be contrary to public policy, and damages are not recoverable *by the child* for any antenatal failure to detect and abort it. This right at common law crystalizes on delivery of the child.[55]

Duty to the employer

Contracts of employment[56] within the National Health Service usually incorporate the General Whitley Council Conditions of Service, which, *inter alia*, set out expressly or by adoption the arrangements in respect of issues of professional conduct and/or competence arising.[57]

Since the NHS and Community Care Act 1990, NHS Trusts which are established thereunder are able to offer their career-grade staff whatever terms and conditions of service they wish.[58]

The Court of Appeal in *Johnstone v Bloomsbury Health Authority*[59]considered whether an express term in a contract, however onerous, has priority over an implied term as to health and safety. The Court of Appeal held by a majority that the well-established principle of contract (ie that implied terms are subject to express terms) should apply (notwithstanding that the NHS is effectively a monopoly employer of junior doctors). It was agreed that the express term in Johnstone's contract as a junior doctor which required him to work an 88-hour week was effectively an exclusion clause purporting to exclude the employing Health Authority from liability for personal injury and fell to considered under the provisions of the Unfair Contract Terms Act 1977. However, the court was not prepared to go into the public arena and debate complex issues of NHS funding.

Consequently, a doctor's duties to his employer (which are over and above those he would otherwise owe) are, subject to statutory provisions, controlled by the contract of employment into which he freely enters. As Legatt L.J. observed in *Johnstone*:[59] 'Those who cannot stand the heat should stay out of the kitchen'. Protection to the employee who whistle-blows is now conferred by the Public Interest Disclosure Act 1998.

Conclusions

If there were to be a single answer to the obstetrician's question, 'How can I avoid entanglement with the law?', I would, without hesitation, say that it must lie in the quality of the relationship between the doctor and his patient. The kind, courteous, sympathetic and considerate doctor who makes the time to listen and talk to his patients is unlikely to find himself charged with a breach of any duty. In the first place, he is less likely to make any serious error in the care of his patient; and secondly, if he does he is less likely to be sued for any incompetence or face a disciplinary tribunal.

'Defensive medicine' is a product of paranoia. If a patient suffers an injury, it is either caused negligently or it is not. No patient can recover damages for an injury resulting from an obstetrician's 'defensive' acts unless that patient shows that the obstetrician, in acting as he did, failed to act in accordance with a recognised body of obstetric opinion *or* that what was done could not withstand critical analysis.[60] One man's 'defensive medicine' is another's prudent discharge of his professional duties.

References

1   Particularly in the case of the obstetrician, this extends to his patient's unborn child.
2   The injury or loss has to be more than minimal.
3   Medical Act 1858 and s.36 and s.38–45 and schedule 4 to the Medical Act 1983 and The Medical (Professional Performance) Act 1995.

4   See R v General Medical Council ex p Toth – Queen's Bench Division (Crown Office List), Lightman J. – 23 June 2000 – limited powers of filtering complaints to GMC.

5   The phrase 'serious professional misconduct' was substituted by the Medical Act 1969 for the phrase 'infamous conduct in a professional respect' in the 1858 Act.

6   Slater v Baker [1767] 2 Wils. 359 – but see Re S, *The Times*, 16 October 1992. There have been several recent cases before the GMC where gynaecologists have been found guilty of serious professional misconduct for removing ovaries without express consent and without medical justification.

7   It is important to note that this applies to obstetricians and gynaecologists whether or not they are employed in the NHS: it is not a sufficient discharge of this duty to leave the matter to the employing authority as though it were that authority's sole responsibility. To this extent, a doctor may be accountable to the PCC of the GMC even in circumstances where, by virtue of having a common employer, he may effectively escape vicarious liability for the negligence of another doctor employee acting on his behalf. (See *infra* on the duty in the contractual relationship.)

8   Action has been taken against those who, by signing certificates or prescriptions, have enabled others to act as though they were registered medical practitioners.

9   This would include the prescription of a drug or an appliance in which they have a direct financial interest or in respect of which an improper inducement has been accepted.

10   Offence under section 2(1) of the Theft Act 1968 – see R v Firth (CA) [1990] 1 Med LR 411. The duty to inform the Health Authority is stressed in the 'Green Book' – *Management of Private Practice in the NHS*, DHS, March 1986.

11   Public Interest Disclosure Act 1998.

12   See the Ritchie Report into Quality and Practice within the NHS arising from the actions of Rodney Ledward (June 2000): '. . . if patient care is to be at the heart of the practice of medicine, then anything which has the potential to place patients at risk must be brought into the open and raised with appropriate clinical or managerial staff'. See www.doh.gov.uk/pdfs//ledwardinquiry.pdf.

13   R v Prentice [1994] QB 302 at 322 (Taylor L.C.J.).

14   Should he fail to do so, he would be liable to a fine not exceeding £1000 – s.10 Coroners Act 1988, as amended.

15   He may only refuse to answer a question with 'lawful excuse'. In practice, he may only refuse where to answer a question might incriminate him – Coroners Rule 1984 r 22; R v Boyes [1861] 1 B & S 311; Rio Tinto Zinc Corpn. v Westinghouse Electric Corporation [1978] AC 547; Rank Film Distributors Ltd v Video Information Centre [1982] AC 380.

16   'This general duty is not subject to dissection into a number of component parts to which different criteria of what satisfy the duty of care apply. . . .' per Lord Diplock in Sidaway v Board of Governors of the Bethlem Royal Hospital and the Maudsley Hospital [1985] AC 871.

17   This is presently being considered by the Royal College of Obstetrician and Gynaecologists' Working Group on maintaining good medical practice.

18   Heafield v Crane [1937] *The Times*, 31 July.

19   Scuriaga v Powell [1979] 123 SJ 406.

20   Emeh v Kensington & Chelsea & Westminster AHA [1985] QB 1012; Udale v Bloomsbury AHA [1983] 1 WLR 1098.

21   Eyre v Measday [1986] 1 All ER 497 (CA).

22   McLennan v Newcastle Health Authority [1992] 3 Med LR.

23   Blyth v Bloomsbury Health Authority (1985). *The Times*, 24th May. See also the GMC *Seeking Patient's Consent* (Feb 1999).

24   Gregory v Pembrokeshire Health Authority [1989] 1 Med LR 81 (CA).

25   Gardiner v Mountfield and Lincolnshire Health Authority [1990] 1 Med LR 205.

26   Hendy v Milton Keynes Health Authority (No. 2) [1992] 3 Med LR 119.

27   Bull and Wakeham v Devon Health Authority [1989] [1997] 4 MLR 117 (CA).

28   Clark v MacLennan and Another [1983] 1 All ER 416.

29   Bovenzi v Kettering Health Authority [1991] 2 Med LR 293.

30   Briody v St Helen's & Knowsley Area Health Authority [2000] Lloyds Med LR 127.

31   Burrows v Forest Health Care NHS Trust (CA) [2000] MLC 0149.

32   See Powell & Another v Boladz & Others [1998] Lloyds Med R 116 (CA).

33   Per Slade L.J. Eyre v Measday [1986] 1 All ER 488 at 495.

34   Thake v Maurice (CA) [1986] 1 All ER 497.

35   A fetus has no independent legal personality. Following birth, however, the infant has legal rights that, before its majority, may be exercised through a 'litigation friend'. The Limitation Act 1980 gives a child at least until the age of 21 years to bring an action. The period may be extended where the requisite knowledge is not acquired until after the age of 18 years. The 'limitation period' within which an action for

personal injuries has to be brought (subject to the overriding discretion of the court to bring an action outside this time) is three years from the date of knowledge. In respect of those with permanent brain damage, an action may be brought at any time on their behalf until three years after their death.

36   The duty of care owed by the obstetrician to an unborn child exists under the ss.1(2)(a) and (4) Congenital Disabilities (Civil Liability) Act 1976. See also: X and Y v Pal and Others [1992] 3 Med LR 195 (Aus NSW CA).

37   See Burton v Islington Health Authority [1992] 3 All ER 833 (CA).

38   See ss.1(2)(a) and (4). See also: X and Y v Pal and Others [1992] 3 Med LR 195 (Aus NSW CA).

39   The child has life for some period (however short), having been separated from its mother.

40   Through a 'litigation friend', who is usually the mother.

41   See Kralj v McGrath [1986] 1 All ER 54, where a mother's compensatory damages were increased by the impact of what had happened to her when her baby died eight weeks after injuries sustained by wholly unacceptable and horrific obstetric care.

42   Subject to a number of exceptions under the Limitation Act 1980.

43   A comparable claim could be brought against a surgeon where a vasectomy has been performed negligently. The standard of care which applies in the therapeutic context (the *Bolam* principle) also applied to contraceptive counselling: Gold v Haringay Area Health Authority [1988] 1 QB 481.

44   But she is under no obligation to, notwithstanding that she is under a general duty to mitigate her loss. (See Emeh v Kensington and Chelsea and Westminster Area Health Authority and Others [1985] 2 WLR 233 [CA].)

45   Allen v Bloomsbury Area Health Authority [1992] 3 Med LR 257.

46   See McFarlane & Another v Tayside Health Board [2000] Lloyds Med LR 1 (HL).

47   Allen v Bloomsbury Area Health Authority [1992] 3 Med LR 257.

48   A child injured by the negligence of the obstetrician has an action on its own behalf – see below.

49   Damages for an unwanted child after a negligent failure of sterilization (or related informed consent) has been distinguished from the foreseeable consequences of a negligent failure to terminate a pregnancy on medical grounds. The *additional* costs of raising a *disabled child* born as a consequence of failing to inform the parents that an antenatal screen suggested fetal abnormality – Rand v East Forest Health Authority [2000] Lloyds Med LR 181 (Newman J.)

50   Otherwise, where the child is handicapped: See Allen v Bloomsbury Area Health Authority [1992] 3 Med LR 257.

51   Subject to the termination of the pregnancy being lawful. See Rance & Another v Mid-Downs Health Authority [1991] 2 WLR 159.

52   See observations on the case of Rand, above.

53   There are no damages for bereavement for the loss of an unborn child. In the absence of a physical injury being suffered, the expectant mother would have to show she suffered a psychiatric injury (McLoughlin v O'Brien [1982] 2 All ER 298; Alcock v Chief Constable of the South Yorkshire Police [1991] 4 All ER 907).

54   No pain and suffering in the delivery of the child over and above that which she would have had in any event.

55   Burton v Islington Health Authority [1992] 3 All ER 833 (CA).

56   See Circular PM(7)11. A proforma for a consultant contract is set out in *The Consultant Handbook*. London: British Medical Association, November 1990.

57   But there is no contractual right: See Higgs v Northern RHA [1989] 1 Med LR 1.

58   The British Medical Association still urges those entering into contracts with NHS Trusts to ensure that the General Whitley Council Conditions of Service and the Terms and Conditions of Service of Hospital Medical and Dental Staff (England and Wales) are incorporated into contracts.

59   Johnstone v Bloomsbury Health Authority [1991] 2 All ER 293.

60   Bolitho & Others v City & Hackney Health Authority [1998] AC 232 (HL).

►2

Liability and Causation in Clinical Negligence Claims

Elizabeth-Anne Gumbel QC

Part 1: Liability

Situations in which clinical negligence may be alleged

There are a number of different situations in which a patient who has suffered personal injury may seek to bring a claim for clinical negligence against an individual clinician. The first task is to establish a relationship between the patient and the clinician that gives rise to a duty of care. The second task is to identify why the clinician is said to be in breach of that duty. The following list illustrates the broad range of circumstances in which a clinical negligence claim may be brought:

(a) Failing to arrange to see a patient when requested to do so and when urgent assessment is required;

(b) When seeing a patient (in a hospital/clinic or at home), failing to examine the patient competently or at all;

(c) After examining a patient, failing to diagnose the patient's condition competently within the expertise of the clinician;

(d) If a diagnosis cannot be made confidently by the initial clinician, failing to refer the patient to an appropriate specialist doctor, hospital/clinic for further investigation, including failing to arrange for the patient's immediate admission to hospital where that is required;

(e) After examining a patient, failing to give the patient competent advice as to his/her condition and the appropriate options for treatment;

(f) Failing to prescribe the correct and/or any treatment for the patient when treatment is required;

(g) Prescribing the wrong treatment for a patient so as to further injure the patient;

(h) Failing to carry out treatment by way of surgical operation or other procedure competently so that the result is to cause additional injury to the patient rather than any benefit;

(i) Failing to follow up the patient after examination or treatment when follow-up is necessary.

The identity of the defendant

The patient with a potential claim first will need to ascertain the correct identity of the defendant who is to be held responsible for the injury.

Every individual clinician owes a duty of care to his patient, and his patient may sue him for breach of duty. In the case of private treatment and of treatment by a general practitioner, the claim is brought against the individual clinician. In the case of National Health Service treatment in a hospital, the claim is brought against the Health Authority or NHS Trust ('the NHS Authority') who is responsible for that hospital.

The NHS Authority is vicariously liable for the acts of all its servants or agents so that if any doctor, nurse, midwife, radiographer, cytologist or other employee is found negligent, the NHS Authority itself will be found liable. This principle was first established in the cases of *Gold v Essex County Council*[1] and *Cassidy v Ministry of Health*.[2] Before these cases, it had been held that the hospital's obligation only extended to selecting competent doctors and nurses and that they could only be liable if they failed to do that.[3]

There is a further situation in which a patient may sue an NHS Authority: where the NHS Authority itself is alleged to be directly liable for its failure to provide the necessary facilities for competent treatment of the patient. Whilst liability is still in respect of the actions of servants or agent of the NHS Authority (who can only act through their servants or agents), the concept of direct liability is different; it applies to the errors of the organization itself rather than individual clinician's errors. An example of an NHS Authority being directly liable to a patient is the case of *Bull v Devon Area Health Authority*.[4] In that case, the NHS Authority was found liable when a consultant obstetrician took 68 minutes to attend to deliver a second twin and the baby suffered brain damage. Delay occurred as the hospital operated on two sites and the consultant obstetrician was required to travel from one site to the other to attend to the patient. The Court of Appeal, in dismissing the Health Authority's appeal, confirmed that:

> ... the system should have been set up so as to produce a registrar or consultant on the spot within twenty minutes, subject to some unforeseeable contingency ... there was an interval of about an hour ... this interval was much too long. Either there was a failure in the operation of the system, or it was too sensitive to hitches which fell short of the kind of major breakdown against which no system could be invulnerable.[5]

Duty of care and standard of care

The test that needs to be satisfied in law to establish negligence in respect of medical treatment, including obstetric treatment, is the same whether it arises from negligent advice, failure to warn, negligent technique in carrying out surgery, development or treatment of subsequent complications or any other complaint. The test is set out in *Bolam v Friern Barnet Hospital Management Committee*:[6]

> The test is the standard of the ordinary skilled man exercising and professing to have that special skill. A man need not possess the highest expert skill; it is well established law that it is sufficient if he exercises the ordinary skill of an ordinary competent man exercising that particular art ... there may be one or more perfectly proper standards, and if he conforms with one of those proper standards then he is not negligent ... a mere personal belief that a particular technique is best is no defence unless that belief is based on reasonable grounds.

The House of Lords followed and applied the *Bolam* test in *Maynard v West Midlands Regional Health Authority*,[7] but pointed out:

> It is not enough to show that subsequent events show that there is a body of competent professional opinion which considers there was a wrong decision, if there also exists a body of professional opinion equally competent, which supports the decision as reasonable in the circumstances . . . a doctor who professes to exercise a special skill must exercise the ordinary skill of his speciality. Differences of opinion and practice exist, and will always exist, in the medical as in other professions. There is seldom any one answer exclusive of all others to problems of professional judgment. A court may prefer one body of opinion to another: but that is no basis for a conclusion of negligence.

In the case of *Sidaway v Board of Governors of the Bethlem Royal Hospital and the Maudsley Hospital*,[8] the House of Lords approved the *Bolam* test as being:

> . . . a rule that a doctor is not negligent if he acts in accordance with a practice accepted at the time as proper by an acceptable body of medical opinion even though other doctors adopt a different practice.

It was stressed in the *Sidaway* case that the *Bolam* test clearly requires a different degree of skill from a specialist in his own special field than from a general practitioner. The qualifications of the doctor carrying out the treatment therefore will be relevant. First, it is necessary to investigate whether the doctor was suitably qualified and experienced to carry out the surgery he undertook at all. Second, if he was so qualified it is necessary to investigate whether or not the standard of the treatment was below that of a competent doctor in the same field.

In *Whitehouse v Jordon*,[9] the House of Lords considered the standard of care of an obstetrician attempting to deliver a baby by forceps. The allegation on behalf of the claimant was that he had been damaged during the forceps delivery by the force that had been applied. It was alleged that the obstetrician had pulled too long , using too much strength on the claimant's head during the attempt to deliver. Further, it was alleged that the obstetrician had continued traction using the forceps after the obstruction of the ischial spines had been encountered so that the claimant's head had become stuck. In the House of Lords, Lord Edmund Davies described how the principle questions calling for decision were as follows: In what manner did Mr Jordan use the forceps? And was the manner consistent with the degree of skill which a member of his profession is required to exercise?

Lord Edmund Davies pointed out that it was unacceptable to ask whether Mr Jordan had committed an error of judgement. He stated:

> To say that a surgeon committed an error of clinical judgment is wholly ambiguous, for while some such errors may be completely consistent with the due exercise of professional skill, other acts or omissions in the course of exercising clinical judgment may be so glaringly below proper standards as to make a finding of negligence inevitable . . . The test is the standard of the ordinary skilled man exercising and professing to have that special skill. If a surgeon fails to measure up to that standard in any respect ('clinical judgment' or otherwise), he has been negligent and should be so adjudged.

In *Loveday v Renton and Wellcome Foundation Limited*,[10] Stuart-Smith L.J. emphasized that, in applying the *Bolam* test, 'the court is not concerned to decide the merits of one practice as opposed to others but only to determine if a respectable and responsible body of medical practitioners would have acted as the defendant acted'.

In any case where a claimant seeks to establish that they have been damaged by the negligence of a medical practitioner, it is for the claimant to prove that (a) on the balance of probabilities, the medical practitioner was negligent in that his treatment fell below the proper standard expected of a practitioner at his level in his field of expertise carrying out the treatment at a specific date; and (b) the damage alleged was caused by the particular treatment, or lack of it, that is alleged to be negligent.

Application of the *Bolam* test to advice

The advice given, or not given, prior to surgery is a frequent cause of complaint and potential litigation. The House of Lords considered in the *Sidaway*[7] the application of the *Bolam* test to advice given prior to treatment (in that case, spinal surgery). Lord Diplock (p. 893D) stated:

> In English jurisprudence the doctor's relationship with his patient which gives rise to the normal duty of care to exercise his skill and judgment to improve the patient's health in any particular respect in which the patient has sought his aid, has hitherto been treated as single comprehensive duty covering all the ways in which a doctor is called upon to exercise his skill and judgment in the improvement of the physical or mental condition of the patient for which his services either as a general practitioner or specialist have been engaged. The general duty is not subject to dissection into a number of component parts to which different criteria of what satisfy the duty of care apply, such as diagnosis, treatment, advice (including warning of any risks of something going wrong) however skilfully the treatment advised is carried out. The *Bolam* case itself embraced failure to advise the patient of the risk involved in electric shock treatment as one of the allegations of negligence against the surgeon, as well as negligence in the actual carrying out of the treatment in which that risk did result in injury to the patient. In modern medicine and surgery such dissection of the various things a doctor had to do in the exercise of his whole duty of care owed to his patient is neither legally meaningful nor medically practicable.

The usual test for establishing negligence applies whatever the purpose for which advice was given. In *Gold v Harringey Health Authority*,[11] the Court of Appeal (in the context of contraceptive advice) reversed the finding of the trial judge who had held that a different test applied to advice given in a non-therapeutic context to that given in a therapeutic context. Stephen Brown L.J. summarized the position:

> In my judgment the test laid down in *Bolam v Friern Hospital Management Committee* as further considered and explained by Lord Diplock in *Sidaway v Board of Governors of Bethlem Royal Hospital* should be applied to the facts of this case. The judge appears to have been persuaded to find a distinction between advice given in a 'therapeutic' and a 'non-therapeutic' context. Such a distinction is wholly unwarranted and artificial.

The extent to which advice in respect of risks needs to be given was further explored in the Court of Appeal in *Pearce v United Bristol Healthcare NHS Trust*.[12] In this case, the claimant, who suffered a stillbirth, complained that she had not been properly advised of the respective risks of induction of labour, Caesarean section and additional delay through total lack of intervention. The Court of Appeal stated:

> Obviously the doctor, in determining what to tell a patient, has to take into account all the relevant considerations, which include the ability of the patient to comprehend what he has to say to him or her and the state of the patient at the particular time, both from the physical point of view and the emotional point of view. There can often be situations where a course different from the normal has to be employed. However, where there is what can realistically be called a 'significant risk', in the ordinary event, as I have already indicated, the patient is entitled to be informed of the risk.

The extent to which there is an obligation to advise patients of the risks of the treatment they are recommended may be affected by the implementation of the Human Rights Act 1998. A recent case in Strasbourg suggests that there may be a breach of Article 8 of the European Convention[13] if an authority fails to provide an individual with the necessary information to make proper decisions about his/her wellbeing, health and home. In *Guerra and Others v Italy*,[14] the European Court found a violation of Article 8 where the applicants were not provided with sufficient information about the risks to their health from pollution from a nearby factory. Similar principles may apply in respect of information about medical treatment now that the Human Rights Act 1998 has come into force.

Recent application of the *Bolam* test by the court

The most recent review of the application of the *Bolam* test by the House of Lords was in the case of *Bolitho v City and Hackney Health Authority*.[15] In this case, Lord Browne-Wilkinson considered the argument put forward on behalf of the claimant:

> ... that the Judge had wrongly treated the *Bolam* test as requiring him to accept the views of one truthful body of expert professional advice even though he was un-persuaded [sic] of its logical force.

It was argued that if this were the position, whenever a defendant could call a truthful witness to say the practice adopted by the treating doctor was in accordance with a body of sound medical opinion, the defendant would succeed in dismissing the claim. This would mean that even if the treatment defied logic it would not be negligent if other doctors also adopted it. Lord Browne-Wilkinson explained the position as follows:

> ... in my view, the court is not bound to hold that a defendant doctor escapes liability for negligent treatment or diagnosis just because he leads evidence from a number of medical experts who are genuinely of the opinion that the defendant's treatment or diagnosis accorded with sound medical practice. In the *Bolam* case itself, McNair J. stated that the defendant had to have acted in accordance with the practice accepted by a 'responsible body of medical men'. Later at p. 588 he referred to 'a standard of practice recognised as proper by a competent reasonable body of opinion' ... in *Maynard's* case Lord Scarman refers to a 'respectable' body of

> professional opinion. The use of these adjectives – responsible, reasonable and respectable – all show that the court has to be satisfied that the exponents of the body of opinion relied upon can demonstrate that such opinion has a logical basis. In particular in cases involving the weighing of risks against benefits, the judge, before accepting a body of opinion as being responsible, reasonable or respectable, will need to be satisfied that in forming their views, the experts have directed their minds to the question of comparative risks and benefits and reached a defensible conclusion on the matter.

Lord Browne-Wilkinson went on to accept in terms that if a professional opinion is not capable of withstanding logical analysis, the judge is entitled to hold that the opinion is not reasonable or logical. That is, ultimately it is the judge – not the expert – who determines whether a medical procedure or practice is acceptable as conforming to the standards expected of a particular type of medical practitioner at a given date. Of course, considerable help will always be required from the expert evidence for the judge to determine the question of acceptability. Lord Browne-Wilkinson considered it was likely to be rare that a judge would reject a genuinely held medical opinion as unreasonable. Nevertheless, there may be cases where this argument succeeds. The fact that the defendant can call evidence supporting the practice adopted is not therefore conclusive to the outcome of the case.

Clearly, it is important that the judge should be provided with literature and other evidence supporting the procedure adopted by the treating doctor in order for him to understand the logical basis of adopting that procedure.

The role of the judge to adjudicate on the opposing medical experts' views and reach a conclusion of his own also was considered in *Penney, Palmer and Cannon v East Kent Health Authority*.[16] This case involved claims by three women whose cervical smears had been reported as negative, and each of whom went on to develop invasive adenocarcinoma of the cervix, which required radical and invasive treatment, including hysterectomy. The trial was on the issue of liability only. Both causation and quantum were reserved. The issue for the judge was whether the primary screeners had been negligent in reading each of the smears as negative, thereby terminating the investigation of those smears (a finding that the smear was 'borderline' or 'inadequate' would have led to it being repeated).

Despite the trial focusing on liability, none of the screeners who had read the smears gave evidence and there was no direct evidence as to the training and management of the screeners. The evidence called on each side was expert evidence from pathologists, a total of five of whom gave evidence.

The defendant called expert evidence to support the proposition that:

> ... the abnormalities to be seen on the slides would not have been recognised as such by a reasonably competent cytoscreener at the time. In those circumstances the classification of the slides as 'negative' could properly have been made by a reasonably competent cytoscreener.

The defendant argued that the evidence was a complete defence within the *Bolam* test. In the Court of Appeal, the defendant argued that the judge had been wrong in failing to apply the *Bolam* test to the issues in the case.

The Court of Appeal analysed the position as follows:

> ... the *Bolam* test has no application where what the Judge is required to do is to make findings of fact. This is so even when those findings of fact are the subject of conflicting expert evidence. Thus in this case there were three questions which the Judge had to answer:
>
> (i) What was to be seen in the slides?
>
> (ii) At the relevant time could a screener exercising reasonable care fail to see what was on the slide?
>
> (iii) Could a reasonably competent screener, aware of what a screener exercising reasonable care would observe on the slide, treat the slide as negative?

As far as the issue of what was on the slides was concerned, the judge could not be expected to determine this without the help of expert evidence; however, once he had heard the conflicting evidence in this respect, it was ultimately a matter for him to determine as a question of fact what the slides showed. Once the judge had resolved this issue, he then needed to answer the second and third questions, applying the *Bolam* test. The Court of Appeal described how at that stage:

> Whether the screener was in breach of duty would depend on the training and the amount of knowledge a screener should have had in order to properly perform his or her task at that time and how easy it was to discern what the Judge had found was on the slide. These issues involved both questions of opinion as to the standards of care which the screeners should have exercised.

The *Bolam* test and the Human Rights Act 1998

The Human Rights Act 1998 directly incorporates the European Convention on Human Rights[17] into English law. In respect of an action against a public authority (which will include NHS Authorities and general practitioners treating NHS patients), an application can be brought under section 6 for breach of a convention right. In considering whether a claimant has an application for breach of Article 2 (the right to life), Article 3 (the right to be protected from inhuman and degrading treatment) or Article 8 (the right to respect for private and family life), the *Bolam* test will have no direct application. Once a breach is proved, the public authority may be liable to pay damages.[18] However, the starting point for the assessment of damages for breach of the provisions of the Act will be the principle of 'just satisfaction' applied by the European Court of Human Rights instead of damages based on full compensation.[19] Further, not every clinical negligence claim will involve a breach of convention rights. Actions in negligence are likely to continue to be pursued by the injured patient and the *Bolam* test likely to continue to apply.

Part 2: Causation

The problem

In essence, to succeed in a claim for clinical negligence the claimant first must prove that the defendant owed him/her a duty of care. Second, the claimant must prove that the standard of clinical care provided was below a competent level. Third, he/she must show that the lack of competent care caused the injury of which he/she complains. Proving causation can be the most difficult aspect of the claim.

One obvious problem in a clinical negligence case is that the claimant usually has a clinical problem before any treatment commenced. It is necessary for the claimant to prove that it was the alleged treatment, or lack of it, that caused the injury and the loss and damage of which he complains.

There are three situations in clinical negligence cases that give rise to different causation issues:

1) The issue of what would have happened if different treatment actually had been given.
2) The issue of what would have happened if different treatment had been offered to the claimant.
3) The issue of what difference competent treatment would have made to the claimant's condition and prognosis.

The balance of probabilities test

If the issue is what would have happened if different treatment had been given, the claimant needs to prove that if he/she had received competent treatment a particular result would have followed.

This is the situation where what the claimant needs to prove is a matter of historical fact. The claimant must prove, on a balance of probabilities, that the result alleged would have resulted after competent treatment. For example, a child injured through mismanagement of the mother's labour and the child's delivery must prove, on the balance of probabilities, that with competent care he/she would have been delivered as a healthy, undamaged baby. If the claimant can prove it is 51% likely that competent care would have led to safe delivery, the claimant will recover damages assessed on the basis of 100% compensation.

In the case of *Hotson v East Berkshire Health Authority*,[20] the claimant suffered a hip injury, which the defendant negligently failed to diagnose. There was an identifiable negligent act on the part of the defendant. However, even with competent diagnosis the claimant would only have had a 25% chance of recovery. That is, on the balance of probabilities, the claimant would have been no better off *with* competent care. The House of Lords stated that unless the claimant could show, on the balance of probabilities, that he would have been better off, he could not recover damages at all.

In a different situation – in the case of *Wilsher v Essex Area Health Authority*[21] – the claimant suffered blindness following treatment in the special care baby unit. It was accepted that there had been negligence in that a junior doctor had inserted a catheter into the claimant's umbilical vein instead of the umbilical artery. There were a number of different factors identified that could have led to the claimant's injury, however, one of which was the administration of excess oxygen. The House of Lords confirmed that it was for the claimant to prove, on the balance of probabilities, that the administration of excess oxygen had caused his injury and that he had failed to do so.

As Lord Reid explained in *Davies v Taylor*:[22]

> When the question is whether a certain thing is or is not true – whether a certain event did or did not happen – then the Court must decide one way or the other. There is no question of chance or probability. Either it did or did not happen. But the standard of civil proof is the balance of probabilities. If the evidence shows a balance in favour of it having happened, then it is proved that it did in fact happen.

The same test applies when the question is, what would have happened with competent treatment? If, on the balance of probabilities, the claimant would have recovered, his recovery is treated as a certainty. If, on the balance of probabilities, he would not have recovered, that failure also is treated as a certainty.

A further complication arises when the alleged negligence involves an omission. In this situation, there is a two-stage test, as explained by the House of Lords in *Bolitho v City and Hackney Health Authority*.[15] Lord Browne-Wilkinson:

> Where as in the present case, a breach of a duty of care is proved or admitted, the burden still lies on the [claimant] to prove that such breach caused the injury suffered ... In all cases the primary question is one of fact: did the wrongful act cause the injury? But in cases where the breach of duty consists of an omission to do an act which ought to be done (e.g. the failure by a doctor to attend) that factual inquiry, is by definition, in the realms of hypothesis. The question is what would have happened if an event, which by definition did not occur, had occurred.

In dealing with the issue of causation in respect of omissions, the claimant has two possible ways of proving that the negligence caused his injury. Where (as in *Bolitho*) the allegation is that a senior doctor ought to have been called, the claimant may prove on the balance of probabilities one of two things: either a) that, had the senior doctor been summonsed, then that particular doctor would have administered such treatment as would have saved the claimant from injury (where causation is proved even if failure by the senior doctor to administer the treatment would not have been negligent within the *Bolam* test); or b) that, had the senior doctor been summonsed, then if he had failed to administer the treatment he would have been negligent within the *Bolam* test.

In practical terms, if evidence is available from the senior doctor who would have been called and he states he would have given the treatment, then the claimant has proved causation. If, on the other hand, the doctor states he would not have given the treatment, then enquiry is necessary as to whether such failure would have been negligent within the *Bolam* test. If it would be negligent, the claimant proves causation; if it would not, he fails to do so.

Absence of choice

The situation can arise where the claimant has, through the defendant's negligence, missed the opportunity to undergo treatment or to avoid a situation or risk. Again, in this situation the claimant must prove, on a balance of probabilities, that he/she would have done something different in the absence of negligence.

In this situation, it is necessary for the judge to answer the hypothetical question, what would the claimant have done if the defendant had given competent advice?

An example of this situation is the case of *Newell and Newell v Goldenberg*,[23] where the issue was what the claimants would have done had they been properly advised of the risks of failure of a vasectomy operation. The claimants needed to prove that, on the balance of probabilities, they would have taken other additional contraceptive measures. The judge found that, had they been given competent advice, they would have been content to take the risk of relying on the husband's vasectomy. The judge found that Mrs Newell would not have undergone surgery, which would in any event have been contra-indicated.

The claimants, having proved breach of duty, received only £500 damages to compensate them for the anxiety and distress of finding Mrs Newell pregnant. They failed in respect of all other heads of damage because they could not prove, on the balance of probabilities, that the outcome would have been different. That is, they could not prove, on the balance of probabilities, that the claimants would have instigated sufficient additional contraception to avoid a pregnancy.

A similar situation arises in cases where the claimant has not been warned of all the risks of surgery but would have made the same choice even with a fuller account of the risks. In these cases, it cannot be shown on the balance of probabilities that the outcome would have been different with competent advice and warnings.

Loss of a chance

A situation may arise where the outcome of the defendant's negligent act depends on the hypothetical action of a third party. Here, the claimant only needs to prove that he/she has lost the chance of achieving a particular result. This chance may be significantly less than 50% but the claimant will only recover damages assessed in the proportion of the lost chance.

In *Anderson v Davis*,[24] the claimant recovered two-thirds of his alleged loss of earnings as a lecturer on the basis that he had had a two-thirds chance of obtaining promotion in this job. In *Doyle v Wallace*,[25] the claimant recovered damages on the basis that she had a 50% chance of becoming a teacher, which was lost as a result of her injury.

Forseeability

The claimant must show, on the balance of probabilities, that the defendant caused the injury. The claimant also must show that it was foreseeable that if the clinician was negligent, the claimant would suffer injury of the type in fact suffered. In *Brown v Lewisham and North Southwark Health Authority*,[26] Lord Justice Beldam set out the position:

> A doctor is obliged to exercise the care and skill of a competent doctor. He must take care in the examination, diagnosis and treatment of his patient's condition to prevent injury to his health from risks which a competent practitioner would foresee as likely to result from his failure to do so. He is not a clairvoyant nor if he tells his patient that

he can find nothing wrong is he liable if his patient has a condition which was not discoverable by competent examination. The public policy of limiting liability of tortfeasors by the control mechanism of foreseeability seems to me to be as necessary in cases of medical as in any other type of negligence. I do not see on what policy ground it would be fair or just to hold a doctor to be in breach of duty who failed to diagnose an asymptomatic and undetectable illness merely because he was at fault in the management of a correctly diagnosed but unrelated condition. In short, it must be shown that the injury suffered by the patient was within the risk from which it was the doctor's duty to protect him.

The test is based on that applied by Lord Bridge in *Caparo Industries PLC v Dickman*,[27] where he pointed out:

It is never sufficient to ask simply whether A owes B a duty of care. It is always necessary to determine the scope of the duty by reference to the kind of damage from which A must take care to save B harmless.

In *Rahman v Arearose Limited and University College London NHS Trust*,[28] the claimant lost the sight in one eye and suffered psychiatric injury after an assault which was followed by negligent medical treatment. Complex issues of causation arose in respect of the responsibility of the respective defendants for the psychiatric injury. Laws L.J. explained that:

... in all these cases the real question is, what is the damage for which the defendant under consideration should be held responsible. ... [the question] in truth can only be understood, in light of the answer to the question, *from what kind of harm was it the defendant's duty to guard the claimant*. Novus actus interveniens, the eggshell skull, and (in the case of multiple torts) the concept of multiple tortfeasors are all no more and no less than tools or mechanisms which the law has developed to articulate in practice the extent of any liable defendant's responsibility for the loss and damage which the claimant has suffered *[emphasis added]*.

Conclusion

Frequently, the factual situation in a clinical negligence case is complex. It may need a number of experts who specialize in different areas to address the standard of care that the claimant has received and the reasons for the poor outcome. The task of the lawyers should be to give clear instructions to the experts so that they can address the issues on liability and causation that the court will need to determine. Whilst the answers to the relevant questions may involve difficult medical analysis, the questions should be relatively easy to state once the factual situation has been analysed correctly by the lawyers. In each case, the questions need to be tailored to the particular facts, but should be directed at eliciting the following:

(1) What happened to the claimant to leave him/her with the injury of which he/she complains?
(2) Did any clinician who treated or failed to treat the claimant fail to act competently within the *Bolam* test?

(3) Would competent treatment, on the balance of probabilities, have avoided some injury?

(4) What would have been the claimant's condition and prognosis with competent treatment?

References

1   Gold v Essex County Council [1942] 2 KB 293.
2   Cassidy v Ministry of Health [1951] 2 KB 343.
3   In Hillyer v St Bartholomew's Hospital [1909] 2 KB 820, Kennedy L.J. expressed the view that a hospital, although responsible for the exercise of due care in selecting its professional staff – whether surgeons or doctors or nurses – was not responsible if they or any of them acted negligently in matters of professional skill and care.
4   Bull v Devon Area Health Authority [1993] 4 Med LR 117.
5   Bull v Devon Area Health Authority [1993] 4 Med LR 117: Lord Justice Mustill, p. 142.
6   Bolam v Friern Barnet Hospital Management Committee [1957] 1 WLR 582.
7   Maynard v West Midlands Regional Health Authority [1984] 1 WLR 634.
8   Sidaway v Board of Governors of the Bethlem Royal Hospital and the Maudsley Hospital [1985] AC 871.
9   Whitehouse v Jordon and Another [1981] 1 WLR 246.
10 Loveday v Renton and Wellcome Foundation Limited [1990] 1 Med LR 117.
11 Gold v Harringey Health Authority [1988] QB 481.
12 Pearce v United Bristol Healthcare NHS Trust [1999] PIQR P53.
13 The Convention for the Protection of Human Rights and Fundamental Freedoms Article 8 provides that 'everyone has the right to respect for his private and family life, his home and his correspondence. There shall be no interference by a public authority in the exercise of the right except as in accordance with the law and is necessary in a democratic society in the interests of national security, public safety or the economic well-being of the country, for the prevention of disorder or crime, for the protection of health or morals, or for the protection of the rights and freedoms of others'.
14 Guerra and Another v Italy [1998] 26 EHRR 357.
15 Bolitho v City and Hackney Health Authority [1998] AC 232; Lloyd's Med Rep 26.
16 Penney, Palmer and Cannon v East Kent Health Authority [2000] Lloyd's Med Rep 41.
17 Convention for the Protection of Human Rights and Fundamental Freedoms.
18 Section 8 of the Human Rights Act 1998 requires the court, in deciding whether to award damages, to take into account the principles in Article 41 of the European Convention and the need for 'just satisfaction'.
19 Section 8 Human Rights Act 1998.
20 Hotson v East Berkshire Health Authority [1987] AC 750.
21 Wilsher v Essex Area Health Authority [1988] 1 AC 1074.
22 Davies v Taylor [1974] AC 207.
23 Newell and Newell v Goldenberg [1995] 6 Med LR 371.
24 Anderson v Davies [1993] PIQR Q87.
25 Doyle v Wallace [1998] PIQR Q146.
26 Brown v Lewisham and North Southwark Health Authority [1999] Lloyd's Med Rep 110 at 118.
27 Caparo Industries PLC v Dickman [1990] 2 AC 605.
28 Rahman v Arearose Limited and University College London NHS Trust [2000] 3 WLR 1184.

▶3

Consent

Robert Francis QC

In this chapter, the principles governing the legal justification for the provision of treatment to a patient are considered. Treatment for these purposes includes any act that involves physical contact with the patient or the ingestion of medication. Therefore, it embraces physical examination and the prescription of medication with the intent that the patient should consume it. We are not concerned here with professional advice, except where it is relevant to the concept of consent

The principles can be stated shortly. No medical treatment may be given to a patient without his/her valid consent or that of another lawful authority. Treatment given without such legal justification is likely to be considered battery in criminal law, and trespass to the person in civil law.[1] Consent given on the basis of inadequate information about the risks involved in the proposed treatment will not be a defence against liability in negligence for a failure to give sufficient information or advice to the patient.[2]

A patient having legal capacity to make such decisions may refuse treatment for good or bad reasons, or for no reasons at all, and cannot be compelled to submit to treatment.[2] On the other hand, patients who lack such capacity or are unable to communicate their decision may – and in some cases, must – be provided with such treatment that is in their best interests to receive. Where the loss of capacity is likely to be permanent or more than temporary, this will include not only treatment necessary to prevent loss of life or a deterioration in health, but any form of treatment which it is in the patient's best interests to receive and which will be needed before there is likely to be any recovery of capacity.[1] Where the incapacitated patient resists such treatment, reasonable restraint may be applied to enable it to be given.[3]

Capacity to consent to or refuse medical treatment

Any adult (ie a person over the age of 18) is presumed to have the capacity to consent to medical treatment. By statute,[4] the consent of any person aged 16 or over has the same status as that of an adult. Children under the age of 16 may possess the relevant capacity, but in their case there is no presumption of it. Any child of any age will have the capacity to give a valid consent to medical treatment if of sufficient maturity and understanding.[5] This general requirement must be understood in the light of more recent authority in relation to the capacity of adults. An adult will lack capacity if he is unable to receive and retain treatment information, or to believe it, or to weigh it in order to reach a decision.[6] A child will need to demonstrate a similar level of ability to establish capacity. In the case of both child and adult, the degree of capacity must be commensurate to the gravity of the decision being taken.[7] In assessing capacity, it must be remembered that it is the ability to make a decision that is to be looked at, not the quality of the decision actually taken. It might be thought that any serious inroad into this principle would run the risk of infringing Article 6 of the European Convention on Human Rights.

Capacity can be lost by adult or child temporarily through unconsciousness, severe pain, phobia or other phenomenon seriously interfering with the patient's decision-making abilities.[8] It should be remembered that the mere presence of fear or pain, etc., does not necessarily deprive the patient of capacity. What must be assessed is their effect on the patient's abilities. One person may be able to withstand severe pain and remain in possession of his/her faculties while another might be rendered helpless by the mere threat of an injection.

The ingredients of consent

Consent sufficient to render lawful the provision of medical treatment is no more and no less than a communication by the patient of his or her agreement to receive the proposed treatment at a time while possessing the legal capacity to give such consent. These ingredients will be considered in turn below.

Proposal of treatment

Even though the process whereby treatment is provided normally will start with the patient presenting him/herself to the doctor in order to request advice and treatment, the first essential step in the process of consent is the proposal by a doctor, or nurse, to provide specific treatment to the patient. In order to be capable of giving rise to a valid consent, the proposal must be accurate, and contain sufficient detail to enable the patient to understand the nature and effect of what is to be done. Obviously, to give a misleading and inaccurate description whereby the patient is materially deceived as to the true nature and effect of the intended treatment will not provide the basis for a valid consent. The information does not, for this purpose, have to disclose every detail and technicality of what is to be done; nor does it have to include any information on the risks of the treatment. However, such information may be necessary to enable the practitioner to fulfil his duty of care to the patient in relation to the provision of professional advice. The sole requirement in relation to the provision of information for the purpose of obtaining a valid consent sufficient to amount to a defence against an action or prosecution for battery is that sufficient information is provided to enable the patient to have a broad understanding of the nature and effect of the treatment.

No particular form of communication of the proposal is required. Thus it may be written, oral, communicated by conduct, or a combination of these. For example, a nurse may explain that she intends to take a blood sample, as she advances towards the patient bearing a syringe. This is likely to be a sufficient communication of her intention, enabling the patient to understand what will happen if he or she proffers an arm.

Communication of consent

As with the proposal for treatment, consent may be communicated in writing, orally, by conduct, or by a combination of these. The consent must refer to the proposed treatment or at least include it. It may refer to treatment which might prove to be necessary but which will not necessarily be adopted. However, consent expressed in vague or general terms may not be valid to cover the actual treatment provided. It is doubtful whether phrases such as 'such further or alternative operative measures as may be found to be necessary during the course of the operation', which were to be found in many standard consent forms until recently, have any effect.

Duration of authority

By definition, consent is given in advance of the proposed treatment. It may be given immediately before the treatment, or weeks before. The consent, if valid when given, will remain in force unless the patient revokes it or unless the circumstances change to remove the basis on which the treatment was agreed. Thus, a consent for an operation under general anaesthetic will continue to apply even after the patient has become unconscious under anaesthetic. On the other hand, if a patient consented to chemotherapy treatment for breast cancer, but before this could be administered it was discovered that the diagnosis was wrong, the consent given under the false belief in the truth of the diagnosis would not justify continuing with the chemotherapy.

Revocation

Consent may be revoked by the patient, if retaining the capacity to do so, at any time before the treatment is given. If it is practicable to do so, treatment must be stopped once it has begun. Revocation may be made in any form in which the consent can be given. Difficulties might arise where the revocation is communicated to someone other than the treating doctor – a nurse, for instance – and is not then passed on. The liability of the doctor might depend on what he/she knew or ought to have known. However, the authority employing the nurse undoubtedly would be liable to the patient for the non-communication of the information to the treating doctor. As with an initial refusal of consent, a patient with capacity can revoke authority for treatment for any or no reason.

A revocation of consent cannot be made once the patient has ceased to have the capacity to make such a decision. However, if circumstances have so changed since the consent was given that it is no longer in the incapacitated patient's best interests for the treatment to be given or continued, the patient would not be obliged to receive it. The doctor's decisions on what to do then would be governed by the rules concerning the treatment of patients lacking the capacity to make their own decisions. He/she would be entitled to provide such treatment as is necessary to save the patient's life or to prevent a serious deterioration in health, or generally is in the best interests of the patient, and is necessary to provide the treatment before recovery of capacity.

Factors nullifying consent

It has already been demonstrated that lack of legal capacity may invalidate consent. Consent also will be vitiated by fraud, duress or undue influence. Thus, a consent obtained by a deception as to the true nature of what was proposed is no consent at all. An authority given by a weakened individual under the oppressive influence of an insistent group of relatives also may be invalid. The effect of strongly expressed views by close family members may have a different effect according to the condition of the patient. An elderly stroke victim may still possess legal capacity to make decisions, but be too debilitated to withstand the pressure exerted by his or her family.

Treatment of patients unable or unwilling to decide for themselves

Adults

The right of an adult patient possessing full capacity to make such a decision to refuse medical treatment is absolute. There is no alternative means of obtaining authority to provide treatment however necessary anyone believes it to be and however unpleasant or offensive the consequences of the treatment not being provided may be. In *Re MB*,[7] it was made clear that respect had to be afforded even to a decision which is 'so outrageous in its defiance of logic or of accepted moral standards that no sensible person who had applied his mind to the question to be decided could have arrived at it'.

An adult patient who has lost the capacity to make a treatment decision through unconsciousness or other disability and who has not made a valid advance refusal of treatment may be provided with such treatment as is immediately necessary to save life or a deterioration in health or is otherwise in his or her best interests. Such treatment has to be provided for these reasons before it is likely that the patient will recover capacity to decide for him or herself. It cannot be emphasized too strongly that it is unlawful to impose treatment on an unconscious patient without his or her consent merely because it is more convenient for the doctor to provide it immediately rather than waiting for the patient to wake up and discuss the matter. In determining the patient's best interests the treating doctor must act in accordance with accepted competent and responsible medical practice. If he does so, he will not subsequently be exposed to liability merely because a different view of the best interests might reasonably have been taken.[9] The prudent doctor normally will consult an available near relative or partner where this is appropriate. However, no relative, spouse or other third party has legal power to consent to treatment of an adult, even where the patient has previously expressed a wish that decisions should be taken by a named individual. The doctor may, however, take into account what is said by such persons in deciding where the best interests of the patient lie.

In cases of socially controversial treatment, such as sterilization or where there is a dispute between interested parties, an application may – and in some cases must – be made to the court for a declaration that the proposed treatment is in the best interests of the patient. The court will consider all the evidence and decide whether what is proposed is indeed so

Children

Children under the age of 16 may have legal capacity to make their own decisions (as discussed above). The consent of such children will provide the legal justification for any form of treatment. Unlike competent adults, they have no absolute right to refuse treatment. However mature and competent a child under 16 years of age may be, a consent provided by a person with parental responsibility will override the refusal.[10] Whether the doctor will wish to impose treatment in such difficult and sensitive circumstances then becomes a matter of medical practice and ethics, not of law. If the consent of neither the parents nor the child can be obtained, recourse may be had to the court, which, in the exercise of the inherent jurisdiction, may authorize the imposition of any form of treatment on the unwilling child. The only consideration for the court is whether it is in the best interests of the child to have the treatment under all the circumstances of the case.

Mistaken belief in consent

If a doctor honestly but mistakenly believes he has the consent of a patient to a procedure, what are the consequences? He might have been misinformed by a junior that the consent had been taken. He may be unaware of the oppressive or misleading circumstances in which the authority was extracted from the patient. It has been suggested[11] that a mistaken belief in the existence of a valid consent is no defence to an action in trespass or prosecution for battery. While there does not appear to be any direct authority on the point, it is suggested that this should not be the position. In just the same way that a mistaken but honest belief in circumstances which, if true, would justify the use of force in self defence, a similar quality of belief as to the existence of an authority to treat should protect the practitioner from a prosecution for assault. The same ought to apply in relation to civil liability in trespass, but, again, there is no legal authority to confirm this. Even if this is correct, there may be liability in negligence if the practitioner has not taken proper care to check the authenticity of the consent.

Making decisions in advance

In practice, nearly all decisions to agree to medical treatment are made in advance of the treatment, whether by a few seconds or, in the case of operations under general anaesthesia, some hours or even days previously. Such decisions remain valid and justify treatment within the scope of the consent unless they are revoked. In the same way, it is possible for a patient to determine in advance that he/she will not authorize particular treatment either at all or in specified circumstances.[12] While most commonly this may take the form of a refusal in advance to authorize blood transfusions or other treatment for religious reasons, a patient with the capacity to make such decisions may in advance prohibit the provision of any specific medical treatment or care. The purpose of such advance refusals is that the patient can ensure that his or her wishes will be respected even if he/she loses the capacity to make decisions whether through unconsciousness or some intervening disability. Such decisions may be made in writing or orally. They can only have application when the patient whose treatment is under consideration is unconscious or lacks the capacity to make a treatment decision. If capacity remains, the doctor will seek authority, as described above, and respect any competent refusal. The law concerning advance refusals is still developing, but the following points are reasonably clear:

▶ At the time the decision is made, the patient must possess the relevant capacity to make it.

▶ The decision must be made free of duress, undue influence or other vitiating factor.

▶ It must have been intended to apply in the circumstances that confront the doctor and patient at the time the treatment is under consideration.

▶ The patient must not have revoked it while competent to make the decision before or at the time the need for treatment arises.

▶ To have practical effect the advance decision must be communicated to the doctors who would otherwise be under a duty to treat the patient in his or her best interests as they judge them to be.

Consent in obstetrics and gynaecology

As in any other type of medical practice, the doctor must obtain the consent of his patient before providing treatment in accordance with the principles summarized above. There are, however, some special considerations in specific areas that deserve separate consideration.

Sterilization

Sterilization may either be the primary purpose of a procedure or the consequence of treatment given for some other purpose. Thus, hysterectomy may be necessary to treat a cancer, but will inevitably lead to the sterilization of the patient. In principle, the law treats both types of treatment in the same way. If the patient is a competent adult, her consent must be obtained to the treatment, and she must be advised of the consequences of it to the extent required by competent medical practice. While in theory such practice might not require a woman to be warned that a therapeutic procedure would have the consequence of sterilizing her, this seems highly unlikely; and in any event, such a practice might lead a court to find that it was not a practice that withstood logical scrutiny. Therefore, gynaecologists would be well advised to ensure that their patients were fully aware of the consequences to their fertility of any proposed treatment. Similarly, where sterilization is the primary object of the treatment the patient ought to be made aware of the risks of failure, and of the prospects, or lack of them, of restoring fertility. Case law would suggest that patients need not be presented with various options for contraception where this is the purpose of the procedure,[13] but it might be questioned whether this now reflects current medical practice.

In the case of adults or children who are incapable of making treatment decisions of this importance for themselves, a very cautious approach must be adopted. The law sees sterilization of those unable to make their own decisions as a matter of particular social concern. Accordingly, no procedure the primary purpose of which is to sterilize a patient unable to make his/her own valid decision should be performed without obtaining a declaration of the court that the procedure is lawful and in the best interests of the patient. There is now a well-established legal procedure for obtaining the court's approval in such cases. The court will expect the doctor proposing the treatment to have reached his conclusion in accordance with a responsible body of medical opinion, but will not necessarily be bound by that opinion. The court will make its own assessment on the evidence before it of the patient's best interests.[14] In the case of children, it will be very rare indeed for the court to authorize a sterilization, particularly if the child may be able to make her own decision on reaching adulthood.[15]

Adults with learning difficulties who are unable to make their own treatment decisions and are proposed for sterilization present particular challenges. The assessment of best interests will take account of the degree of risk to which they are exposed by not being sterilized, whether there is any less radical alternative, and whether there is any significant risk of pregnancy in any event. It is unlikely that the court will authorize such a procedure merely because there is a remote or speculative possibility of conceiving.[16]

When the treatment proposed is for a disease but will have the side effect of sterilization, no application to the court is necessary in the case of patients unable to make their own decision.[17] Current legal practice does not regard such cases as raising the particular social sensitivities as arise in the 'non-therapeutic' cases.

Abortion

It has been held that no application to the court is required for a declaration in the case of abortions for mentally incompetent patients.[18] The safeguards of the Abortion Act 1967 are thought to be sufficient, but it may be questioned whether this is so. The decision to terminate a pregnancy can be a very difficult one for those fully in possession of their faculties. The existence of grounds for termination under the Act does not necessarily mean that the procedure is in the patient's best interests. Therefore, it is suggested that in any case where there is particular difficulty or dissent, an application to the court would be prudent. It surely would be better to run the risk of paying the costs of an unnecessary application to court rather than facing litigation for a termination retrospectively said not to be in the patient's best interests.

Caesarean section

Obstetricians owe a duty to two patients at the same time: the mother and the baby yet to be born. Those duties may conflict where the mother will not agree to treatment necessary to save the baby. For a number of years, the courts granted declarations authorizing the delivery by Caesarean section to be imposed on unwilling patients in the interests of themselves or their baby. In one case, the mother was competent to make her own decision, but this was over-ridden in a hearing lasting less than 20 minutes.[19] In other cases, applications were made without any representation of the patient and without any formal evidence being tendered. The court was prepared to act on information relayed by telephone; with no opportunity for cross-examination of the witness.[20] This practice was brought to a halt by the Court of Appeal in two landmark cases: *Re MB*[8] and *St George's Healthcare NHS Trust v S.*[21] The court laid down guidelines, which should be followed in cases of patients in need of surgical delivery who lack capacity. They should be read in full by any practitioner confronting this type of case, and can be summarized as follows:

▶ Any concern about a patient's capacity should be identified as soon as possible and an appropriate assessment of it made by a suitably qualified doctor; in serious or complex cases, this should be an independent psychiatrist. The assessment should include consideration of the patient's capacity to manage her property and affairs. The assessor must be made aware of the legal criteria for capacity.

▶ Where the patient has made a valid advance directive, she should be treated in accordance with it; where there is doubt about its validity, a court application should be made for a declaration.

▶ In the absence of such a directive, the patient must be cared for according to the responsible Health Authority's judgement of her best interests.

▶ If a declaration is to be sought and the patient is thought to be unable to manage her property and affairs, the Official Solicitor must be informed to allow appropriate court representation to be arranged.

▶ Any court application must be supported by accurate and relevant information about the reasons for the proposed treatment, the risks involved, any alternatives, and the patient's reasons for refusal, if known.

▶ No declaration will be granted without the patient or her representative having notice of the proceedings and an opportunity to put her case.

Where a declaration or other court order is made, its terms must be communicated quickly and accurately to the patient.

References

1   *In: Re F (Mental Patient: Sterilisation)* [1990] 2 AC 1.
2   *Sidaway v Board of Governors of the Bethlem Royal Hospital and the Maudsley Hospital* [1985] AC 871.
3   R *v* Bournewood CMH MHST [1999] 1 AC 58.
4   Family Reform Act 1969, s.8.
5   *Gillick v West Norfolk and Wisbech AHA* [1986] AC 112.
6   *B v Croydon HA* [1995] FCR 332; *Re MB (Medical Treatment)* [1997] Med LR 217; [1997] 2 FLR 426.
7   See *Gillick* (above); *Re T (Adult: Refusal of Medical Treatment)* [1992] 4 All ER 649.
8   *Re MB* (above).
9   *Re SL* (Adult Patient) (Sterilization) [2000] 2 FLR 452.
10   *In: Re R (A Minor) (Wardship: Consent to Treatment)* [1992] Fam 11; *In: Re W (A Minor) (Medical Treatment: Courts Jurisdiction)* [1993] Fam 64.
11   Staughton L.J., in *Re T (Adult: Refusal of Treatment)* [1993] Fam 93, 122
12   *Re T (Adult: Refusal of Treatment)* [1993] Fam 95; *Airedale NHS Trust v Bland* [1993] AC 789.
13   *Gold v Haringey HA* [1988] QB 481; [1987] 2 All ER 888.
14   *Re SL* above.
15   *In: Re B* (A Minor) (Wardship: Sterilization) [1988] AC 199.
16   *In: Re A* (Medical Treatment: Male Sterilization) [2000] 1 FLR 193.
17   *In: Re E* (A Minor) (Medical Treatment) [1991] 2 FLR 585; In: Re GF (Medical Treatment) [1992] 1 FLR 293.
18   Re SG (Adult Mental Patient: Abortion) [1991] 2 FLR 329.
19   *In: Re S (Adult: Refusal of Treatment)* [1993] Fam 123.
20   *See Thameside and Glossop Acute Services NHS Trust v CH*; *Rochdale Healthcare NHS Trust v C* [1996] 1 FLR 762; *Norfolk and Norwich Healthcare NHS Trust v W* [1996] 2 FLR 613; *Re L*, 5 December 1996 (unreported).
21   St. Georges Healthcare NHS Trust *v* S [1999] Fam 26.

►4

Procedure: The Civil Procedure Rules

Martin Spencer

In this chapter, I shall consider the progress of a typical action for clinical negligence under the Civil Procedure Rules (CPR). Introduced on 26 April 1999 as the culmination of the Woolf reforms, the CPR have now been in force for over a year, and have implemented the recommendations of Lord Woolf's report, *Access to Justice.*[1]

The Clinical Negligence Pre-action Protocol

With the implementation of the CPR, two Pre-action Protocols also were implemented: the Personal Injury Pre-action Protocol and the Clinical Negligence Pre-action Protocol (CNPAP). The concept of Protocols has, of course, long been well known in medical circles, with the existence of Protocols in many areas of clinical care. In relation to litigation, the rules of court have themselves always provided the standard for litigators once proceedings have been issued. However, the laying down of *pre-action* standards of conduct is a new, and in my view highly welcome, concept for litigators. Too often in the past, claimants' lawyers kept their Defence counterparts in the dark as to what was happening in relation to an adverse clinical event. They gathered evidence – sometimes over years – and then, often shortly before the expiry of the limitation period, they issued proceedings and sprung these like a trap on the healthcare provider and its lawyers. Instead of being a final resort, litigation was all too often the first resort.

For their part, healthcare providers often were slow to acknowledge their errors, and when a complaint was made the shutters were put up: little was provided by way of explanation and an already difficult situation was thereby aggravated. Sometimes, it was years before the victim of a medical accident found out what had really happened, and the subsequent litigation was blighted by being conducted many years after the events with which it was concerned.

The primary purpose of the CNPAP is to make litigation a *last* resort, only reverted to when all other avenues to resolve the dispute have been explored and have failed. However, its ambitions go wider than simply addressing the pre-action conduct of the lawyers on each side. Unlike the Personal Injury Pre-action Protocol, the CNPAP takes matters up at an earlier stage, before lawyers are involved at all. Its stated aim is to change the relationship between *patients* and *healthcare providers* and to dispel the mistrust that has hitherto characterized healthcare disputes. I quote from the CNPAP:

> It is clearly in the interests of patients, healthcare professionals and providers that patients' concerns, complaints and claims arising from their treatment are resolved

as quickly, efficiently and professionally as possible. A climate of mistrust and lack of openness can seriously damage the patient/clinician relationship, unnecessarily prolong disputes (especially litigation) and reduce the resources available for treating patients. It may also cause additional work for, and lower the morale of, healthcare professionals. At present there is often mistrust on both sides . . .

To achieve its ambition to dispel such mistrust, the CNPAP seeks to encourage openness, timeliness and awareness of options – openness through early communication and exchange of information, timeliness by obtaining information at an early stage, and awareness of options so that litigation becomes the last resort, not the first.

The Protocol provides good practice commitments for both healthcare providers and for patients and their advisers. The first step under the Protocol is obtaining the health records, which must be provided within 40 days of their request. If the healthcare provider cannot comply with this deadline, it should give an explanation as soon as it is aware of the difficulty. If the deadline is not complied with, the patient is entitled to make an application for pre-action disclosure under CPR Part 31.16. Once the health records are to hand, the patient is in a position to instruct an expert to advise on whether he or she has a valid claim; it will be rare in a clinical negligence context that a patient will be able to proceed to make a claim without a supportive expert report, which should address both negligence and causation. Assuming that the expert is supportive, the next stage is the Letter of Claim. This is an important and formal document that effectively turns the patient and healthcare provider into, respectively, the claimant and defendant. It sets out the alleged facts, the main allegations of negligence, the injuries sustained and gives an outline of the financial loss incurred. The intention is that the healthcare provider is given sufficient information to enable it to commence its own investigations and to evaluate the claim, including in financial terms. The CNPAP provides for a moratorium on the issue of proceedings for three months whilst the healthcare provider is given a chance to investigate the claim, but receipt of the Letter of Claim itself must be acknowledged within 14 days.

At the same time as sending the Letter of Claim, the claimant also may make an offer to settle. This is optional, but it is formally recognised in CPR Part 36.10 in that the court may later take the offer into account when making any order as to costs.

Within three months of the Letter of Claim, the healthcare provider should make its response, both to the Letter of Claim and, where appropriate, to the offer to settle. Indeed, even where the claimant has not made an offer to settle, the healthcare provider itself may make such an offer at the stage of response. The response should set out clearly the defendant's position: whether the claim is admitted, or partly admitted, or denied and, if denied, why; responding in detail to the allegations of negligence.

Thus, before proceedings are ever brought, the issues between the parties should have been explored in some detail and each side should have knowledge of where the other stands in relation to the claim. The CNPAP further encourages the parties to explore alternatives to legal action, such as following the NHS complaints procedure or alternative dispute resolution. The last resort, therefore, clearly is the bringing of an action in the courts for clinical negligence, and, under the CPR, the court will look critically at whether the parties complied faithfully with the CNPAP before resorting to litigation. If they did not, there are sanctions, including in respect of any orders for costs subsequently made. The CNPAP is now an important and integral part of any clinical negligence action. It has had the effect of causing much fewer claims to reach the courts, and it means that the courts should now only be burdened with the more serious claims, or those which are defended in principle.

Failure to comply with the Protocol may lead to sanctions being imposed at a later stage. There are such sanctions within the CPR themselves (see, for example, Part 3.1[5] and 3.9) and also in the Practice Direction which accompanies the Protocol. Thus, the Practice Direction suggests that the court may make an order:

▶ that the party in default pay all of the costs or part of the costs of the proceedings, even on an indemnity basis;

▶ awarding the claimant interest for a shorter period, or at a lower rate, than it would otherwise have done;

▶ ordering the defendant to pay interest on damages at a higher rate than it would otherwise have done, though not exceeding 10% above base rate.

Litigation under the CPR

The CPR, when introduced on 26 April 1999, effectively put a nuclear bomb under the civil litigation process. More than a century of lawmaking, encapsulated within the Supreme Court Practice for the High Court and the County Court Practice for the County Court, was virtually swept away, the intention being to make a clean start. Lawyers had to learn a new language: plaintiffs were no longer plaintiffs but 'claimants', parties were no longer given 'leave' but 'permission', and children and patients now bring proceedings through their 'litigation friend' rather than a 'guardian *ad litem*'. At the heart of the CPR is the 'overriding objective' contained in Part 1 – namely, to enable the court to deal with cases justly by:

▶ ensuring that the parties are on an equal footing;

▶ saving expense, by dealing with cases proportionately;

▶ ensuring that cases are dealt with expeditiously and fairly; and

▶ allotting to the case an appropriate share of the court's (limited) resources.

The lawyers are no longer trusted with the exclusive conduct of the litigation; too often in the past, this meant unnecessary and unreasonable delay whereby not just the parties to the case but all litigants were affected. From being reactive, the court now takes a proactive approach through its powers of 'case management': it will take a case by the scruff of the neck and lay down a procedural timetable whether the parties like it or not. Whilst previously an action would only come before a judge at the instigation of one of the parties, the bringing of a claim now sets off a process whereby the court will arrange case management conferences of its own accord, and the lawyers will need to persuade the court that their conduct of the case is reasonable and appropriate, given the issues and the amount at stake. The court expects the parties to cooperate with each other, to explore settlement at every possible opportunity, and only to expend costs where justified. For clinical negligence cases, one of the most important developments is the power of the court to limit the number and disciplines of experts, encouraging the parties to agree to the instruction of joint experts wherever possible.

The 'track' system

As part of its case-management powers, the court now allocates every claim brought to a particular management track: the small-claims track (generally for claims worth less than £5000); the fast track (for claims worth between £5000 and £15 000); and the multitrack (for claims over £15 000). For personal injury claims, however, the normal rule is varied: where the damages claimed for pain, suffering and loss of amenity exceed £1000, the claim will be allocated to the fast track and not the small-claims track even if the overall value is less than £5000. The allocation of a case to a particular track has consequences for the way in which the case is dealt with subsequently. Small claims are resolved in a relatively informal manner, with strictly limited possibilities of appeal. Fast-track claims are subject to a strict timetable whereby a trial date is set at an early stage and directions are given to enable the trial to proceed on the allocated date or within the allocated trial period. The trial itself will not last more than one day. In practice, most cases of clinical negligence will be allocated to the multitrack. The significance of this is mostly negative in that the case thereby is not subject to the restrictions and streamlining of the small-claims track and fast track; there is a greater flexibility in the multitrack to enable the court to adapt to the more varied and complicated cases that are dealt with. The Practice Direction accompanying Part 29 (PD 29, 2.6[1]) provides that professional negligence claims are considered suitable for trial in the Royal Courts of Justice, and this will automatically entail allocation to the multitrack.

The statement of case

A claim is now started by the court issuing a claim form at the request of the claimant under CPR Part 7, this being equivalent to the old Writ. At the same time, or within 14 days of issue, the claimant also must serve Particulars of Claim. This is one of the documents that now comprise the 'Statement of Case', which also includes the claim form, the Defence and the reply (if any). The intention is that the language used in these documents (formerly known as 'pleadings') should be simple, setting out plainly the factual ingredients of the parties' case. In personal injury actions (which will include actions for clinical negligence) the Particulars of Claim must state the claimant's date of birth and brief details of the personal injuries sustained. There also must be attached a Schedule of Loss and a medical report where the claimant relies on such evidence. If the claim arises out of a patient's death, the Particulars of Claim must state that the claim is brought under the Fatal Accidents Act 1976, and give details of the dependants, their dates of birth and the nature of the dependency claim (see Practice Direction 16, paragraphs 4 and 5).

The CPR also make provision for what should be contained in the Defence. It is no longer acceptable simply to 'not admit' and 'deny' the allegations in an unhelpful fashion that gives no clue as to the real nature of the Defence. Under Part 16.5, the defendant must state which allegations in the Particulars of Claim he denies *and his reasons for so doing*, setting out, if appropriate, his version of events where they differ from the claimant's. Thus, in a clinical negligence claim, it is suggested that a defendant will, before serving the Defence, have taken statements from the clinicians involved, thus enabling the defendant to set out in the Defence an accurate version of what is contained in the medical notes, correcting any misinterpretations on the part of the claimant. The defendant also will wish to justify the treatment of the claimant or deceased, thereby answering fully the allegations of negligence. In this regard, the merits of the CNPAP can be seen: with the three-month moratorium on proceedings after the Letter of Claim, the defendant should have had time to investigate the claim and obtain the necessary statements. No longer should the situation arise where a defendant is suddenly faced with proceedings out of the blue in circumstances whereby it has had no opportunity to investigate the matter and is thereby effectively forced to issue a Defence that is a blanket denial, giving away as little as possible. If this situation should arise, the court is likely to investigate how it came about, and will probably make penal cost orders accordingly.

A further innovation introduced by the CPR is that important documents such as Particulars of Claim and Defences have to be verified by a Statement of Truth (see Part 22). This requirement underlines that the pleadings are no longer simply part of the procedural games that lawyers play, but are actually important documents intended to convey information upon which the court can rely. In some cases, they even may be used as evidence. It is a contempt of court to sign a Statement of Truth without an honest belief in the truth of the facts stated. If a lawyer signs the Statement of Truth (as he may do under Practice Direction 22, paragraph 3.1), he should not do so lightly, but first should obtain his client's authority, having explained the significance of it.

Evidence: general

The court has the power, under the CPR, to control the evidence that is put before it. This power is contained in CPR Part 32.1, which states the following:

(1) The court may control the evidence by giving directions as to:
  (a) the issues on which it requires evidence;
  (b) the nature of the evidence which it requires to decide those issues; and
  (c) the way in which the evidence is to be placed before the court.
(2) The court may use its power under this rule to exclude evidence that would otherwise be admissible.
(3) The court may limit cross-examination.

These provisions are far-reaching and are an important feature of the court's case-management powers. No longer is the calling of evidence in the exclusive control of the parties. Generally, at trial facts that need to be proved by the evidence of witnesses will continue to be proved by the oral testimony of those witnesses in public; but at any other hearing, the evidence will be in writing. The Rules provide for the requirement to serve witness statements for use at trial as had become the norm before the CPR. With the requirement for statements of case to contain Statements of Truth, they too may be used as evidence in interim applications.

The new rules in relation to evidence have resulted in a change in the way trials are now often conducted. Judges will intervene more readily in controlling and limiting the evidence with a view, for example, to controlling the length of a trial. At the start of the trial, the parties may expect the judge to lay down or ask the parties to propose a timetable, with set time limits for cross-examination of the witnesses. Similarly, counsel may be restricted in the time that they are accorded for making submissions at the end of the trial.

Expert evidence

In any clinical negligence action, expert evidence is likely to be of crucial importance. No expert who now agrees to act for a party in such a claim can afford to be ignorant of the provisions in CPR Part 35. To be an expert involves a commitment that may well interfere with the expert's clinical duties and this is the price an expert must be prepared to pay if he is to fulfil his duties to the court.

What is an expert? This is defined in CPR Part 35.2 as 'an expert who has been instructed to give or prepare evidence for the purpose of court proceedings'. This is important because a firm of solicitors may use an expert to give internal advice or a preliminary view of a case. Such a person is not subject to the disciplines of the CPR.

The duties of an expert were comprehensively set out first in *The Ikarian Reefer*[2] of which decision – before implementation of the CPR – no expert could afford to be ignorant (although many in fact were). The most important principle is that an expert's duty lies not to the party who happens to instruct him, but to the *court* (CPR Part 35.3). One consequence of this is that the expert will draw to the court's attention all matters which he/she considers to be material to the issues before the court, whether or not favourable to the interests of the instructing party. Nor can the expert make biased assumptions in relation to the way in which the factual evidence will emerge – for example, by assuming that the evidence of the clinicians will be preferred to the evidence of the claimant, or *vice versa* (at least, without justifying such assumptions).

The form and content of an expert's report are laid down in the Practice Direction accompanying CPR Part 35. It should be addressed to the court, not to the instructing party, and it should contain, among other things, a summary of the conclusions reached, a statement that the expert understands his duty to the court and has complied with that duty, and a Statement of Truth. The consequences of verifying a report without an honest belief in the truth of the report are the usual ones under Part 32.14:

proceedings for contempt may be brought. Moreover, it is difficult to see how such an expert would survive his own profession's disciplinary procedures. This only goes to emphasize that provision of an expert report is a serious matter with important responsibilities and consequences. Previously loyalties, which sometimes existed between certain solicitors and medical experts, may have to be reassessed. The report also must state the substance of all material instructions, written and oral, on the basis of which the report was written.

The emerging case law shows how seriously the courts are taking the provisions in the CPR on the impartiality of experts. In *Stephens v Gullis*,[3] an expert was prevented from giving evidence on the basis that his report did not comply with the requirement of Part 35. The judge said:

> Mr Isaac, not having apparently understood his duty to the court and not having set out in his report that he understands it, is in my view a person whose evidence I should not encourage in the administration of justice.

The court has the power to restrict expert evidence, and an expert may only be called with the court's permission (CPR Part 35.4). A party may put written questions to an expert for the purpose of clarifying the report (CPR Part 35.6), and the court may direct that evidence on a particular issue be given by a single joint expert. At any stage, the court may direct a discussion between experts to identify the issues and reach agreement thereon, if possible. An agreement by a clinician to provide expert evidence thus entails a commitment to make time available for such discussions where necessary.

Finally, a new provision which again emphasizes the expert's duty to the court gives an expert the right to ask the court for directions to assist him in carrying out his function as an expert (see CPR Part 35.14).

Offers to settle and payment into court

Offers to settle and payments into court are dealt with comprehensively in CPR Part 36. The Rules are designed to encourage the parties to make such offers and payments as early as possible, with the provision of penal consequences should an offer/payment prove to have been a good one which ought to have been accepted. A major development is the claimant's offer to settle. Where such an offer is made, but is declined, and then the claimant equals or exceeds the offer made, the court is given the power to award interest on the whole or part of any sum of money awarded to the claimant at a rate not exceeding 10% above base rate for some or all of the period, starting with the latest date on which the defendant could have accepted the offer without needing the court's permission (usually 21 days). Additionally, the court may order that the claimant be entitled to his costs on an indemnity basis from such date.

A further important provision relates to the recognition of offers to settle made before the commencement of proceedings (see CPR Part 36.10). Thus, a defendant may offer to settle a claim, and this will be recognized in the later proceedings provided that the defendant makes a Part 36 payment (ie a payment into court) within 14 days of commencement of proceedings of not less than the sum offered before the proceedings began.

Where a claimant fails to beat a defendant's Part 36 payment or offer, as before implementation of the CPR, the consequence is that the claimant can expect to be ordered to pay the defendant's costs. However, the CPR make one important change: previously, after a payment into court, the claimant had 21 days to accept, but if he failed to do so, the order to pay the costs would date back to the date of the payment in (whilst he would have his own costs from the date of acceptance if this was within the 21 days). Now, where a claimant fails to beat a Part 36 payment, the court will order the claimant to pay the defendant's costs incurred 'after the latest date on which the payment or offer could have been accepted without needing the permission of the court' unless it considers it unjust to do so (CPR Part 36.20). Again, this should encourage defendants to make early Part 36 payments rather than payments in shortly before trial, given that many of the highest costs are often incurred in the immediate pre-trial period.

The rules in relation to Part 36 offers and payments are more flexible than before, and the court has a consequent discretion in how to deal with them. Thus, CPR Part 36.5(3) provides that a Part 36 offer must state whether it relates to the whole of the claim or to part of it, or to an issue that arises in it (and if so, to which part or issue). Clearly, if an offer to settle a particular issue is declined and then the offeror equals or betters the offer made, the court would wish to reflect that offer in the costs order made, for example by ordering the offeree, even though the overall eventual winner, to pay the costs that arose in relation to the issue in question. To take an example, an issue of contributory negligence might arise which the defendant offers to settle on a 50% basis, but which the claimant declines. If the claimant is then held to be 60% to blame for the injury, but wins an issue in relation to damages and thereby beats a Part 36 payment into court, he might nevertheless be ordered to pay the costs of the trial which related to the negligence issue. Equally, a claimant's Part 36 offer could be broken down into its constituent parts, enabling the defendant to accept the offer in relation to, for example, general damages for pain and suffering and past loss, leaving future loss as the only live issue between the parties. If the offer is declined, however, and then the claimant equals or betters the figures in relation to general damages and past loss, but loses overall because, for instance, he loses an issue on expectation of life, he nevertheless may retrieve some of the post-payment in costs in relation to the issues on which he succeeded. In principle, the court, in making its order, will seek to do what is just, in accordance with the overriding principle.

Costs

CPR Parts 43–48 deal with costs and are enormously detailed, beyond the scope of this chapter. In general, though, the court is given a wide discretion over costs, including whether they are payable by one party to another, the amount of the costs and when they are to be paid. Costs are clearly an important aspect of all litigation. Usually, the parties will try to agree the amount of costs to be paid by the losing party, but if agreement cannot be reached, the court will assess the costs. Costs may be assessed on different bases, depending upon who is asking for the assessment. Thus, a losing party who has to pay may ask the court to assess how much he must pay to the other side – known as a 'party and party' assessment. This is not the same as the 'solicitor and client' assessment which the court may make when assessing how much a solicitor is entitled to be paid for work done for his own client.

The consequence of these different bases for assessment is that there may be a shortfall between what the solicitor is entitled to be paid and what the other side is ordered to pay. The successful party will then have to make up the difference, usually from the damages that he is awarded. The court may, however, sometimes order the costs to be paid on an 'indemnity' basis (often as a punitive measure), in which case there should be no such shortfall. As well as there being awards for the costs of the proceedings generally, separate individual awards of costs may be made at various stages of the litigation. Thus, the court can order a party to pay the costs of a particular unsuccessful application, even where that party is otherwise successful overall. Where the court decides that costs have been wasted unnecessarily, it may make a 'wasted costs' order against the lawyers involved, so that it is the lawyers who have to pay the costs rather than the litigants.

The general rule continues to be that the unsuccessful party will be ordered to pay the successful party's costs. But the court is empowered to make a different order having regard to all the circumstances including:

▶ the conduct of the parties;

▶ whether a party has succeeded on part of his case, even if he has not been wholly successful; and

▶ any payment into court or admissible offer to settle made by a party that is drawn to the court's attention, whether or not made in accordance with Part 36 (CPR Part 44.3[4]).

The conduct to be taken into account includes the following:

▶ Conduct before *and* during the proceedings, and in particular the extent to which the parties followed any relevant Pre-action Protocol.

▶ Whether it was reasonable for a party to raise, pursue or contest a particular allegation or issue.

▶ The manner in which a party has pursued or defended his case or a particular allegation or issue.

▶ Whether a claimant who has succeeded in his claim, in whole or in part, exaggerated his claim.

In relation to clinical negligence cases, failure to follow the CNPAP will be an important factor, particularly if it has resulted in the costs being inflated or unnecessary costs being incurred.

References

1   *Access to Justice*. The Final Report of the Right Honourable Lord Woolf. London: HMSO, July 1996.
2   *The Ikarian Reefer* [1993] 2 Lloyds Rep 68.
3   *Stephens v Gullis* [2000] 1 All ER 527.

▶5

Expert Evidence

Roger V Clements

It is the function of the expert to explain technical matters so as to assist the court in understanding the issues; but uniquely amongst witnesses, experts are permitted to express their opinion about matters before a court, often to give an opinion on the principle issue. The responsibilities of the expert witness are correspondingly great.

Who is an expert?

In considering negligence, the court will need to understand the standards to be expected of a doctor in the circumstances of the case. The expert must have the specialized knowledge and experience relevant to the facts under investigation. He must be independent – he should neither be in a therapeutic relationship with the claimant, nor should he be closely connected with the defendant doctor or hospital. He will need particularly to bear in mind the date of the case and apply only those standards which were appropriate to that time.

In causation, the expert's role is somewhat different. Here, the court will not be interested in what was known *at the time* of causation; rather, the best view currently available as to the association between the allegedly negligent act and the injury.

Duties of the expert

The expert's duty, irrespective of the side that calls him, is to the court. That has always been so and has been repeatedly emphasized by the courts, most notably in recent years by Cresswell J. in the *Ikarian Reefer*.[1] That duty has now been formally codified in part 35 of the Civil Procedure Rules (CPR) (see Chapter 4). The principle themes dominating Part 35 are:

▶ The overriding duty of the expert to the court.

▶ The proportionality of cost to the value of the claim.

Rule 35.3 sets out the duty of an expert to help the court, a duty that overrides any obligation of the expert to those instructing or paying him. The expert's duty to the court is clear, but the expert also has a duty to the client who instructs and pays him. *The Draft Code of Guidance for Experts*[2] draws a distinction between those experts who are instructed solely in an advisory capacity (advice) and those who are instructed to prepare evidence for the purpose of court proceedings (report). Every expert, when first approached, is adviser to the client. In many instances, that remains his only role. If the expert's opinion is unfavourable to the instructing side, he is unlikely to be asked to prepare evidence for a court. Once he is so instructed, he becomes an expert within the definition of Part 35 (35.2). Where the expert is able to support the case of the party instructing him, the case will inevitably be based on his opinion. In an adversarial system, the expert necessarily becomes part of the legal team and will be expected to advise on the conduct of the case, not only on the presentation of expert evidence for his 'side' but also in challenging the evidence produced by experts on the other side.

The tension between these roles extends throughout the course of litigation.

Privilege

Traditionally, the dialogue between expert and instructing solicitor has been protected by legal privilege; that privilege has been qualified by the CPR. The report prepared for the court must include the substance of all material instructions (whether written or oral) and must summarize the facts and instructions given to the expert upon which those opinions are based. These instructions will not be protected by privilege and may under certain circumstances be disclosed to the court if the court is 'satisfied that there are reasonable grounds to consider the statement of instructions given ... to be inaccurate or complete'. At present, there is still some uncertainty concerning the precise interpretation of this rule.

Training

Doctors often believe that they have only to use their ordinary medical skills in order to be expert witnesses. Most, however, know little about the law and less about procedure. Experts ignorant of the law within which they operate are a menace to the courts, for they waste time addressing the wrong questions and applying the wrong standards. There is no longer any excuse for this – there is ample training available for those who wish to avail themselves of it. The Expert Witness Institute[3] runs a full training programme, including a course in basic law for experts.

Procedure

Procedure differs somewhat for experts called by the claimant and by the defendant. In the case of a claimant, the expert is usually instructed very early in the proceedings; indeed, the claimant does not know whether she has a case until expert opinion has been obtained. Experts for the defendant, on the other hand, are not usually instructed until after the letter of claim and sometimes not until after proceedings have been issued.

Instruction

The Draft Code of Guidance for Experts[2] enjoins the expert not to accept instructions unless they are clear. The information required by the expert when first approached should include the following:

▶ The identities of the parties;

▶ The nature and extent of the expertise called for;

▶ The purpose of requesting the advice or report;

▶ The track;

▶ The court;

▶ The time scale;

▶ The fees – when they are to be paid; and by whom they are to be paid.

The records

It is essential to see all of the relevant records. If the notes are incomplete, the expert must so advise the instructing solicitor. The records usually will be produced in photocopy and the standards for such copies are set out in the Pre-action Protocol. It is the expert's responsibility to check that the records are complete and that every page has been faithfully copied. Not infrequently, the left margin is missing from the photocopy or is spoiled by the punching of holes or binding so as to obscure important times and dates. Such pages should be rejected. Large documents such as partograms should be provided in their original A3 format and not divided (with the inevitable omissions) into A4 slices. This advice applies with particular force to cardiotocograms (CTGs). There is a general reluctance on the part of defendants to photocopy CTGs in continuity and they are often provided in A4 segments, sometimes cobbled together with sellotape. This is no longer satisfactory and should be rejected. Professional copies can be made, in the UK, by The Times Drawing Office (15 Maddox Street, London W1; Tel: 020 7629 7500), and in Dublin by J D Hackett & Co. Ltd. (17 Lower Baggot Street, Dublin 2; Tel: 00 353 1 676 0301; Fax: 00 353 1 661 4092; e-mail: jdh@iol.ie).

A serviceable copy often can be made by feeding the original through an old-fashioned domestic fax machine. It is folly for the expert to base his opinion on inadequate copy.

It is essential that *every document* is examined in detail. It is my personal practice to put the documents into strict chronological order before examining them. It is a distinct advantage if the hospital records are paginated at an early stage; only in this way can the expert's advice or report be made intelligible to the lawyers – by appropriate reference to the page numbers.

The consultation

It is an essential pre-requisite for a claimant's expert to interview the claimant whilst in possession of all the medical records so as to compare her version of events with the written records. Only in this way can the claimant's view be obtained reliably. Where her memory is different from the medical records, the expert may take the opportunity to clarify the important points of difference. He should refrain from offering an opinion on such matters but confine himself to outlining the areas of apparent conflict. In relation to consent and advice, it will not be possible to ascertain the claimant's understanding without such an interview. Similarly, it is a distinct advantage for the defence expert to interview the doctors concerned, but in my experience of acting for defendants, there is a marked reluctance to allow the expert to interview the treating doctor.

The first report

It is not possible for an expert called to give evidence on breach of duty, whether by claimant or defendant, to produce only one report in a medical negligence case that comes to trial. The initial advice has as its purpose the guidance of counsel in drafting or rebutting the particulars of claim. The first advice is inevitably a 'one-eyed' document, for when first instructed the expert has only one side of the story. It will not be until after the exchange of lay-witness evidence that the expert has a binocular view.

Traditionally, the expert's first draft (advice) foreshadowed the report ultimately produced for the court, and often required little modification when the full facts of the case became clear, after lay-witness evidence had been exchanged. Now, with the restriction on public funding of claims and the introduction of conditional-fee arrangements (CFAs), the first advice to a claimant may be no more than a brief overview based on a limited core bundle of papers; advice which allows the claimant's legal advisers to decide whether further funding, either from the public purse or by CFA, is appropriate. Guidelines have now been introduced[4] for such screening reports in clinical negligence cases.

The covering letter

The letter accompanying the report may include a concise and simplified view of his overall assessment of the case. It also should indicate where further information or opinion is required and outline the purpose for which the advice is made and the use to which it may be put. If the document is not intended as a report for disclosure, as is usually the case, it is important to state that fact unequivocally in the covering letter.

Conference

The earlier the expert is involved in a meeting with solicitors and counsel, the better. Time spent in conference is well worth the time and expense, as it saves both in the long run.

The statement of case

Statements of case are exchanged so that each side may know the other party's case. The particulars of claim and the defence define the allegations and limit the areas of dispute. No evidence can ultimately be given that does not relate to these allegations. A medical report describing the injuries suffered by the claimant must accompany the particulars of claim. This will usually be entirely factual with no opinion on liability.

After the exchange of statements of case, each side can ask the other for clarification; that clarification will often require further expert input.

The final report

The requirements of a report to be disclosed to the court are set out clearly in Part 35 of the CPR. The expert (35.10) must state that he both understands his duty and has complied with it. In *Access to Justice*[5] (III.13.35), Lord Woolf suggested that the report should be supported by a declaration; many of the points to be covered in that declaration are spelled out in the Practice Direction (1.2), although the precise wording is not prescribed. It is for each expert to determine the precise nature of the declaration that accompanies his report but a model has been suggested by the Expert Witness Institute.[6]

For the purpose of court proceedings, an expert report must:

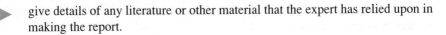

- be addressed to the court,
- give details of the expert's qualifications, and
- give details of any literature or other material that the expert has relied upon in making the report.

Where there is a range of opinion, the expert in the report must:

- summarize the range of opinion, and
- give reasons for his own opinion.

The report must contain a summary of the conclusions reached and it must set out the substance of all material instructions and be verified by a statement of truth. The statement of truth is set out in the Practice Direction and must be followed precisely.

The construction of a report should follow a recognizable pattern with an index and numbered lines or paragraphs. The first and largest part of the report should be detailed reconstruction of the events in question and a careful analysis of all of the relevant medical records. The reconstruction should be couched in terms that an intelligent educated layman would understand. Where there are two versions of events, one by the claimant and one by the hospital records, they should be set out and attention drawn to the difference.

In the second part of the report, the expert should go on to explain the technical matters involved. Such explanatory material may be separated conveniently from the main report into appendices. These should be illustrated liberally to improve understanding.

A third part of the report should relate the case in point to this technical explanation. It should give a critical appraisal of the conduct of the case.

Finally, the expert should give an unequivocal assessment of the standards of care and, if he believes these to have been defective, should set out clearly the areas in which care fell short of a reasonable standard. In this discussion, he should be careful to avoid the term 'negligence' since this is a question of law and might be misunderstood by doctors. In any event, it is for the court to decide after hearing evidence what is acceptable to the profession and hence whether the care was negligent.

In forming his opinion on the standards of care, the expert will refer to standard textbooks, to identify what is an acceptable standard. Where there is research evidence, national or college guidelines, these too may be helpful. Learned scientific papers published shortly before the events in question are likely to be of more value to the defendant than the claimant. Textbooks on the other hand are common coinage and a practitioner ought to be at least as well informed as the postgraduate textbook current at the time.

In causation, it is not necessary that the references quoted should antedate the accident. The very highest level of current knowledge is required to assess causation, irrespective of what was known about causation at the time of the accident.

Questions to experts

Once reports have been exchanged, rule 35.6 of the CPR allows a party to put written questions to the expert of another party about his report. The questions may be put only once and must be within 28 days of service of the expert's report. They 'must be for the purpose only of clarification of the report'. In practice, 'clarification' seems to enjoy a very broad interpretation. No time limit is set in the rules for the answers to the questions but the *Code of Guidance* suggests 28 days.

Sometimes, such questions involve a great deal of additional time for the expert. Before embarking on this work, the expert must ascertain from those instructing him who is responsible for the fees incurred.

Experts' discussions

The courts had previously the power to order discussions between experts but those powers were seldom used. Now, codified in Part 35 of the CPR (35.12) experts' discussions have become the rule. Procedural judges order discussions in most if not all of medical negligence cases in the expectation that it will narrow points of difference between the experts. If trial is not avoided, the time spent in court is much reduced. In November 1999, the Clinical Disputes Forum (CDF)[7] published draft guidelines,[8] which were revised and republished in July 2000.[9] The guidelines, in common with the *Code of Guidance*, emphasize the importance of the agenda to success of the enterprise. The agenda must be detailed and must be agreed in advance by the lawyers of both sides, and should consist, as far as possible, of closed questions; that is, questions that can be answered with 'yes', 'no' or a number.

The most successful meetings are face to face. Whenever the value of the claim justifies it, every effort should be made to get the experts in the same room. At the end of the meeting, a statement should be signed by all those attending, leaving no room for subsequent disagreement about what was agreed. The resulting document will be helpful to the lawyers and to the courts but the rules state unequivocally (35.12[5]) that 'the agreement shall not bind the parties unless the parties expressly agreed to be bound by the agreement'. It is usually advisable to have separate agenda and discussions between experts in different disciplines.

During the CDF consultation on experts' discussions, the most controversial aspect was the attendance of lawyers. The working party initially was reluctant to encourage the presence of lawyers, and they were conscious of a judicial inclination against it. Nevertheless, as the result of consultation the working party changed its view because there appeared to be more advantages than hazards. The main advantages were the maintenance of client confidence and the ability, afforded to the lawyers, to understand the reasoning behind the experts' decisions. The working party therefore recommended a default position in which the lawyers should attend but recognize that in some cases the parties will agree that they should not and the court may so order.

The single joint expert

Expert evidence is expensive. The CPR set out to ration expert evidence, to limit the number of experts called by each side and, where ever possible (35.7), to use a single joint expert (SJE). Whilst the court has the power, under the CPR, to impose a SJE upon the parties, there does not seem at present to be any tendency for the courts to use this power in medical negligence litigation. Increasingly, however, the courts are encouraging and persuading the parties to agree joint experts. There is no enthusiasm on either side for the appointment of single experts for the main issues of liability. There is, however, an increasing willingness to allow them in tangential matters (such as neuroradiology in cerebral palsy) and in quantum. The *Code of Guidance*[2] sets out the principles underlying the conduct of the SJE. At every stage, the conduct of the SJE should be governed by the principles of fairness and transparency. Nothing must be shared with one party without also being shared with every other party in the dispute. All instructions to the SJE *must* be in writing. At the beginning of the case, the SJE must ascertain that he has instructions from both sides and that those instructions are clear. Ideally, a joint letter of instruction should be written but if both sides insist on instructing the expert separately, the expert must make sure that there is no conflict and that each side is aware of the details of the others' instructions. It is not possible to combine the role of adviser with that of SJE, and if already appointed as adviser, the expert should decline SJE instructions. Any advice given to a party must be copied to all parties; if the SJE is invited to attend a conference with counsel, an opportunity should be offered to the solicitors for the other parties to attend that part of the conference attended by the SJE. It is essential that, at the very beginning, the SJE should obtain in writing a clear undertaking for either or both parties for the payment of his fees.

In most cases, the SJE's report will be accepted by both parties. Occasionally, it may be necessary for him to give oral evidence, in which case he may be cross-examined by either or both parties before the court.

Evidence in court

Only rarely does medical malpractice litigation come to trial. Experts who have written scores of reports may never have the experience of their opinions being tested in court. In the days immediately before the trial, the expert should read again the essential court papers. The most important single precaution is to re-read the final report that must form the basis of the evidence to be given orally. Inevitably, minor (perhaps even major) errors will appear for the first time. This is the time to note them, for all is still not lost. Having re-read his own final report, the expert should read the final report of the experts on the other side, identifying the strengths and weaknesses of both cases. His views should by now have been thoroughly tested by counsel in conference so that he is fully aware of the arguments likely to be advanced by the other side and also of the extent to which those arguments can be resisted. It is essential that, before going into the witness box, the expert should have a personal 'court bundle' with which he is familiar, so that, in the heat of cross-examination, important references are ready to hand.

Immediately after the oath, the expert usually will be asked to produce a curriculum vitae and perhaps to summarize it before the court. The curriculum vitae should emphasize those aspects of the expert's own career which are relevant to the case in question.

The first part of oral evidence is the easy bit – examination-in-chief – the opportunity for the expert to go through the final report explaining in as much detail as is necessary for the judge to understand the issues. The pace at which the expert gives evidence should be determined by the judge. The evidence is for the judge and it matters little whether anybody else hears it; it is essential that the judge should not only hear it but have the opportunity to understand it at a speed commensurate with the judge's only requirements to note it. Judges will usually take down the critical part of the evidence in long hand. The expert should address the judge and watch what he does with his hands. If the judge is not writing, it suggests that the judge either knows what he is being told already or thinks it insufficiently important to write down.

In cross-examination, opposing counsel will challenge the expert. In this exercise, counsel will be assisted by his own expert, who will be sitting behind him and providing the ammunition for the questions. The attack may take a number of forms, perhaps attempting to discredit the witness' standing, undermining his status and experience, questioning the relevance of the authorities upon which he relies or just goading him into anger so as to provoke exaggeration and excess. The temptation for the expert is to engage in argument with opposing counsel, arguments which may become heated and which may lead to indiscreet answers. It is only the judge whose opinion matters; defeating opposing counsel is *not* the object of the exercise.

Answers must be addressed to the judge. It is useful discipline always to turn towards the judge before answering counsel's questions. If this produces a brief pause then so much the better. If the question does not permit the answer 'yes' or 'no', the experts should feel under no compulsion to give way to counsel's insistence that it should be so answered. Questions in cross-examination often contain several propositions each one of which has to be considered separately. It is entirely proper, under such circumstances, to turn to the judge and explain that the question demands three separate answers and the expert intends to give three separate answers. If the question contains an assumption that is not true, that too must be explained to the judge. The false assumption should be addressed calmly and then rejected. Sometimes, counsel will put hypothetical questions to the expert. The answer given should make it clear that the hypothesis is understood but that it is only a hypothesis, and it may be helpful after the answer to the question to add 'but that is not this case'.

Sometimes, counsel's challenge is appropriate and the expert must concede. It is important to concede gracefully and accept it when an alternative point of view might reasonably prevail. Obstinacy in the face of convincing argument will not impress the judge. Finally, when cross-examination is finished, the expert and counsel will have an opportunity for re-examination. Sometimes, at the very end of the expert's evidence, the judge will ask questions. These questions often are the key to the case. They indicate the area in which the judge believes he needs to investigate. The answers assume considerable importance.

When the opposing experts are giving evidence, counsel will usually need skilled assistance in mounting a challenge and, during cross-examination, will need his own expert sitting in front of or behind him so as to feed questions and challenge wrong answers. In fulfilling this function, the expert is again acting as adviser and is exercising his duty to the party who called him.

References

1   National Justice Campania Naviera SA v Prudential Assurance Co. Ltd. (*The Ikarian Reefer*) [1993] 2 Lloyd's Rep 68. Clinical Risk 1999; 5(4):135–136.
2   Draft Code of Guidance for Experts under the Civil Procedure Rules 1998 (CPR). Clinical Risk 1999; 5(5): 168–172.
3   The Expert Witness Institute, Africa House, 64–78 Kingsway, London WC2B 6BG, UK. Website: http://www.EWI.org.uk.

4   Tansley G. Guidelines for screening reports. Clinical Risk 2001; 7(1): 14.
5   *Access to Justice*. Final report of the Right Honourable Lord Woolf. London: HMSO, July 1996.
6   Clements RV. The New Civil Procedure Rules: Part 35. Clinical Risk 1999; 5(3): 90–92.
7   Clinical Disputes Forum. Website: http://www.clinical-disputes-forum.org.uk/.
8   Consultation on guidelines on experts discussions in the context of clinical disputes. Clinical Risk 1999; 5(6): 205–208.
9   Guidelines on experts' discussions in the context of clinical disputes. Clinical Risk 2000; 6(4): 149–152.

►6 ⟋

Leading Cases

James Watt

Duty of Care

McKay v Essex Area Health Authority [1982] QB 1166

A pregnant mother contracted rubella during the early months of pregnancy. Although blood tests had been undertaken by the Health Authority, the diagnosis was not made, and the baby was born with significant disabilities. An action was brought on behalf of the child alleging that there had been negligence in not treating the mother for rubella, and in not advising her that she could have an abortion. This was an action for 'wrongful life' since it could not be alleged that the defendant's conduct had caused the child's injuries, but that the child had been allowed to 'enter into life' with severe incurable injuries.

The Court of Appeal held that there was no duty of care owed to *the child* to advise the mother of the serious consequences for the child of exposure to rubella and of the desirability of an abortion, although such a duty was owed to the mother. Therefore, there could be no claim by the child. In effect, the child's claim was for a right to be aborted, which was contrary to public policy as a violation of the sanctity of human life.

'Wrongful life' claims are to be distinguished from 'wrongful birth' claims, which involve an action by a parent where it is claimed that a birth should not have taken place. This includes failed sterilization operations, failure to warn that a sterilization operation may not succeed, failed abortions, and failure to advise a mother of the risk that her baby is likely to be born with serious disabilities, thus depriving her of the ability to choose whether or not to have an abortion.

Burton v Islington Health Authority; De Martell v Merton & Sutton Health Authority [1992] 3 All ER 833

For many years, unlike the position in other jurisdictions, there was no case in which a decision had been sought respecting a possible duty of care to an unborn child. In these two cases, in which the children were born before 22 July 1976, damages were claimed for negligent treatment while the children were in the womb. It was asserted by the defendants that no duty of care was owed to the children at the time the injuries were inflicted.

The Court of Appeal held that a child can recover damages at common law for a pre-natal injury. As damage to a fetus is within the foreseeable risk of harm that could arise from a defendant's negligence, the cause of action arises when the fetus is born injured when the child acquires the legal personality to be able to sue.

The Congenital Disabilities (Civil Liability) Act 1976 came into force on 22 July 1976. It confers a right of action on a child who is born alive and disabled in respect of the disability, if it is caused by an occurrence which affected either the parent's ability to have a normal, healthy child, or affected the mother during pregnancy, or affected the mother or child in the course of its birth, causing disabilities that would not otherwise have been present. A defendant is liable to the child if he is or would – if sued in time – have been liable in tort to the parent, and it is no answer that the parent has suffered no actionable injury. The Act applies only to children born *alive*.

Breach of duty

Bolam v Friern Hospital Management Committee [1957] 2 All ER 118

In 1954, Mr John Bolam was admitted to hospital suffering from depression and was advised by his consultant psychiatrist to undergo a course of electro-convulsive therapy (ECT), a well-established form of treatment capable of alleviating depression.

The procedure involved passing an electric current through the patient's brain, and it was likely that the patient would have convulsions during the treatment. Moreover, a remote possibility existed that the patient might suffer fractures. Some psychiatrists had gone as far as to use relaxant drugs, a practice that had begun the previous year, 1953. Others favoured a measure of manual restraint of the patient. Mr Bolam's consultant fell within another group who, concerned about what were described as mortality risks from the use of relaxant drugs, provided them only when there were particular reasons for their use. He was not in favour of manual restraint.

The risk of fractures was not explained to Mr Bolam when he signed the consent form. Although the first course of ECT proceeded without incident, during the second course, which was properly administered, the patient suffered gravely from the dislocation of both hip joints. He had fractures of the pelvis on each side as the head of each femur was driven through the acetabulum during the procedure.

The patient's principal allegations were as follows: First, the consultant had failed to warn him of the risk of the very injuries from which he had suffered and therefore had deprived him of the opportunity of deciding whether or not to undergo the treatment. Second, the treatment had been given negligently. He should have been protected from the risk of fracture by the use of relaxant drugs, or, if no drugs were used, some manual control should have been provided (and not just having the patient lying with a pillow under his back and his lower jaw supported on a mouth gag by a male nurse, which were the arrangements for this patient).

The issue to be decided was whether the patient's consultant had been negligent in failing to take precautions against the risk of fracture, either by the use of relaxant drugs or by arranging manual restraint of the patient. Although there was impressive expert evidence to support the use of the relaxant drugs, much was said about the risks of mortality associated with them, and examples were given. There was a firm body of opinion against using relaxant drugs as a routine. It was thought by the experts that manual restraint might increase rather than diminish the risk of fracture.

During the course of his summing up, the judge adopted the views expressed by a judge in a Scottish case some two years earlier. The judge said:

> A doctor is not guilty of negligence if he has acted in accordance with a practice accepted as proper by a responsible body of medical men skilled in that particular art . . . A doctor is not negligent if he is acting in accordance with such a practice merely because there is body of opinion which takes a contrary view.

The jury returned their verdict for the defendant.

Although this case remained a decision at first instance, it will be seen from the cases referred to below just how much significance the House of Lords has attached to the '*Bolam* test', as set out above by the judge.

Whitehouse v Jordan [1981] 1 All ER 267

The defendant, a senior registrar, took charge of the claimant's delivery after she had been in labour for a considerable time. The consultant's notes had indicated that delivery might be difficult and that a 'trial of forceps' would have to be attempted before a Caesarean section was undertaken. Although during the trial of forceps the defendant pulled six times, with the mother's contractions, there was no progress on the fifth and sixth pulls and the baby was then delivered swiftly by Caesarean section. The child suffered brain damage from asphyxia.

The claim was primarily on the grounds that the defendant 'had pulled too long and too hard' during the trial of forceps, causing the brain damage. In evidence, the claimant insisted that she had been 'lifted off the bed' by the application of the forceps and while the judge acknowledged this to have been clinically impossible he found the defendant's actions to have been negligent.

The Court of Appeal reversed this judgment, however, on the grounds that the finding of negligence arose from an unjustified interpretation of the factual evidence and also (*per* Lord Denning) that if the defendant had pulled too long and too hard, this was no more than an error of judgment, and not negligent. The claimant's appeal to the House of Lords was dismissed unanimously, but not before criticism of Lord Denning's observation was made clear: Lord Edmund-Davies saying that reference to an error of judgment was wholly ambiguous, as while some errors could well be consistent with the exercise of professional skill, others might be so below the proper standard that a finding of negligence must follow.

In a reference to the *Bolam* test, Lord Edmund-Davies made it clear that if a surgeon fails to measure up to the standard of the ordinary skilled man exercising and professing to have that skill in any respect ('clinical judgement' or otherwise), he will have been negligent.

Maynard v West Midlands Regional Health Authority [1984] 1 WLR 634

Just as *Whiehouse v Jordan* was the first case in which the House of Lords expressed a clear view about the standards to be applied relating to treatment, so this case was the first to reach the House directed to questions of diagnosis.

The patient had a chest complaint and two consultants, a physician and a surgeon, thought that the most likely diagnosis was tuberculosis. The patient had swollen glands in the mediastinum which was not accompanied by lesions in the lungs; there was a possibility that she was suffering from Hodgkin's disease, which could be fatal unless treatment was given early. The doctors decided to take a biopsy without waiting for the result of a test that could show whether or not she was suffering from tuberculosis. During the biopsy the patient suffered an inherent risk of such surgery: damage to the left laryngeal recurrent nerve, resulting in paralysis of the left vocal cord.

At first instance, the primary facts were not in dispute; nor was it alleged that the surgery was carried out negligently. The question was whether it was wrong and dangerous to have taken the biopsy when the most likely diagnosis was tuberculosis.

The judge, having heard distinguished expert evidence from both sides, found for the claimant, primarily because he had particularly liked the evidence of one of the experts called on her behalf whilst complimenting the other experts on the quality of their evidence.

The Court of Appeal did not care for the judge's approach, and allowed the defendant's appeal by a majority, regarding themselves as able to re-interpret the expert evidence from the transcript of the trial, particularly as there had been no dispute about the facts. The claimant obtained leave to appeal from the House of Lords.

The House of Lords unanimously dismissed the appeal. Lord Scarman was satisfied in this case that the Court of Appeal was justified in its conclusions. In the realm of diagnosis, he confirmed that 'the test is the standard of the ordinary skilled man exercising and professing to have that special skill'. Lord Scarman was troubled by the judge's expressed 'preference' for one distinguished professional opinion over another. He stated that such a 'preference' is not sufficient to establish negligence in a practitioner whose actions have received the seal of approval of those whose opinions, truthfully expressed and honestly held, were not preferred. He said:

> ... in the realm of diagnosis negligence is not established by preferring one respectable body of professional opinion to another. Failure to exercise the ordinary skill of a doctor (in the appropriate specialty, if he be a specialist) is necessary.

Sidaway v The Board of Governors of the Bethlem Royal Hospital and the Maudsley Hospital [1985] AC 871; [1985] 1 All ER 643

In this case, the claimant sued after she suffered disabilities following a neurosurgical operation intended to alleviate pain in her neck, right shoulder and arms. She claimed not that the surgery performed was negligent, but that the neurosurgeon had been negligent in failing to warn her of the risk of damage to either the spinal cord or to nerve roots, particularly as the operation which gave rise to the claim was the second undergone by the patient. .

The neurosurgeon died before the case was heard. The patient insisted that her surgeon had given no warning of any kind before the operation, but was not believed by the judge. He found that she had not been told that the operation was one of choice rather than of necessity, that she had been told that a nerve root might be disturbed and the consequences, but not about the risk to the spinal cord. He applied the *Bolam* test and found for the defendant. The Court of Appeal agreed.

This was the first case to be brought to the House of Lords concerning allegations of negligence over an issue of consent. While the appeal was dismissed unanimously, Lord Scarman differed from his colleagues about the nature and amount of information required to be given to a patient to enable the patient to give an 'informed consent'. Lord Bridge (with whom the other three Law Lords agreed) said that there were three parts to a doctor's professional function: diagnosis, advice and treatment. So far as the provision of information to a patient was concerned, he preferred to apply the *Bolam* test to the question of what a patient should be told

Bull v Devon Area Health Authority [1993] 4 Med LR 117

A mother gave birth to twins in hospital. In part because the hospital operated on two sites, there was an interval of 68 minutes between the birth of the two children, the second of whom suffered hypoxia, which led to brain damage caused by the delay in his birth. The medical evidence showed that no more than 20 minutes should have passed between the birth of the first and the second twin.

There had been a substantial delay in summoning expert obstetric assistance to the birth of the second twin, and the Health Authority was held to be liable for having implemented an unsatisfactory and unreliable system for calling expert assistance in an emergency. Such an emergency as occurred was foreseeable, and the Health Authority had an inadequate system for dealing with the known risks that such an emergency was likely to create. Further, there was no reason why this kind of duty should be limited to obstetric services. It would apply to any service offered by a hospital in which a foreseeable emergency might arise.

Bolitho v City and Hackney Health Authority [1997] 4 All ER 771; [1997] 3 WLR 1151

The patient was two years old when he was admitted to hospital suffering from croup. The senior house officer (SHO) who had seen him on an earlier admission examined him again and arranged for him to be nursed on a one-to-one basis. The next morning, he was much better and was seen later by the consultant on his ward round, who was not concerned by his condition. The boy ate a large lunch.

At about 12.40 hours, the nurse summoned the Sister as the boy's colour was very poor and his respiratory sounds 'awful'. Sister asked the Senior Registrar to see the boy at once. Neither she nor the SHO did so at any time. On her return from her telephone call to the doctor, Sister was surprised to see the boy walking about the ward 'with a decidedly pink colour'. At 14.00 hours, the boy had another episode of respiratory difficulty, which was reported to the Senior Registrar by phone. Again, the patient appeared to recover completely. At 14.30 hours, however, the boy became distressed and the nurse summoned the cardiac arrest team because the patient's respiratory system had become completely blocked. He suffered a cardiac arrest, and, as it took between nine to ten minutes to revive him, severe brain damage resulted.

The negligence claim came to trial after the patient had died. The judge accepted the evidence from the Sister about the sequence of events that had occurred. The Senior Registrar was in breach of her duty of care to the patient having neither attended nor having arranged for a suitable deputy to see the patient. As negligence had been established, it had to be decided whether the cardiac arrest would have been avoided if a suitable doctor had attended. By the end of the trial, it was agreed by the parties first that intubation to provide an airway would have ensured that respiratory failure would not have led to cardiac arrest, and second, that intubation had to have taken place before 14.30 hours.

The judge accepted the Senior Registrar's evidence that if she had seen the boy at 14.00 hours, she would not have intubated him, but would have sought to ensure that speedy intubation could have taken place if necessary.

Eight medical experts, five for the claimant and three for the defendant gave evidence on the question of whether a competent doctor should have intubated if he or she had attended the patient at any time after 14.00 hours. The judge found that all the experts were distinguished and truthful. One of each of the experts for either side was particularly impressive and diametrically opposed. The judge held that the Senior Registrar, if she had attended and not intubated the child, would have demonstrated a proper level of competence. He followed Lord Scarman in the *Maynard* case (see above) and gave judgment for the defendants.

The Court of Appeal agreed with the judge by a 2-1 majority, and the House of Lords upheld the judgment unanimously. The House once more confirmed that the standard of care in medical negligence cases was to be decided by a responsible, reasonable and respectable body of medical opinion (the *Bolam* test); although in rare instances, the court will reject such a body of opinion if it is illogical. The House indicated that the *Bolam* test does not apply in determining causation.

Penney, Palmer and Cannon v East Kent Health Authority [2000] Lloyds Rep Med 41

These three women had cervical smears reported as negative but went on to develop invasive adenocarcinoma of the cervix, requiring very extensive and radical treatment.

The patients' case was tried initially on the issue of liability. The judge had to decide whether the primary cytoscreeners who had examined the slides had been negligent in deciding that the smears were negative. None of them gave evidence, but extensive and conflicting expert evidence was given. The Court of Appeal sustained the judge's finding at first instance that the primary cytoscreeners had been negligent, and with reference to the *Bolam* test, (a) confirmed that it was generally applicable as the cytoscreeners were exercising skill and judgement in determining what report they should make; but (b) it applied subject to the qualification that expert evidence which the defendant's conduct accorded with sound medical practice had to be capable of withstanding logical analysis.

Causation

Barnett v Chelsea Hospital Management Committee [1969] 1 QB 428

Three nightwatchmen attended hospital, clearly appearing to be ill, and complaining of vomiting. The casualty officer did not see the men and advised them to go home and see their own doctor. Five hours later, however, one of the men died from arsenic poisoning.

The court held that the casualty officer was negligent as he had not seen or examined the patients. The medical evidence indicated that it could not be said that but for the doctor's negligence the deceased would have lived, because the medical evidence made it plain that even if the claimant had received prompt treatment it would not have been possible to diagnose the condition and to administer an antidote in time to have saved him. Therefore, the negligence did not cause the death.

This is an example of the 'but for' test of causation. If the claimant would not have been damaged *but for* the defendant's negligence, the negligence is one cause of the damage. If the damage would have occurred in any event, the defendant's behaviour is not a cause.

Hotson v East Berkshire Health Authority [1987] 2 All ER 909

The claimant was 13 years old when he dropped 12 feet from a rope he was swinging from on to muddy ground, landing on his seat. He was taken to hospital, where only his left knee was X-rayed and he was discharged home with an elastic knee bandage. After five days of excruciating pain and no assistance from his family doctor, he was re-admitted and his hip X-rayed, when an acute traumatic fracture separation of the left femoral epiphysis was found.

Emergency treatment by traction with manipulation under general anaesthetic was given, together with reduction and pinning of the fracture. A major threat from the fracture was interference with the blood supply to the epiphysis, the spongy extremity of the upper femur whose surface is covered with cartilage, which slots into the cavity of the acetabulum to form the hip joint. The risk was that the interference with the blood supply would cause avascular necrosis, resulting in a displaced hip, pain, restriction in mobility and general disability and a virtual certainty of the development of osteoarthritis in the joint. The patient went on to suffer avascular necrosis

It was common ground that the hospital had been negligent in sending the boy home when he was first brought to hospital, and quantum of damage needed to be addressed. At first instance, the judge held that immediately after the accident there was a 75% chance that the patient's disability would have occurred without any negligence by the hospital. He therefore awarded 25% of the damages to which the claimant would otherwise have been entitled.

Although the Court of Appeal agreed with the trial judge and dismissed the defendant's appeal, the House of Lords thought quite differently. The House said that the basic question to be answered was 'did the breach of duty cause the injury to the claimant or did it not?' In order to prove causation of the avascular necrosis, the claimant had to show that, had there not been negligence, he would have had a better than 50% chance of making a virtually full recovery. The judge had found that the avascular necrosis was caused by the separation of the left femoral epiphysis when the boy hit the ground after his fall. Therefore he was not entitled to any damages for the severe permanent disability. The appeal by the defendants was therefore allowed.

Wilsher v Essex Area Health Authority [1988] AC 1074

This case, when finally decided by the House of Lords, confirmed that where negligence can be established, the onus remains on the claimant to prove that the damage suffered by a patient was caused by the negligence which occurred.

Martin Wilsher was born three months prematurely weighing only 1200 g. He would have had only a one in five chance of survival without the special care he received. He had a stormy time, and was close to death. The fear of brain damage was always present. He required extra oxygen for 11 weeks. Ultimately, he developed sufficiently to be discharged with no impairment to his intelligence. He suffered one grave handicap, however – virtual blindness.

Proceedings were brought alleging that the blindness had been caused by retinopathy of prematurity (then called retrolental fibroplasia or RLF) because he had received an excessive supply of oxygen the monitoring of which had been negligently managed.

An element of negligence had occurred when a doctor failed to notice that a catheter had been inserted into an umbilical vein rather than into an artery resulting in inaccurate monitoring.

When this, and a subsequent error were corrected, it was appreciated that the patient had had excessive oxygen for about 8–12 hours. The excess oxygen was taken as being the cause of the patient's blindness (save for one dissenting judgment in the Court of Appeal) until the case reached the House of Lords. On the factual and expert evidence, RLF was not the only prospective cause of the patient's blindness. Prematurity, hypercarbia, intraventicular haemorrhage, apnoea, or patent ductus arteriosis could have brought it about. The House of Lords held that it was wrong of the judge effectively to have required the defendants to prove that the RLF was not caused by the excess oxygen administered, and affirmed the requirement for the claimant to prove causation of damage as well as the breach of duty which had been found against the defendants.

Loveday v Renton & Wellcome Foundation Ltd. [1990] 1 Med LR 117

This case was the lead action in a group of some 200 claims made on behalf of small children who, it was alleged, had suffered permanent brain damage following pertussis vaccination. The trial was based on a preliminary issue: *Can or could pertussis vaccine used in the United Kingdom and administered intramuscularly in normal dosage cause brain damage or death in young children?*

The claimant argued that negligence arose when a doctor vaccinated in breach of guidelines and would be liable for any resulting brain damage, and also that the court was not to decide whether expert opinion 'was well founded' but to discover the 'preponderance of confluence' of medical opinion. The claimants case centred on clinical case reports, and the 'widely held belief' that the vaccine could, if only rarely, cause permanent brain damage.

The judge refused to accept these arguments, applying the *Bolam* test to the first point, and made clear that it was the task of the court to determine the factual issue by weighing and evaluating the evidence to discover whether the claimant had discharged the burden of proof of causation. The case reports did no more than raise the hypothesis of whether or not the vaccine could cause brain damage in children where the onset of serious illness occurred between 24 and 72 hours after vaccination. He found for the defendants in a most extensive and comprehensive judgment.

Sterilization/vasectomy

Thake v Maurice [1986] 1 All ER 497

The male claimant underwent a vasectomy, but became fertile after re-canalization. Thus, the female claimant became pregnant. Although the defendant had given both claimants a detailed demonstration of the procedure and its effects, he had failed to give his usual warning that there was a slight risk that the male claimant might become fertile again. A majority in the Court of Appeal held that, on an objective interpretation, the defendant (who was liable to the claimant in contract as well as in tort, as this was a private operation) had not given a contactual guarantee that the operation would make the male claimant irreversibly sterile. Nonetheless, the defendant was liable in negligence. He had said that he had failed to give his usual warning about the slight risk of re-canalization. There was no expert evidence before the court and the claimant was entitled to rely on the defendant's evidence of a departure from his own usual practice regarding a warning.

Lybert v Warrington Health Authority [1996] 7 Med LR 71

The claimant became pregnant whilst awaiting a hysterectomy. She was told that although a hysterectomy could not be performed during what was to be her third delivery by Caesarean section, a sterilization could be carried out. She signed a consent form, was delivered of a healthy child and sterilized. Contraception was abandoned. Fifteen months later, the claimant became pregnant again, and gave birth to a healthy boy.

At first instance, the judge found for the claimant, and the Court of Appeal agreed. Otton L.J. held *inter alia* that:

1) there was a duty to ensure that a proper and effective system to provide a warning to a patient was in place;
2) the judge was entitled to decide that a sufficiently clear and comprehensible warning was never given;
3) it was likely that the claimant and her husband would have heeded a proper warning;
4) in view of the mother's history, it was to be expected that the claimant would have used additional contraception while waiting for the hysterectomy.

Gold v Haringey Health Authority [1987] 2 All ER 888

In 1979, the day after the birth of her third child, the claimant underwent a sterilization, which failed. She subsequently had a fourth child. She alleged that the defendants were negligent in failing to warn her of the risks that the sterilization procedure could fail to render her sterile.

The evidence showed that the failure rate for female sterilization was in the range of 20–60 per 10 000, with operations carried out immediately after birth at the higher end of the range. By contrast, the failure rate for vasectomy was five per 10 000.

The trial judge found that the risks of failure were not explained to the patient. The defendant had provided no advice about the possibility of vasectomy, or explained the relative failure rates for the two procedures. The medical experts were unanimous in saying that they would have warned about the risks of failure of sterilization, but acknowledged that a substantial body of responsible doctors would not have given a warning in 1979. Applying the *Bolam* test, it could be said that the defendant was not negligent, but the judge drew a distinction between advice given in a therapeutic context, and that given in a contraceptive context. In the former, there was a responsible body who would not have given a warning, but, he said, there was no such body of opinion in the latter case. Therefore, he found for the claimant.

The Court of Appeal reversed the finding. The court refused to accept that any distinction should be drawn between therapeutic or non-therapeutic advice. Such a distinction would be a departure from the *Bolam* test, which 'does not depend on the context in which any act was performed, or any advice given. It depends on a man professing skill or competence in a field beyond that possessed by the man on the Clapham omnibus'. Therefore, the defendant was not liable because there was a responsible body of medical opinion which, in 1979, would not have given a warning.

Pearce v United Bristol Healthcare Trust [1999] PIQR P 53

The claimant suffered a miscarriage on December 4 1991. Her estimated date of delivery had been November 13 1991. On November 27, she was examined by a doctor. The baby was still viable. He advised that medical intervention was inappropriate, having discussed the risks of induction and the disadvantage of Caesarean section. No reference was made by the doctor to the increased risk of still birth from the passage of time after November 27 (which was no more than between 0.1% and 0.2%).

The judge dismissed a claim by the patient, and the Court of Appeal agreed, holding that the *Bolam* test is to be applied to the giving or failure to give advice by a doctor. Where a patient alleges that she has been deprived of the opportunity to take a proper decision about her treatment, if there is a significant risk which would affect a reasonable patient's judgment, then it is the doctor's responsibility to tell the patient.

In this case, the expert evidence indicated that the risk created by the passage of time was not significant.

Quantum

McFarlane v Tayside Health Board [1999] 3 WLR 1301

In 1989, the claimants, who lived in Scotland, decided that Mr McFarlane would have a vasectomy as the couple had four children. In October 1989, the operation proceeded satisfactorily and after the patient had provided two samples of sperm, he was advised by letter that it was now safe to abandon contraception. This advice was wrong. In mid-June 1992, Mrs McFarlane gave birth to another healthy child, Catherine. Although she was at once accepted into the family, the parents took proceedings in Scotland. Mrs McFarlane claimed £10 000 for her pain and distress occasioned by her pregnancy and childbirth, and the couple claimed £100 000 for the cost of bringing up Catherine.

Both claims were dismissed at first instance, but on appeal, the Second Division of the Court of Session allowed both the claimants' appeals.

The defenders appealed to the House of Lords. This was the first time that a claim relating to a negligent sterilization had come to the House, although a number of such cases had been before the Court of Appeal, which had allowed both of the claims in earlier actions.

Lord Steyn analysed the results of such claims made all over the developed world. Four of the five Law Lords ultimately agreed that the mother's claim was entirely justified, and allowed it, but the couples' claim for the cost of bringing up Catherine was a claim for economic loss. Lord Steyn said that the parents' claim could be allowed applying the notion of 'corrective justice' but he preferred to invoke 'distributive justice', which he acknowledged to be a moral theory. Applying this theory, he considered that tort law does not permit parents of a *healthy* unwanted child to claim the costs of the child's upbringing from a Health Authority or a doctor, and so that claim was dismissed.

Thus, the result in this case overturned the earlier Court of Appeal decisions concerning the maintenance and upbringing of a child. The question of what should be awarded to a child born in these circumstances but with mental and/or physical disabilities was not addressed by the court.

Consent

F v West Berkshire Health Authority [1989] 2 All ER 545

The patient was a woman aged 36 years, with a serious mental disability. A voluntary patient in a mental hospital, she had formed a relationship with a male patient. The psychiatrists believed that the patient would not understand the meaning of pregnancy, labour or delivery, and, if she did give birth, would be unable to look after a baby. They said that it would be disastrous for her to have a child. Other contraceptive methods were considered to be unreliable and/or to involve a risk of harm to her physical health. Therefore, it was thought prudent for her to be sterilized. However, because of her mental disability she could not consent to an operation, and no wardship jurisdiction could be invoked because she was physically over the age of majority.

Ultimately, the House of Lords invoked the principle of *necessity* to provide a solution. Treatment necessary to preserve the life, health or wellbeing of the patient may be given lawfully without consent. It was said that an operation or other treatment performed on adult patients incapable of consenting would be lawful if it was in the best interests of the patient. It would be in the patient's best interest 'if, but only if, it is carried out in order either to save their lives or to ensure improvement or prevent deterioration in their physical or mental health'.

Although the statement about the range of treatment rendered lawful by the observation above about the patient's best interests is very broad, and could be said to cover almost everything which a doctor might think of doing to a patient, Lord Brandon clearly was concerned not to place unjustified restraint on the defence about the performance of treatment to or operation on a patient which the patient needed and to which he was entitled. The same argument was deployed to justify the adoption of the *Bolam* test as the right standard for measuring the patient's best interests: 'If doctors were to be required, in deciding whether an operation or other treatment was in the best interests of adults incompetent to give consent, to apply some test more stringent than the Bolam test, the result would be that such adults would, in some circumstances at least, be deprived of the benefit of medical treatment which adults competent to give consent would enjoy. In my opinion it would be wrong for the law, in its concern to protect such adults, to produce such a result'.

Particularly in the light of the comprehensive guidelines set out by the Court of Appeal in *Re MB* [1997] 8 Med LR 217; [1998] 3 All ER 673 (see pages 70 above, and below), great care must be taken before providing any treatment without the agreement of the court, save in defined circumstances.

Treatment will be lawful if it is the best interests of the patient if, but only if, it is carried out either to save her life or to ensure improvement or prevent deterioration in her physical or mental health. In the case of a patient whose incapacity is only temporary, a doctor should do no more than is reasonably required, in the best interests of the patient, before she recovers consciousness, and she can be consulted and her consent sought to such further treatment, including such operation as may be advisable.

Re T (Adult: Refusal of Medical Treatment) [1992] 4 All ER 649

The patient had been brought up as a Jehovah's Witness, but was not a baptized or practising member of the faith. When 34 weeks pregnant, she was injured in a car accident. The possibility of a blood transfusion arose, but after a private conversion with her mother, the patient told the medical staff that she did not want a blood transfusion. After the patient had been delivered by emergency Caesarean section, her condition deteriorated, and she was admitted to intensive care, where the consultant wished to give a blood transfusion.

The patient was placed on a ventilator and remained sedated and in a critical condition until after an emergency hearing before the judge, when a blood transfusion was given. The judge had granted a declaration that the giving of the transfusion would not be unlawful. At a second hearing, the judge said that the patient had neither consented to nor refused consent to the transfusion, and it was therefore lawful for the doctors to do what they regarded as being in the patient's best interests.

The Court of Appeal agreed. Lord Donaldson M.R. stated that the basic rule in the case of a competent patient is that she has an absolute right to choose whether to consent to medical treatment, or to choose one treatment rather than another on offer. (See *Re S* [Adult: Refusal of Medical Treatment] [1992] 4 All ER 671, below.) This right exists 'notwithstanding that the reasons for making the choice are rational, irrational, unknown or non-existent'. It does not follow that because adult patients have the right to choose that they have necessarily exercised that right. In this case, Lord Donaldson said that in his view, sufficient evidence existed to justify a finding that T was not in a physical or mental condition to have the capacity to consent or refuse consent to treatment; and in any event, the influence of her mother was such as to vitiate T's decision. Doctors faced with a refusal of consent have to give very careful consideration to the patient's capacity to decide at the time when the decision was made. A patient's capacity may be temporarily reduced. The doctors should consider whether at the time the decision is made the patient had the capacity commensurate with the gravity of the decision which he purported to make. The more serious the decision, the greater the capacity required.

Lord Donaldson also said that where a patient has been subjected to the influence of a third party, the real question was, 'Does the patient really mean what she says or is she merely saying it for a quiet life, to satisfy someone else, or because the advice and persuasion to which she has been subjected is such that she can no longer think and decide for herself?' In other words, was the decision expressed in form only, not in reality?

Re S (Adult: Refusal of Medical Treatment) [1992] 4 All ER 671

In this case, a mature woman aged 30 refused, on religious grounds, to consent to delivery by Caesarean section. The patient had been admitted to hospital with ruptured membranes; she was in spontaneous labour and had been so since admission. If the patient did not undergo delivery by Caesarean section, her baby could not be born alive, and there was a grave risk to the mother's life.

On an emergency application to the judge, Sir Stephen Brown P. granted a declaration that it would be lawful to perform the operation and any necessary consequential treatment despite S's refusal of consent, because the treatment was in the 'vital interests' of the patient and the unborn child.

The legal basis for the judge's decision is quite unclear and follows no authority. In *Re T* (above), Lord Donaldson, when stating the basic proposition that a competent patient had a right to choose whether to accept or reject medical treatment, said, 'The only possible qualification is a case in which the choice may lead to the death of a viable foetus and, if and when it arises, the court will be faced with a novel problem of considerable legal and ethical complexity'. A case from the United States also was referred to, in the mistaken belief that the court had ruled that a competent patient could be compelled to undergo a delivery by Caesarean section.

Re MB (1997) 8 Med LR 217; [1998] 3 All ER 673

The patient was admitted to hospital in spontaneous labour. Her footling breech presentation resulted in clear advice to her that she should be delivered by Caesarean section. The patient fully understood the advice and was prepared to agree but could not tolerate the use of a needle to induce anaesthesia. She also firmly rejected induction using a facemask. In addition to advice from her consultant obstetrician and consultant anaesthetist, her GP visited her in hospital and she was seen by a consultant psychiatrist. She remained adamant that she could not accept the induction of anaesthesia, and so an application was made to the court, but not before arrangements had been made for the patient to be legally represented by solicitors and leading counsel. The judge heard the hospital's application by telephone (in the hearing of the patient's representative), and after he granted a declaration that induction of anaesthetic would be lawful, the patient appealed to the Court of Appeal which sat the same night at 23.00 hours. The Court of Appeal heard argument from the patient and the hospital at length and dismissed the patient's appeal at about 01.30 hours the following day. Thereafter, the patient submitted to the induction with a good grace, and was safely delivered. Later, the Court of Appeal, in a reserved judgment, provided detailed guidance about the proper steps to be taken including application to the court if the issue of consent to a procedure cannot be resolved by advice to the patient. The guidance is set out in Chapter 3, page 34, and is of particular importance to patients and obstetricians.

Foreseeability

Brown v Lewisham & North Southwark Health Authority [1999] Lloyds Med Rep 110

After quadruple coronary artery by-pass surgery in London, the patient was discharged eight days later to return to hospital in Blackpool. He developed a deep-vein thrombosis (DVT) in his left leg, which was not recognized until after his re-admission to the Blackpool hospital 10 days after his original surgery. Heparin, which had been given earlier, was re-started. The patient suffered an adverse reaction to the heparin known as thrombocytopenia and thrombosis (HITT) and on the same day the heparin was stopped. The patient's underlying condition was not recognized. Because of a justified concern that the patient might suffer a fatal pulmonary embolism, the anti-coagulent therapy with heparin and warfarin was started again. After another two days, the complete occlusion of the common iliac vein in the patient's left leg occurred, leading to swelling, gangrene and a mid-thigh amputation of the leg. The patient claimed damages for the loss of his leg.

The Court of Appeal upheld the judge's finding at first instance. that it was not negligent not to have diagnosed the DVT while the claimant was in the London hospital. Because the claimant had had a chest infection while in the London hospital, he should not have been discharged to Blackpool, and this was negligent, but this failure did not cause the loss of his leg because (1) even if he had remained in the

London hospital, he would not have been diagnosed earlier nor would the treatment have been different from that provided in Blackpool, and (2) the journey itself did not materially affect the development of the DVT. The burden of proving a causal link between the fault of the defendant and the claimant's injury rests with the claimant.

Consent to treatment: minors

Re B (A Minor) (Wardship: Medical Treatment) [1981] 1 WLR 1421

In this case, a child born with Down Syndrome had a blockage of the intestine requiring an operation to remove it. The patient would die unless the operation was carried out. If the operation was, as expected, to be successful, the patient's life expectation would be 20–30 years. Her parents thought it better that she should die, and declined to give their consent to the operation. The Court of Appeal held that the issue was whether the operation was in the best interests of the child.

Templeman L.J. said that the court might decline to permit life-saving medical treatment where the result would be that the child's life would be so awful that the child should be allowed to die. In this case, if no doubt existed that the child would have the normal life span and suffer the normal difficulties of a child with Down Syndrome, the duty of the court was to decide that the child should live. The exercise to be undertaken by the court was to weigh the quality of the child's life.

Gillick v West Norfolk and Wisbech Area Health Authority [1985] 3 All ER 402

A circular had been issued by the Department of Health and Social Security (DHSS) to Health Authorities, advising that a doctor who was consulted by a girl under the age of 16 at a family planning clinic would not be acting unlawfully if the doctor prescribed contraceptives for the girl, provided that the doctor was acting in good faith to protect the girl from the harmful consequences of sexual intercourse. The circular also made it clear that the principle of confidentiality between doctor and patient applied to a girl under the age of 16, and although a doctor ought to try to persuade the girl to involve her parents about the question of contraceptives, the doctor could, in exceptional circumstances, prescribe contraceptives without contacting the girl's parents or seeking their consent.

The claimant, a devout Catholic, had five daughters under 16 years of age. She sought a declaration that (1) the advice in the circular was unlawful because it amounted to advice to doctors to commit the offence of causing or encouraging unlawful sexual intercourse with a girl under the age of 16, contrary to the Sexual Offences Act 1956, s.28, or the offence of being an accessory to unlawful sexual intercourse with a girl under 16, contrary to s.6 of the Act; and (2) that a doctor could not give advice and treatment to any child of the claimant under the age of 16 without the claimant's consent, because that would be inconsistent with her parental rights.

The House of Lords rejected the claimant's application for a declaration. The claim that a doctor would be committing an offence contrary to the 1956 Act was not accepted because where a doctor exercised a *bona fide* judgement that contraception was in the best interests of a minor patient to protect her from the consequences of sexual intercourse the exercising of that judgement would negate the mental element of the offences. A majority of the House also concluded that a girl under 16 did not lack the legal capacity to consent to contraceptive advice and treatment merely because of her age. Lord Scarman said that as a matter of law, a minor child below the age of 16 has the capacity to consent to medical treatment when the child achieves a sufficient understanding and intelligence to enable him or her to understand fully what is proposed. That is a question of fact.

Part II
The Principles of Risk Management

▶7

CNST Standards for Obstetrics

David R Knowles

Background

The Clinical Negligence Scheme for Trusts (CNST) was established on 1 April 1995 as a direct consequence of NHS Trusts' anxieties about their ability to manage and pay medical negligence claims.

When the first Trusts were established in 1991, one of the new 'freedoms' was to pay their own medical negligence claims. Up to that point, most claims had been paid either by top-sliced Regional Health Authority funds or from the residual cash transferred to the NHS when the medical defence organizations ceased to provide indemnity for hospital doctors.

The Treasury initially envisaged that if a Trust was unable to pay a claim from revenue, it could do so by extending its 'external financing limit' (ie its borrowing capacity). This was not deemed to be a workable proposition by most Trusts and there was a national call for the establishment of some kind of risk-sharing pool, or for commercial insurance to be permitted. In an effort to seek the optimal solution, the Department of Health sought bids from potential service providers.

The first contract for the CNST in England was awarded to two firms (The Medical Protection Society [MPS] and Willis Corroon Limited) for the management of claims and for the formal establishment of a process of clinical risk management. The scheme was based on a voluntary risk-sharing pool from which all claims after 1 April 1995 would be paid. A separate scheme – the Existing Liabilities Scheme – was also established to fund claims arising from incidents before April 1995. Both schemes would be managed by a special Health Authority (the National Health Service Litigation Authority [NHSLA]) The initial contract for legal services provided by the MPS was not renewed, but Willis still provides the risk management services.

Incentives

The risk management system introduced at the time consisted of a set of defined standards at three levels, with significant financial incentives for achieving them. A Trust achieving the level shown below would receive a discount on their contribution. While initially Trusts assessed themselves, soon this was shown to be unworkable, and a team of assessors was appointed to visit every Trust.

The discount scale of contribution to the Scheme for attainment of the specified level was established and is illustrated in Table 7.1.

Table 7.1 Discount scale of contribution to the CNST

Level attained	Discount
No progression from base position	0%
Level 1	10%
Level 2	20%
Level 3	25%

The original prospectus stated that 'it is hoped that by the promotion of best practice in Risk and Claims Management, the Scheme will provide members with the tools to make real advances in patient care'. While this intention has been realized in many instances, the financial driver has also played a major role in ensuring progression through the system.

Application in obstetrics

From the outset, the importance of good risk management in obstetrics has been recognized. While all standards apply to most acute specialties (especially surgical ones), obstetrics is the only acute specialty that has had its own set of specific standards from the start.

Standards

The current standards were revised and reissued in June 2000.[1] Within each standard, there are a number of more detailed criteria. For each standard, there is an overview of the general intention and key references are included. For each criterion, there is a statement of:

▶ the level at which it applies;

▶ the source on which it is based;

▶ guidance on achieving compliance;

▶ how verification will be checked; and

▶ cross-links with other standards.

Unlike the previous version of the standards in obstetrics,[2] the current version makes explicit the weighting given to the importance of each individual criterion within the standards as a whole. These standards were drawn up using the following sources: guidance from the Department of Health and from Royal College reports; recommendations made by the four Confidential Enquiries; and specific issues raised by assessors, members, or the technical advisors to the Scheme.

The main standards applicable to all Trusts are as follows:

1 The Board has a written strategy in place that makes their commitment to managing clinical risk explicit. Responsibility for this strategy and its implementation is clear.
2 A clinical incident reporting system is operated in all medical specialties and clinical support departments.
3 There is a policy for the rapid follow-up of major clinical incidents.
4 An agreed system of managing complaints is in place.
5 Appropriate information is provided to patients on the risks and benefits of the proposed treatment or investigation, and the alternatives available, before a signature on a consent form is sought.
6 A comprehensive system for the completion, use, storage and retrieval of health records is in place. Record-keeping standards are monitored through the clinical audit process.
7 There are management systems in place to ensure the competence and appropriate training of all clinical staff.
8 A clinical risk management system is in place.
9 There are clear procedures for the management of general clinical care.
10 There are clearly documented systems for management and communication throughout the key stages of maternity care.

It should not be forgotten that the standards described above are, in the main, also applicable to maternity services. The specific standards or features within them that many Trusts find particularly difficult to achieve are as follows:

▶ Standard 3, which defines the criteria for effective clinical incident reporting.

▶ 5.2.2: There is a policy/guideline stating that consent for elective procedures is to be obtained by a person competent and capable of performing the procedure.

▶ 6.1.1: There is a unified health record which all specialties use.

▶ 7.2.1: All medical staff in training attend a specific induction appropriate to the specialty in which they are working.

▶ 7.2.2: Clinical risk management is included in the general induction arrangements for all healthcare staff.

▶ 7.2.3: The Trust has clear policies for addressing shortfalls in the conduct, performance and health of clinical staff, and staff are made aware of this.

▶ 7.2.4: The Trust has an induction system covering all temporary (ie locum, bank or agency) clinical staff to ensure that such employees are competent to perform the duties of their post.

▶ 7.2.5: Medical staff in training can demonstrate that they are technically competent to undertake their duties.

▶ 7.2.6: The Trust has a clear policy requiring a consultant to have attended a relevant training programme before embarking upon techniques which are new to him/her and which are not part of an Ethical Committee approved research programme.

▶ 7.2.7: Training programmes are in place to ensure that staff operating diagnostic or therapeutic equipment can do so in a safe and effective manner.

▶ 7.3.1: Ninety per cent of eligible staff have attended basic life-support training in the past 12 months.

▶ 7.3.2: There is a section on clinical risk management in the medical staff handbook incorporating key policies and procedures.

▶ 7.3.3: Staff who operate diagnostic or therapeutic equipment are technically competent to undertake their duties.

▶ 9.3.2: There are specific clinical procedures, pathways or guidelines for each specialty.

It is worth noting that the requirements described above would be regarded as basic in any industry other than healthcare. In most Trusts, the lack of clinical management processes and clear definitions of clinical policy makes it hard for them to comply with the basic control mechanisms required by the CNST.

The additional criteria for maternity are as follows:

▶ 10.1.1: The arrangements are clear concerning which professional is responsible for the woman's care at all times.

▶ 10.1.2: There are referenced, evidence-based multidisciplinary policies for the management of all key conditions/situations on the labour ward. These are subject to review at intervals of not more than three years.

▶ 10.1.3: There is an agreed mechanism for direct referral to a consultant by a midwife.

▶ 10.1.4: There is a personal handover of care when medical shifts change.

▶ 10.1.5: There is a labour ward forum or equivalent, to ensure that there is a clear documented system for management and communication throughout the key stages of maternity care.

▶ 10.1.6: All clinicians should attend six-monthly multidisciplinary in-service education/training sessions on the management of labour and cardiotocogram (CTG) interpretation.

▶ 10.2.1: There is a lead consultant obstetrician and clinical midwife manager for labour ward matters.

▶ 10.2.2: The labour ward has sufficient medical leadership and experience to provide a reasonable standard of care at all times.

▶ 10.3.1: Emergency Caesarean section can be undertaken rapidly and in a short enough period to eliminate unacceptable delay.

▶ 10.3.2: There is a personal handover to obstetric locums, either by the post-holder or senior member of the team, and *vice versa*.

The more mechanistic and easily achieved features are 10.1.2, 10.1.3 and 10.2.1. Those that have proved more difficult in practice include 10.1.5, 10.1.6 and 10.3.2.

Many of the standards are based upon RCOG guidelines (for example 10.2.2) but the level of detail has been increased in the interests of assessment and of translating a concept into a working system. The feature states:

> In order to provide safe care at all times, sufficient staff of appropriate seniority must be readily available. It is the view of the CNST that over time there will be a greater involvement of Consultants throughout the 24-hour period as this will result in better organisation and clinical decision making.

Specifically:

> Consultant supervision should be available for the Labour Ward for a minimum of 40 hours per week of scheduled sessions.

And:

> A Doctor of at least three years experience in obstetrics (or the Consultant on call) should be available within 30 minutes. This Standard crosslinks with the requirement for emergency Caesarean Section to be available within 30 minutes.

And:

> A Specialist Registrar level-one minimum should be resident on the Labour Ward at all times, or available within five minutes.

[as with the RCOG standards, specific reductions are permitted for smaller units]
At least one standard – 10.3.1 – goes beyond current guidance:

> In view of the importance of speed in emergency Caesarean Section for fetal distress it is important that the time taken to organise the staff, equipment and operative facilities is minimal. When a decision is taken to perform a Caesarean Section as an emergency, the person taking the decision should indicate clearly the urgency with which it needs to be carried out (e.g. immediate, within 30 minutes, up to three hours) and should record the time the decision was taken. The interval between decision and delivery should be routinely recorded for all such procedures and subject to an annual review. Where the Standard is not met on a regular basis remedial measures are set in place.

The verification of attainment of this feature is particularly specific where the guidance states the following:

> It is anticipated that this will be the subject of continuous Directorate audit. The Assessor will expect to see these audit records for all emergency Sections for fetal distress. Where the interval is greater than the Standard set by the trust the review of the reasons why this occurred and the remedial action(s) taken (if necessary) will also be available.

The requirement for continuous audit of a basic system and the requirement to introduce change when the local standard is not achieved are new and welcome developments.

Compliance

At first glance, reading through the standards described above one might assume that almost every Trust would be expected to have all these simple measures in place as a matter of basic clinical organization. Unfortunately, the reality is somewhat different: in July 2000, while the Scheme had a very high uptake amongst Trusts with almost all Trusts joining it, the achievement was as illustrated in Table 7.2.

Table 7.2   Levels of attainment by Trusts in the Scheme

Level of achievement	Number achieving	% of members
No progression	88	23
Level 1	265	68
Level 2	35	9
Level 3	1	0.25

Source: CNST, August 2000

This state of affairs five years after the introduction of a basic scheme aimed at minimal levels of professional organizational competence is indicative of the risks that patients may suffer within NHS hospitals. A recent pilot study into medical mismanagement in the UK,[3] has shown that 6.7% of all patients are affected. It is self-evident that despite the real progress that has been made, there is a substantial way to go before anyone involved can feel proud of the system.

On the other hand, the experience within hospitals is that the publishing of the standards, coupled with mandatory external three-year inspection, is driving change. This is particularly true when a Trust has had its attainment level reduced with consequential significant financial penalty due to increased contribution.

Progress in attainment of these useful standards has been surprisingly slow, as noted above; however, it is hoped that the current criticism of poor clinical practice, and the government and professional initiatives intended to strengthen clinical governance, will ensure a higher degree of compliance and thus a greater degree of safety for the patient than in the past.

The future

The CNST has, in many senses, exceeded expectation. At the outset, it was anticipated that about half the Trusts would join the Scheme, but the overwhelming majority joined and remained in the Scheme.

In 2000, the CNST was one of many organizations charged with driving up clinical standards. One might suggest that if these disparate organizations were jointly managed, with a common agenda, progress might be faster; but on the other hand, the CNST, with less than 10 staff, is currently achieving progress, while much larger, newer and more costly organizations have yet to prove themselves. The financial carrot offered by the CNST may indeed prove more effective than the stick held by others.

References

1 *Clinical Risk Management Standards*, version 01. London: NHSLA, June 2000.
2 *CNST Manual of Guidance.* London: NHSLA, 1977.
3 Smith J. Study into medical errors planned for the UK [News]. *BMJ* 1999; 319: 23.

▶8

Clinical Risk Management and the Analysis of Clinical Incidents

Charles Vincent and Kieran Walshe

Introduction

This chapter provides a general introduction to clinical risk management. First, we introduce some basic principles of risk management, and consider its development in the NHS in relation to the rise in litigation and the growing understanding of the scale of harm to patients. An important aspect of risk management is the investigation and analysis of adverse outcomes, and we provide both an outline conceptual framework and a short obstetric example. A close analysis of clinical incidents leads to a broader understanding of risk management and how it might develop in the future, which we discuss in a concluding section. This chapter is necessarily short, and many important issues are addressed only briefly. However, we have provided a number of references on key issues. The related issue of risk management standards is covered by David Knowles in Chapter 7, while Roger Clements covers specific risk management issues in obstetrics in Chapter 9.

Principles of clinical risk management

Clinical risk management was developed initially as a means of controlling medical negligence litigation. In the United States, early risk management strategies were dominated by attempts to reform the legal system and stem the rising costs of compensation. Gradually, however, the need to examine systematically the underlying clinical problems became apparent, together with the need to care for injured patients rather than simply treating them as potential litigants.[1] The introduction of risk management has therefore been driven by anxiety about litigation. However, it has the potential to act as a gateway to a problem of much greater importance – that of injury to patients – which current quality initiatives have not addressed adequately.

Clinical risk management can be defined either in terms of its form or its function – through the processes involved or the outcomes it is intended to produce.[2] It has become conventional to do the former, and to conceptualize risk management in three main processes or stages: identifying risk; analysing risk; and controlling risk. Risk is seen, in broad terms, as exposure to events that may threaten or damage the organization. Risk management involves balancing the costs of risk (or the consequences of such exposure) against the costs of risk reduction. In this classical, and narrow, definition of risk management, used widely outside healthcare, the process can be characterized as financially driven and organization-centred. It is driven financially, in that the costs of risk exposure and risk reduction predominate in decision making and other considerations or issues are therefore less important. It is organization-centred, in that the process is focused on protecting the organization and its interests against risk, and the interests or concerns of other stakeholders are not necessarily explicitly recognized. To the outside observer, this way of describing risk management makes it sound as if it has much in common with traditional insurance.

In healthcare, these issues remain important and sometimes, regrettably, still dominate discussions of risk management. However, we will argue for a broader view of risk management, with strong parallels to the patient safety initiatives now being developed in the United States and Australia.[3] In this broader view, the primary aims of clinical risk management are improving quality and protecting patients.[1,4] Clinical risk management, then, is one of a number of organizational systems or processes aimed at improving the quality of healthcare, but one which is primarily concerned with creating and maintaining safe systems of care. While the processes may be the same – identifying, analysing and controlling risk – the purpose is quite different and much more in keeping with the aims and values of clinical practice.

The need for clinical risk management

Although in some countries, such as the United States, systems for risk management in healthcare have been commonplace for two decades or more,[5] it was not until the late 1980s that such arrangements began to develop in the British National Health Service (NHS). Indeed, the past ten years have seen a growth of interest in clinical risk management internationally, with substantial developments in many countries in Europe and elsewhere.

The main impetus for the development of clinical risk management in the UK has come from the rising incidence and costs of litigation for clinical negligence against healthcare organizations. In 1975, there were about 500 claims a year across the NHS; by 1992, this had risen to around 6000 claims.[6] In 1975, the total cost of claims to the NHS was around £1 million; by 1996, claims for clinical negligence cost the NHS about £200 million. Costs are predicted to reach £500 million per annum by 2001,[7] with obstetric claims representing over half of the financial burden.

Estimating the eventual costs of current claims in progress is difficult, but it has been suggested that these costs amount to £1–2 billion. Although these costs will be spread across a number of years, they still represent a substantial future commitment of NHS resources.

Even at their present levels, however, the costs of clinical negligence litigation to the NHS do not, by themselves, explain the growing recognition of the need for clinical risk management. After all, these costs still only represent about 0.75% of total NHS spending each year, and clinical negligence litigation is focused mainly in a few clinical areas (such as obstetrics, gynaecology, accident and emergency, and orthopaedics). In many areas of the NHS, negligence litigation is much rarer or even virtually unknown. Furthermore, research elsewhere[8] has suggested that there is at best a tenuous link between litigation and adverse events, showing that very few negligent adverse events actually result in litigation. Indeed, many instances of litigation are not based on actual adverse events.[8] In the NHS, the rise of risk management is part of a wider and growing interest in quality management and improvement, reflected in a succession of government and professional initiatives[9] aimed at ensuring that healthcare organizations have robust and effective systems for assuring the quality of care they provide. Risk management has also benefited from a growing realization within the NHS of the scale and severity of iatrogenic injury to patients in advanced healthcare systems, and the need to do more to protect patients and prevent adverse events (see *An Organisation with a Memory*[10]).

Adverse events in healthcare

Iatrogenic effects of drugs and other treatments have been recorded in many studies, although not always labelled as such. However, it is only comparatively recently that the overall scale of injury to patients has become apparent. The Harvard Study[8] found that adverse events (ie occasions when patients are unintentionally harmed by treatment) occurred in almost 4% of admissions in New York State. For 70% of these patients, the resulting disability was slight or short-lived, but in 7% it was permanent, and 14% of patients died as a result – in part – of their treatment.[8] Therefore, in this study serious harm came to around 1% of patients admitted to hospital. Similar findings have been reported from studies carried out in Colorado and Utah in 1992. A recent Australian study revealed that 16.6% of admissions resulted in an adverse event, of which half were considered preventable.[11] A British pilot study of 1000 patient records suggested that 10% of patients admitted to British hospitals may suffer adverse events, and with 8.5 million admissions to English hospitals each year this suggests 850,000 adverse events per annum.[10]

The financial costs of adverse events in terms of resources and reduced efficiency are unknown, but it is likely that they are vastly greater than the immediate costs of litigation. An operation with an adverse outcome, for instance, may lead to at least one further operation, a longer stay in hospital, additional outpatient appointments and so on. In Australia, adverse events were estimated to account for 8% of all hospital bed-days.[11] In Britain, each adverse event led to an additional eight days in hospital, suggesting a total cost to the NHS of £2 billion per annum in extra bed-days, over half of which is preventable.[10] In addition, adverse events involve substantial costs in the form of long-term care, disability payments and other benefits, which are likely to far outweigh the costs of individual hospitals.

Adverse events also involve a huge personal cost to the people involved – both patients and staff. Many patients suffer increased pain, disability and psychological trauma, often compounded by a protracted, adversarial legal process. Staff may experience shame, guilt and depression after making a mistake, with litigation and complaints imposing an additional burden.[1]

Over the past decade, there has been a much greater recognition of the costs and consequences of adverse events, highlighted by a growing attention to the quality of healthcare, and this in itself has promoted the development of risk management. In addition, a series of high-profile system failures in which major lapses in the quality of care have resulted in serious injuries to patients have done much to raise public awareness about the risks of healthcare, and professionals' and managers' awareness of the need for risk management[12] The rise of risk management should be seen as part of a wider move within the NHS towards modern and effective systems for quality improvement.

The rise of risk management in England in the 1990s

Until the late 1980s, no NHS organizations had a formal risk management function. Many had some of the components or apparatus of risk management in place (for example, most had some form of incident or accident reporting), many had health and safety committees and advisors, some had clinical pharmacists who collated data on medication errors and reactions, and most had people responsible for managing complaints and litigation. But these components were rarely connected, or made to work together, and there was little ownership at a corporate level of these processes or systems by senior managers and clinicians. The essentials of risk management – linked processes for identifying, analysing and then controlling risk – were definitely not in place.

In 1995, however, the Clinical Negligence Scheme for Trusts (CNST; see Chapter 7) was established, and the introduction of national standards for risk management made it less a matter for individual Trust discretion and more a national requirement that NHS Trusts should have such systems in place.

Risk management was given further impetus with the introduction of clinical governance.[13] Defined officially as 'a framework through which NHS organisations are accountable for continuously improving the quality of their services and safeguarding high standards of care by creating an environment in which excellence in clinical care will flourish', clinical governance represents an explicit assertion that NHS organizations are responsible for the quality of clinical care they provide, and that those who lead them must ensure that systems for quality improvement are in place and are being used, and will be held accountable if they do not. Clinical governance is, in effect, an endorsement of the ideas of whole-system quality improvement which have been increasingly influential in healthcare in the UK and elsewhere.[14,15] National guidance on clinical governance[16] states explicitly that systems for managing risk and adverse events should form a central component of arrangements for clinical governance in NHS organizations.

Risk management in NHS Trusts: the emerging picture

Research undertaken in 1998[17] demonstrated that most NHS Trusts had moved at least some way towards developing the systems for risk management envisaged in the CNST standards, and that some had made rapid progress in establishing risk management as part of their organization. At that time, over 99% of the NHS Trusts taking part in the research had a named member of the Board who took responsibility for clinical risk management. Most NHS Trusts (96%) had some form of senior group or committee tasked with leading on clinical risk management across the Trust, although the remit and makeup of these groups varied very widely. Most NHS Trusts (85%) also had a nominated individual who took day-to-day responsibility for clinical risk management across the Trust – a clinical risk manager. However, this role was almost always combined with other roles and responsibilities. Risk management was less evident in clinical areas or directorates. Under half (44%) of NHS Trusts had named individuals in each clinical directorate or service area with responsibility for clinical risk. Only about one in eight NHS Trusts (13%) reported that they had some kind of group taking responsibility for clinical risk in all clinical directorates.

Incident reporting

NHS Trusts had made use of two main tools for risk management: incident reporting and risk assessment. Most Trusts (96%) had some form of system for clinical incident reporting in place.[17] Of those, over three-quarters (79%) indicated that their clinical incident reporting systems were being used across all clinical directorates or service areas, with the remainder using incident reporting in some areas only (such as those perceived to be at higher risk than others, such as obstetrics or anaesthetics). There was, however, little consensus about what sort of clinical incidents should be reported. Perhaps for this reason, the numbers of incidents being reported varied very widely – the annual total ranged from two to 5000, with an average of 803.[17] The majority of Trusts (63%) reported that the numbers of clinical incidents being reported were rising; only 3% thought that numbers of incident reports were falling. But many attributed the rising rate of reports to an increased awareness among clinicians of the need to report clinical incidents, and a greater willingness to do so, rather than to any underlying change in the quality of care.[17]

Trusts captured a substantial set of information about each clinical incident – including details of patients and staff involved, where and when it happened, what the incident was, and often what action had been taken following the incident. All Trusts said that someone was responsible for reviewing every incident report – usually the clinical risk manager, but sometimes also a manager in the area where the incident occurred. Most Trusts (91%) had a system for filtering out the few most serious and urgent incidents and subjecting them to some form of senior clinical and managerial review. Only half of Trusts used some form of risk-severity scoring to rate all clinical incidents to try to separate the important from the trivial and identify those that needed to be followed up. And only 16% of Trusts always provided feedback to the person who reported an incident on what had happened as a result

Clinical incident reporting is essentially reactive: when something happens and is reported, a risk may be identified and dealt with. But it may be unnecessary and undesirable to wait for risks to reveal themselves and only to take action once some damage has been done. Clinical risk assessment is a proactive process in which information is collected about an organization or clinical service in order to identify what clinical risks might exist. Risk assessments may draw on data from clinical incident reporting, but are also likely to use other sources of information such as surveys, interviews and comparative data from elsewhere. In order to meet the more advanced CNST standards (ie Level 2), NHS Trusts were required to carry out a Trust-wide clinical risk assessment. The research found that just over half of NHS Trusts (56%) had carried out some form of risk assessment in the previous 12 months.

Investigation and analysis of clinical incidents

Adverse outcomes, and sometimes near misses, are often reviewed in morbidity and mortality meetings. Usually, however, several incidents are reviewed during a meeting, with little opportunity to review a case in detail. Often only the immediate and most obvious departures from good practice can be identified. Such meetings are usually confined to a single department, so it can be difficult to resolve more general issues such as interdepartmental conflicts or wider problems of hospital policy. The advent of clinical risk management as a hospital-wide activity offers the chance for detached investigation of a selection of serious or potentially serious incidents. Few risk managers or clinicians carry out such investigations, unless involved in major enquiries, but there is enormous potential for organizational learning. In aviation and other high-risk enterprises, the investigation and analysis of incidents is a major driver of safety initiatives.

So why *do* things go wrong? Human error is blamed routinely for disasters in the air, on the railways, in complex surgery and in healthcare generally. However, quick judgements and routine assignment of blame obscure a more complex truth. The identification of an obvious departure from good practice is usually only the very first step of an investigation. While a particular action or omission may be the immediate cause of an incident, closer analysis usually reveals a series of events and departures from safe practice, each influenced by the working environment and the wider organizational context. While this more complex picture is gaining acceptance in healthcare,[18-20] it is seldom put into practice in the investigation of actual incidents.

A protocol for the investigation and analysis of clinical incidents

In series of papers,[18,21-25] the Clinical Risk Unit has developed a process of investigation and analysis of adverse events for use by researchers. A collaboration between researchers and risk managers was then established to adapt the research methods for routine use in clinical practice. A protocol for the investigation and analysis of serious incidents was developed for use by risk managers and others trained in incident analysis. The protocol gives a detailed account of the theoretical background, process of investigation and analysis, with detailed case examples. As with a clinical guideline, the protocol provides a step-by-step guide to the systematic investigation and analysis of any clinical incident. Here, we can only introduce the main ideas and present a section of a case analysis to illustrate the methods in practice; however, a full account is available elsewhere.[18]

Research foundations

The theory underlying the protocol and its application derives from research in settings outside healthcare. In the aviation, oil and nuclear industries, for instance, the formal investigation of incidents is a well-established procedure.[26] Studies in these areas and in medicine have led to a much broader understanding of accident causation, with less focus on the individual who makes the error and more on pre-existing organizational factors. Such studies have also illustrated the complexity of the chain of events that may lead to an adverse outcome.[18, 22, 24, 27–29] The root causes of adverse clinical events may lie in factors such as the use of locum doctors and agency nurses, communication and supervision problems, excessive workload and educational and training deficiencies.

Essential concepts and an overview of the process

The method of investigation implied by the model is first to examine the chain of events that leads to an accident or adverse outcome, and consider the actions of those involved. The investigator then, crucially, looks further back at the conditions in which staff were working and the organizational context in which the incident occurred.

The first step in any analysis is to identify the 'care management problems' – are actions or omissions by staff in the process of care. These may be slips, such as picking up the wrong syringe, lapses of judgement, forgetting to carry out a procedure, or, rarely, deliberate departures from safe operating practices, procedures or standards (see Table 8.1).

Care management problems have two essential features: care deviated beyond safe limits of practice; and this deviation had a direct or indirect effect on the eventual adverse outcome for the patient. (In cases where the impact on the patient is unclear, it is sufficient that the care management problem had a potentially adverse effect.)

For each care management problem identified, the investigator records the salient clinical events or condition of the patient at that time (eg bleeding heavily, blood pressure falling) and other patient factors affecting the process of care (eg patient very distressed, patient unable to understand instructions).

Table 8.1 Examples of care management problems

- Failure to monitor, observe or act
- Delay in diagnosis
- Incorrect risk assessment (eg of suicide or self harm)
- Inadequate handover
- Failure to note faulty equipment
- Failure to carry out pre-operative checks
- Not following an agreed protocol (without clinical justification)
- Not seeking help when necessary
- Failure to supervise adequately a junior member of staff
- Incorrect protocol applied
- Treatment given to incorrect body site
- Wrong treatment given

Having identified the care management problems, the investigator then considers the conditions in which errors occur and the wider organizational context. The investigator uses this framework for each care management problem (Table 8.2), both during interview and afterwards, to identify the factors that led to that particular problem. For example:

▶ Individual factors may include lack of knowledge or experience of particular staff

▶ Task factors might include the non-availability of test results or protocols

▶ Team factors might include poor communication between staff.

▶ Work environment might include high workload, inadequate staffing or limited access to vital equipment.

Any combination of these might contribute to the occurrence of a single care management problem, and they may be specific to that occasion or more general features of the unit. For instance, there may be a failure of communication between a

Table 8.2 Framework of factors influencing clinical practice

Factor types	Influencing contributory factors
Institutional context	Economic and regulatory context NHS Executive CNST
Organizational and management factors	Financial resources and constraints Organizational structure Policy standards and goals Safety culture and priorities
Work environment factors	Staffing levels and skill mix Workload and shift patterns Design, availability and maintenance of equipment Administrative and managerial support
Team factors	Verbal communication Written communication Supervision and seeking help Team structure (consistency, leadership, etc)
Individual (staff) factors	Knowledge and skills Competence Physical and mental health
Task factors	Task design and clarity of structure Availability and use of protocols Availability and accuracy of test results
Patient factors	Condition (complexity and seriousness) Language and communication Personality and social factors

From Vincent et al.[23]

doctor and a nurse, contributing to a care management problem. This may be an isolated occurrence or a longstanding inter-professional problem with clear implications for the safe and effective running of that unit or hospital.

The investigation process

A series of steps, described fully in the protocol itself and the *British Medical Journal* webpages accompanying it, are followed.[30] Briefly, the case records and any statements are reviewed. Structured interviews with key members of staff are then undertaken to establish the chronology of events, the main care management problems and their respective contributory factors, as perceived by each member of staff. The key questions are: What happened (the outcome and chronology)? How did it happen (the care management problems)? Why did it happen (the contributory factors)? In the analysis phase, an agreed chronology and a full list of care management problems is produced. For each problem, both specific and – where applicable – general contributory factors are identified.

Table 8.3 A summary of the investigation process

All investigations comprise a series of steps, which should be followed as a matter of routine when an incident is investigated:

1   Ascertain that a serious clinical incident has occurred and ensure it is reported formally. Alternatively, identify an incident as being fruitful in terms of organizational learning.
2   Trigger the investigation procedure. Notify the senior members of staff who have been trained to carry out investigations.
3   Investigators will establish the circumstances as they initially appear and complete an initial summary. Decide which part of the process of care requires investigation and prepare an outline chronology of events. Identify any obvious care management problems.
4   Interview staff using the following structured approach:
    ● Establish the chronology of events
    ● Revisit the sequence of events and ask questions about each of the care management problems identified at the initial stage
    ● Use the framework to ask supplementary questions about the reasons for the occurrence of each care management problem.
5   If new care management problems have emerged during the interviews add them to the initial list. Re-interview if necessary.
6   Collate the interviews and assemble a composite analysis under each of the care management problems identified at the start. For each one identify both specific and, where appropriate, general contributory factors.
7   Compile the report of the events, listing the causes of the care management problems, and make recommendations to prevent recurrence.
8   Submit report to senior clinicians and management according to local arrangements.
9   Implement the action arising from the report and monitor progress.

Case example: death of a baby following a difficult delivery

This case example is discussed fully elsewhere[30] and only presented here to illustrate the analytical methods, in particular the role of the contributory factors. In brief, the mother had one previous child, and slight shoulder dystocia was noted at the birth of this first child. The possibility of shoulder dystocia in the delivery of the second child was anticipated by the consultant, and plans were made: in particular that the pregnancy should not progress beyond six days after the due date and no attempt should be made at a difficult mid-cavity instrumental delivery. In the event, the plan was not communicated fully, and a series of problems occurred. Ultimately, the baby was asphyxiated, with the head delivered and the shoulders obstructed, and died within a few hours. The principal care management problems identified were as follows:

▶ The care plan was formulated but not communicated

▶ There was inadequate fetal monitoring in the first and second stages of labour

▶ There was inadequate pain control in the first stage of labour

▶ There was a delay in management in the second stage of labour.

For any senior obstetrician reviewing this case, identification of these problems is relatively straightforward. Here, however, we focus on the contributory factors, which are seldom considered in detail. Each of these care management problems was analysed separately. Only the second – inadequate fetal monitoring – is shown, with the contributory factors, in Figure 8.1. A number of contributory factors influenced the care given in this stage of labour, operating at several different levels of the framework. Staff faced a very distressed patient who did not easily accept their recommendations. Scalp electrode removal was not covered by a unit policy, the midwives were distracted because of the mother's distress, the consultant's care plan was not seen because the notes were not retrieved, and the maternity unit was disrupted because of building works. Only some of these factors had more general implications for the running of the unit, specifically concerning the retrieval of notes, cardiotocograph training and policies on the removal of scalp electrodes.

Subsequent to the analysis of this case and discussion of the implications, a number of changes were made to the organization and policies of the unit. These included the following:

1 A new protocol was designed, stipulating that where there was a conflict between information provided by different types of monitoring equipment, best practice would be to assume the worst case and seek medical advice.
2 An individual training programme was provided for specific members of staff.
3 A programme of further education was provided for all midwives in the assessment and management of shoulder dystocia.
4 There was a review and eventual replacement of all outdated fetal monitoring equipment.

Benefits of a systematic investigation

A structured and systematic approach means that the ground to be covered in any investigation is, to a significant extent, already mapped out. The protocol helps to ensure a comprehensive investigation, and facilitate the production of formal reports.

Care management problem
Fetal monitoring of the first and second stage of labour by cardiotocogram (CTG)

Clinical context and patient factors
Painful and relatively short first stage of labour. Fetal heart rate difficult to monitor and CTG scalp electrodes placed on head at 07.15 hours. Cervix fully dilated at 08.05 hours. Patient became very distressed and unable to co-operate. Episiotomy recommended but resisted. Argument involving husband for several minutes. Episiotomy done. Scalp electrode removed as head crowning at 08.15 hours. CTG prior to removal shows marked decelerations of heart rate and a slowing trend.

Contributory factors

Specific	General
Work and environmental factors Maternity building undergoing extensive building works whilst still in use. Normal geography disturbed	None
Team factors Notes not retrieved from library promptly. Care plan set out by Consultant not seen. Unit normally staffed and workload average	Shift change procedures, need to ensure records recovered fast
Individual factors Midwives failed to heed slowing heart rate on the CTG as they were distracted by the mother's distress and resistance to advice	CTG awareness and training
Task factors Midwives not aware of possible dystocia. Delay between crowning and complete delivery. Scalp electrode removal not covered by policy	Lack of clear policy guidelines

---

Organizational management and institutional context factors
Unit had been without a Head of Midwifery Services for two years. Functions carried out by G-grade supervisors

---

Fig. 8.1. Care management problems and contributory factors.

While the process may initially appear complicated and time consuming, our experience is that using the protocol actually speeds up complex investigations by focusing the investigators on the key issues and bringing out the systemic factors that must ultimately be the target of the investigation. These systemic features are those that are addressed when long-term risk-reduction strategies are implemented.

We have noted that even very experienced clinicians find that following a systematic protocol brings additional benefits in terms of comprehensiveness and investigation expertise. Clinicians are accustomed to identifying the problematic features in the management of a case, and so can easily identify the care management problems. However, the identification of contributory factors and the realization that each problem may have a different constellation of contributory factors are less familiar tasks. A systematic approach pays dividends when exploring these. The protocol does not attempt to supplant clinical expertise. Rather, the aim is to utilize clinical experience and expertise to the fullest extent.

The impact of clinical risk management

Assessing the impact of clinical risk management in the NHS is difficult. The impacts that might be anticipated or expected, such as improved quality and safety, reduced levels of risk, the prevention of some adverse events, avoidance of potential litigation and so on, are very difficult to measure. Moreover, the time scale for such changes may be long, and there may be many other influences or confounding factors. Nevertheless, research undertaken within NHS Trusts in 1998[17] suggested that NHS Trusts had seen some important changes as a result of the development of clinical risk management. First, there had been some impact on the way that cases of clinical negligence are managed. Half of Trusts reported that at least some claims had been identified first through their incident reporting arrangements, and they described advantages such as better documentation of events, faster settlement of claims, and damages minimization, which resulted from such advance warning of claims. Second, over half (54%) of Trusts reported that some clinical audit had been initiated as a result of risk management activities (such as incident reporting and risk assessment). Third, and most importantly, almost three-quarters (74%) of NHS Trusts reported that their clinical risk management systems had brought about some changes in clinical practice. Those changes were very varied in nature, and some examples drawn from the research are described in Table 8.4. Many of them concerned either the introduction of new policies, procedures, guidelines or protocols designed to define more clearly the way that care should be managed or delivered. Some also concerned changes to the way information was recorded, designed both to provide a more consistent and complete record and to improve interprofessional communication.

Looking further ahead, we can see that the wide range of factors implicated in analysis of single incidents will need to be addressed in quality and safety initiatives. Safety programmes in industry, involving socio-technical systems with many similarities to medicine, target the tasks, teams and conditions of work, rather than the staff.[23] Safety needs to be addressed both at the level of the particular clinical process, as it already is in clinical audit, and at the interpersonal and organizational levels. Audits need to be supplemented by broader analyses of organizational and system features. Where tasks can be specified clearly, greater standardization, clear guidelines and less reliance on the vagaries of human memory and vigilance are essential. Team and communication failures have been strongly implicated in many accident analyses and remedial measures can be cheap and straightforward. Systems also have been developed in industry to monitor the conditions of work and the associated organizational factors and decisions that give rise to these conditions. The background conditions that predispose to risk and unsafe practice are monitored directly and routinely to assess not the health of a patient, but the health of a unit – in essence, the unit's vital signs.

Table 8.4 Examples of changes in practice resulting from clinical risk management in NHS Trusts

- Use of bed rails and other measures to prevent falls
- Equipment and arrangements for manual handling changed
- Introduction of pre-operative clinics
- Consent practices changed
- Guidance issued on managing/using syringe drivers
- New prescription sheets introduced
- Management of suspected aortic aneurysms in A&E changed
- Training provided for use of tracheostomy tubes
- Move away from use of mercury thermometers
- Specimen labelling and transport tightened up
- Swab counting procedure in theatres improved
- Policy on use of heparin introduced
- X-rays taken in A&E now quickly reviewed by radiologist
- Procedure used for female sterilization changed
- Syringes labelled when drugs drawn up but not used immediately
- CPR trolleys audited regularly
- Consultant responsible for labour ward identified
- All cardiac monitors changed due to fault
- Better policy for informed consent to treatment
- Development of patient information leaflets that cite risks as well as benefits
- Creation of a pump bank for all infusion pumps used to administer analgesia
- Theatre booking changed – more evenly spaced, enabling better use
- Central referral point for 'at risk children', with needs of child and *not* the client paramount
- Development of new policy for managing serious untoward events
- Children in A&E now seen by more experienced medical staff only

Conclusions and future directions

Over the past decade, clinical risk management in the NHS has been transformed from something of a sideline for a few interested clinicians and managers to a core function in most NHS Trusts. That pace of development has not been without its costs, as clinicians and managers with limited experience of risk management have been required to put systems in place before they necessarily knew what was needed or what would work. Nevertheless, it is an impressive achievement. It seems that now we are moving on from that initial phase of rapid expansion, into a more mature period of consolidation and integration.

In consolidating the progress that has been made, more consideration should be given to the effectiveness of the systems of risk management that have been put in place. While a great deal of time and resources have been invested in ensuring that NHS Trusts comply with the CNST risk management standards, and those standards have widespread acceptance and high face validity, there is little empirical evidence that compliance will result in reduced risk, fewer clinical negligence claims, improved quality, and so on. More research is needed to evaluate approaches to clinical risk management and systems such as incident reporting, so that our future decisions about what risk management arrangements to put in place can be better informed.

There is no doubt that clinical risk management has become established in the NHS largely because of the pressures of litigation for clinical negligence, and few people would argue that such rapid progress would have been made without the stimulus of a litigation crisis. As a result, risk management activities can sometimes seem to be overly concerned with litigation and its consequences for the organization, and not as focused on quality improvement and patient safety as they might be. Perhaps the real test of maturity in clinical risk management systems and processes is whether they succeed in escaping their origins in negligence and litigation and become real contributors to patient safety and quality improvement. Recognition of the true human and financial costs of adverse events is an important first step. In the future, our ideas of risk in healthcare might be less immediately concerned with individual instances of suboptimal clinical practice, and more directed at larger and more significant risk issues, such as the safety and reliability of processes of care and the risks associated with routine clinical practice.[2] In other words, risk management might move its attention from the outliers of clinical practice which are often rare, unusual or idiosyncratic cases from which little can be learnt, to the mainstream of clinical practice where even small changes might make a substantial difference to the quality of care for many patients.

The protocol and methods described herein are, we consider, simply a first step in developing a science of investigation and analysis of clinical incidents. Clinical expertise and experience will always be vital to any serious investigation, but could be considerably enhanced by methods that explore the wider organizational context. The next step in the research process is to review methods of investigation in other high-risk domains, such as aviation and nuclear power, and methods already in use in healthcare. Following this more formal evaluation, a revised method will be possible, followed by the gradual evolution and successive refinement of the methods. Formal methods are likely to be increasingly in demand as the Commission for Health Improvement (CHI) begins to publish reports of its own investigations into serious NHS incidents. One of the Commission's longer-term tasks is to formalize its own methods of investigation and develop guidelines for use in the NHS.

In the future, the connections between clinical risk management and other systems for quality improvement need to be made more explicit and meaningful. The concept of clinical governance is predicated on this idea of greater integration, in which current rather disparate and stand-alone systems of quality improvement are brought together to create a coherent whole which is more than the sum of its parts. By linking existing data and information systems, and joining up quality improvement, staff and other resources, a more robust and effective approach to quality improvement that incorporates clinical risk issues can be created. In the future, this may mean that the risk management function in NHS organizations becomes less separately identifiable than it has been up to now, but more effective in achieving quality improvements.

References

1   Vincent CA. Risk, safety, and the dark side of quality. *BMJ* 1997; 314: 1775–1776.
2   Walshe KMJ. The development of clinical risk management. In: Vincent CA, ed. *Clinical Risk Management*, 2nd edn. London: BMJ Publications, 2001.

3   Kohn LT, Corrigan JM, Donaldson MS, eds. *To Err is Human. Building a Safer Health System*. Institute of Medicine Report. Washington: National Academy Press, 1999.

4   Vincent CA, ed. *Clinical Risk Management*, 2nd edn. London: BMJ, 2001.

5   Mills DH, von Bolschwing GE. Clinical risk management: experiences from the United States. In: Vincent CA, ed, *Clinical Risk Management*. London: BMJ; 1995: 3–17.

6   Dingwall R, Fenn P. Risk management: financial implications. In: Vincent CA, ed, *Clinical Risk Management*. London: BMJ, 1995: 73–87.

7   NHS Executive. FDL(96)39. *Clinical Negligence Costs*. London: NHS Executive, 1996.

8   Brennan TA, Leape LL, Laird NM, Herbert L, Localio AT, Lawthers AG *et al*. Incidence of adverse events and negligence in hospitalized patients. *New England Journal of Medicine* 1991; 324: 370–376.

9   Taylor D. Quality and professionalism in health care; a review of current initiatives in the NHS. *BMJ* 1996; 312: 626–629.

10   Department of Health. *An Organisation with a Memory*. Report of an Expert Group on Learning from Adverse Events in the NHS. London: The Stationery Office, 2000. (URL: http://www.doh.gov.uk/orgmemreport.)

11   Wilson RM, Runciman WB, Gibber RW, Harrison BT, Newby L, Hamilton JD. The Quality in Australian Health Care Study. *Medical Journal of Australia* 1995; 163: 458–471.

12   Smith R. All changed, changed utterly. *BMJ* 1998; 316: 1917–1918.

13   Department of Health. *The New NHS: Modern, Dependable*. London: Department of Health, 1997.

14   Berwick D. A primer on leading the improvement of systems. *BMJ* 1996; 312: 619–622.

15   Blumenthal D, Kilo C. A report card on continuous quality improvement. *Milbank Quarterly* 1998; 76(4): 625–648.

16   Department of Health. *A first class service: quality in the new NHS*. London: Department of Health, 1998.

17   Walshe K, Dineen M. *Clinical Risk Management: Making a Difference?* Birmingham: NHS Confederation, 1998.

18   Vincent CA. How to investigate and analyse clinical incidents: Clinical Risk Unit and Association of Litigation and Risk Management protocol. *BMJ* 2000; 320: 777–781.

19   Leape LL. Error in medicine. *JAMA* 1994; 272: 1851–1857.

20   Reason JT. Understanding adverse events: human factors. In: Vincent CA, ed. *Clinical Risk Management*. London: BMJ, 1995: 31–54.

21   Vincent CA, Bark P. Accident analysis. In: Vincent CA, ed. *Clinical Risk Management*. London: BMJ, 1995: 391–410.

22   Stanhope N, Vincent CA, Taylor-Adams S, O'Connor A, Beard R. Applying human factors methods to clinical risk management in obstetrics. *British Journal of Obstetrics and Gynaecology* 1997; 104: 1225–1232.

23   Vincent CA, Taylor-Adams S, Stanhope N. A framework for the analysis of risk and safety in medicine. *BMJ* 1998; 316: 1154–1157.

24   Taylor-Adams SE, Vincent C, Stanhope N. Applying human factors methods to the investigation and analysis of clinical adverse events. *Safety in Science* 1999; 31: 143–159.

25   Vincent C, Stanhope N, Taylor-Adams S. Developing a systematic method of analysing serious incidents in mental health. *Journal of Mental Health* 2000; 9: 89–103.

26   Reason JT. Adverse events: the human factor. In: Vincent CA, ed. *Clinical Risk Management*, 2nd edn. London: BMJ, 2001.

27   Reason JT. *Human Error*. New York: Cambridge University Press, 1990.

28   Cooper JB Newbower RS, Kitz RJ. An analysis of major errors and equipment failures in anaesthesia management considerations for prevention and detection. *Anaesthesiology* 1984; 60: 34–42.

29   Eagle CJ, Davies JM, Reason JT. Accident analysis of large scale technological disaster: applied to anaesthetic complications. *Canadian Journal of Anesthesia* 1992; 39: 118–122.

30   Vincent CA, Taylor-Adams S, Chapman EJ, Hewett D, Prior S, Strange P, Tizzard A. *A Protocol for the Investigation and Analysis of Clinical Incidents*. London: RSM Press, 1999. (Available from Association of Litigation and Risk Management, Royal Society of Medicine, 1 Wimpole Street, London W1G 0AE, UK.)

9

Risk Management in Obstetrics and Gynaecology

Roger V Clements

Risk

The risk of harm arising from a clinical encounter is related directly to the severity of the illness, the age of the patient and the degree of urgency; it is inversely related to the skill and experience of the healthcare provider. Paradoxically, though logically, complaints and claims are inversely related to severity and urgency, and are more likely to arise in non-urgent social interventions. The high profile of obstetrics and gynaecology in litigation is created partly by patient expectation. If a previously fit and healthy young woman seeking social intervention to control fertility or to have a baby is injured in the process, she is much more likely to complain or sue than is the patient being treated for severe illness.

Thus, in gynaecology the common areas of complaint and litigation occur in the context of sterilization, abortion and family planning. Cancer patients are proportionately less likely to sue, for their expectation of outcome is already impaired. Previously fit women, on the other hand, who believe that a screening programme has let them down are more likely to express anger if they develop the disease the programme was designed to prevent.

Hysterectomy is often performed for relatively trivial reasons and the poor outcome is understandably greeted with considerable surprise and disappointment. If in the presence of normal anatomy the surgeon cannot complete the operation without damage to the ureter or bladder, he/she may afterwards find it difficult to justify. Was it necessary in the first place? Was the surgeon's expertise and experience sufficient to the task? In all types of gynaecological surgery, but particularly in the newer minimal access procedures, the common theme is of doctors operating beyond their training and experience

In obstetric malpractice litigation, three themes predominate:

1 Communication
2 Delay
3 The cascade of events.

Consent issues are usually about failure to communicate adequately with the patient, to understand her wishes and to provide her with sufficient information to make a choice. But there are also communication issues between staff, both vertically and horizontally, within the labour ward setting. In this context, it is essential that if a midwife does not obtain a satisfactory clinical response from a junior doctor she should be empowered (and feel empowered) to go above the head of the junior doctor to someone more senior – to the consultant if necessary – so as to make sure that a proper clinical decision is made. Delay is ubiquitous in obstetric malpractice – delay in making observations and in interpreting those observations, and delay in making decisions to intervene and in implementing those decisions. Birth asphyxia litigation is usually about delay above all else.

But obstetric disasters are not achieved by one end-player. They are usually the result of a cascade of events, a series of indecisions or wrong decisions starting in the antenatal period, usually with the absence of any decision at all, continuing in the labour ward. Complicated (or 'high-risk') obstetrics – involving twins, vaginal breech delivery, vaginal birth after Caesarean section (VBAC) and delivery of the macrosomic baby – need planning, beginning in the antenatal clinic. On admission, there is further opportunity to assess risk factors but it may be more difficult later in labour when events move fast. The junior doctor or midwife left with a complex vaginal delivery that ends in disaster is not usually the only person to have made a mistake; indeed, they are often simply faced with the culmination of a series of errors and omissions made by more senior colleagues.

In addition to these general themes, in obstetric practice there are a number of familiar clinical circumstances in which injury to mother or baby is common, leading to complaint and sometimes litigation:

- Perinatal asphyxia
- Abuse of Syntocinon
- VBAC
- Shoulder dystocia
- Anal sphincter injury
- Consent.

Perinatal asphyxia

The cost of cerebral palsy claims dwarfs all other categories of litigation. Although only 10–15% of cerebral palsy cases can, on present medical knowledge and understanding, be linked to birth events, this minority sometimes results from substandard care. More than a decade ago, the criteria for linking intrapartum asphyxia with cerebral palsy with 'anything approaching a reasonable medical certainty' were set out by Freeman and Nelson;[1] but, of course, the court does not require anything approaching a reasonable medical certainty. The claimant must prove to the court that *on the balance of probabilities* causation of cerebral palsy flowed from the breach of care.

Recently, a concerted effort has been made by a group of paediatricians and obstetricians, chiefly from Australia and New Zealand,[2] to define the prerequisites for proving a causal relation between acute intrapartum events and cerebral palsy. However, the 'consensus statement' has not met with universal approval and appears to have some fundamental flaws.[3]

The appropriate risk management response is not about creating causation hurdles for the injured claimant but about preventing injury. For the minority of babies whose cerebral palsy is acquired during labour, the most common mechanism is asphyxia. In litigation, attention focuses on detection of intrapartum asphyxia and its prevention. Traditionally, the condition of the fetus has been assessed by auscultation of the fetal heart and examination of the liquor amnii. Because meconium in the liquor is a poor predictor of fetal asphyxia, particularly in the term baby, attention has focused on the fetal heart:

> ... there is no evidence that intermittent auscultation using a Pinard stethoscope is of any value in intrapartum care.[4]

Historically, the first attempt to improve fetal monitoring was by fetal scalp blood sampling, but the method is 'time consuming and inconvenient to perform, and uncomfortable for the mother',[4] not to mention the poor quality control and the often paradoxical results. In a medico-legal context, there is often criticism of the defendants for relying on fetal scalp samples which were self-evidently wrong or which were relied upon despite continuing abnormalities on the cardiotocograph (CTG). It must be understood clearly that the information about fetal pH is only valid *at the time of the sample* and has no predictive quality. In circumstances (such as breech delivery) where a period of hypoxia is inevitable during birth, it is doubtful whether fetal blood sampling has any place at all.[5]

The enthusiasts for fetal blood sampling argue that its proper use reduces unnecessary operative delivery if the diagnosis of fetal distress relies only upon observations of the fetal heart rate. However, meta-analysis[4] fails to show any clear advantage and currently the method is employed only in a minority of district general hospitals.

At present, the best opportunity to study the health of the fetus in labour is provided by electronic fetal monitoring (EFM). In the mid-1980s, the Dublin Study[6] led to the widespread acceptance within the profession of the improbable notion that listening to the baby some of the time is as good as listening to the baby all of the time. More recent studies[7,8] have shown a significant reduction in deaths attributed to hypoxia with electronic fetal heart monitoring and a substantial and highly significant reduction in the incidence of neonatal seizures. In spite of these studies, at present there is no consensus that EFM is mandatory in all labours. There is acceptance that in 'abnormal' labour, during augmentation and in the presence of abnormal heart rates there is a need for EFM as it gives most information concerning fetal welfare. The Clinical Negligence Scheme for Trusts (CNST, see Chapter 7) insists on a rolling programme of CTG training for all labour ward staff

Failure to understand, interpret and react to an abnormal CTG is the commonest accusation of the claimant in cerebral palsy cases. The CTG 'monitor' confers no protection on the baby. To be effective, the monitor must be interpreted by staff who are trained adequately. In the context of clinical risk management, the single most important challenge to the maternity services is the 24-hour provision of midwifery and obstetric staff capable of interpreting the CTG and reacting appropriately to the abnormal trace. It is often argued that experts differ on the interpretation of CTGs. Indeed they do, but that has little to do with the realities of litigation where barn door abnormalities so often are ignored, making it impossible to defend a claim.

Abuse of Syntocinon (oxytocin)

So often the apparent cause of the asphyxial injury is the abuse of oxytocin; midwives and junior doctors are empowered by liberal labour ward protocols to use oxytocin for the augmentation of labour without apparently any understanding of the dangers of abuse. The drug is used in the multigravida with as much freedom as in the primip, in breech presentation as well as cephalic, and most particularly in the multip who has a scar from previous Caesarean section.

Vaginal birth after Caesarean section

Labour following a Caesarean section differs only in one respect from other labours; it carries the risk of rupture of the Caesarean section scar. The incidence of rupture is widely quoted as less than 1%[9] but in fact incidences of 0.3–2.0%[10] can be found in the literature. It seems likely that the true incidence is under-reported. The consequences of scar rupture may be severe for both mother and baby; the principle issues arising in such circumstances are usually:

1   Consent
2   Abuse of Syntocinon.

Before setting out on a trial of vaginal delivery where the mother has a Caesarean section scar, it is essential that she be informed of the risk. Since rupture of the scar is the *only* increased risk, that information must be specifically provided. In retrospect, in cases where the scar has ruptured with an adverse outcome it is likely that the parents will say that had the risks been put to them they would have chosen elective Caesarean section. That argument can only be met if a proper discussion with the patient beforehand has been annotated and an adequately informed decision recorded. In advising the mother of the risks, it is reasonable to stress the dangers inherent in delivery by Caesarean section provided only that the risk of *elective* Caesarean section is explained, for that is the true comparison. The risk of elective Caesarean section to the baby is negligible; there are no reliable figures for risk to the mother of serious morbidity but the mortality is of the order of 1:10 000, a similar order of risk to that involved in driving a motor car.

Meta-analysis has not shown convincing evidence that Syntocinon used appropriately increases the risk of scar rupture. That is very different from the conclusion that Syntocinon is entirely safe in VBAC. The use of Syntocinon figures prominently in litigation following scar rupture, and if the drug is to be used at all it must be employed with extreme caution. One of the myths surrounding scar rupture is that there are warning signs that presage the disaster. The literature does not support that view; neither does anecdotal experience, save only that in many cases that come before the courts hyperstimulation can be detected on the tocograph in the period leading up to scar rupture.

Shoulder dystocia

The large number of claims for Erb's palsy following shoulder dystocia is a cause of concern to the Litigation Authority. Whilst obstetric brachial plexus palsy is the commonest injury to follow shoulder dystocia, it is not the most severe. Asphyxial damage to the baby, intrapartum death and soft tissue damage to the mother are also occasionally subjects of litigation. Until the publication of a specialist textbook on the subject,[11] general obstetric and midwifery texts were not always coherent in their advice to obstetricians and midwives confronted with this most terrifying of all obstetric dilemmas.

Shoulder dystocia and its prediction and management are discussed in Chapter 13.

Anal sphincter injury

There are no reliable figures for the incidence of anal sphincter injury following vaginal birth. Figures of 0.6–2.3% are quoted.[12] There is no evidence base to show the protective effect of episiotomy because the literature does not distinguish adequately between medio-lateral and midline episiotomy. It is seldom possible for the claimant to discharge the burden of proof that a third degree tear occurred through lack of skill or care. The accusation is usually that, an anal sphincter injury having occurred, the repair of it was defective. Sphincter injuries are missed because women are not properly examined in the third stage of labour. The injury goes unrecognized and is only subsequently repaired when the patient, weeks or months after the event, complains of anal incontinence. In the past decade, the follow-up of women after primary repair has revealed a disappointingly high incidence of imperfect continence. Until recently, it was difficult to discharge the burden of proof that had the sphincter been repaired at the time of the injury she would on the balance of probabilities have had her continence restored. A recent meta-analysis[13] has demonstrated that 66% of women regained full continence after primary repair but only 49% after secondary.

Consent

Consent is the subject of Chapter 3 and will not be dealt with here in detail. There are, however, some aspects of consent in the context of obstetrics and gynaecology that are different and need to be considered

In expressing the relationship between the healthcare professional and the patient, consent is a somewhat negative concept; the positive expression of that relationship is *choice*. Most of our patients, both in obstetrics and gynaecology, are fit young women either having uncomplicated pregnancies or seeking minor interventions to improve the quality of life or to control fertility. The emphasis should be upon facilitating patient choice, providing sufficient information for the woman to decide which method of management is most acceptable to her. In obstetrics, as elsewhere, the obsession with the consent form and the need to have it signed often proves a distraction from the real business of informing the patient and allowing her to make the choice. In any event, in the context of labour ward treatment the consent form is of little assistance.

When a gynaecologist obtains consent for an elective procedure, the process is no different from that in any other branch of surgery. The patient must be given sufficient understanding to enable her to make a choice in circumstances where she is free to exercise choice. The introduction of the term 'informed consent' is unhelpful in this regard. If the phrase means anything at all (and what is uninformed consent?), it is a term of art relating to the standard applied by the courts in other developed countries. That standard – ie the standard of the prudent patient – applies throughout the developed world except in the British Isles. In these islands, the courts still apply the test of the responsible doctor. In other words, the amount of information required to be given is that which any reasonable doctor would give in the circumstances – the same test as for treatment.[14] At least that was the case before *Bolitho*.[15] It remains to be seen to what extent the courts will apply the risk-benefit analysis to the question of information in the context of consent. It might, for instance, apply in the case of VBAC where the court might take the view that even if other doctors did not warn of the risk of rupture of the uterus, a risk-benefit analysis would show that such practice would fail to measure up to a reasonable standard.

The circumstances in the labour ward prevent the imparting of critical information in sufficient quantity within a reasonable timescale to meet any objective analysis. In circumstances such as prolapsed cord or severe antepartum haemorrhage, there is simply no time or opportunity to explain the treatment options in detail to a terrified woman. It may be argued (and has been so argued in the courts) that a woman in labour, in severe pain and under the influence of drugs is not competent to give consent in any event.[16] Consent for obstetric procedures presents special difficulties to both doctor and patient. Some of it can be overcome by antenatal education and the imparting of information at a time when there is no crisis. Many emergency situations can be foreseen, and good management should aim to create the circumstances so that (because complications have been anticipated) when the need to intervene *does* arise, the tension associated with the emergency is reduced. But it is unrealistic to suppose that all emergencies can be foreseen. The obstetrician and the midwife should seek to build up such a degree of trust in a patient that she will be able to accept emergency advice given in her best interests.

References

1   Freeman AM, Nelson KB. Intrapartum asphyxia and cerebral palsy. *Paediatrics* 1988; 82: 240–249.
2   McLennan A. A template for defining a causal relation between acute intrapartum events and cerebral palsy. International consensus statement. *BMJ* 1999; 319: 1054–1059.

3   Dear P, Rennie J, Newell S, Rosenbloom L. *Clinical Risk* 2000; 6(4): 137–142.
4   Steer PJ, Danielian P. Fetal distress in labour. In: DK James, PJ Steers, CP Weiner, B Gonik (eds.) *High-Risk Pregnancy: Management Options*, 2nd edition. WB Saunders Company, 1999: Chapter 64.
5   Gibb DMF, Arulkumaran S. Cardiotocographic interpretations: clinical scenarios. In: *Fetal Monitoring in Practice*, 2nd edition. Oxford: Butterworth–Heinneman, 1997: Chapter 8.
6   McDonald D, Grant A, Sheridan-Pereira M, Boylan P, Chalmers I. The Dublin Randomized Controlled Trial of intrapartum fetal heart rate monitoring. *American Journal of Obstetrics and Gynaecology* 1985; 152: 524–539.
7   Vintzileos AM, Nochimson DJ, Guzman ER *et al*. Intrapartum electronic fetal heart monitoring versus intermittent auscultation: a meta-analysis. *Obstetrics and Gynaecology* 1995; 85: 149–155.
8   Thacker SB, Stroup DF, Peterson HB. Efficacy and safety of intrapartum electronic fetal monitoring: an update. *Obstetrics and Gynaecology* 1995; 86: 613–620.
9   Dickinson JE. Previous Caesarean section. In: DK James, PJ Steer, CP Weiner, B Gonik (eds.) *High-Risk Pregnancy: Management Options*, 2nd edition. WB Saunders, 1999: Chapter 67.
10 ACOG Committee Opinion if Vaginal Delivery after a Previous Caesarean Birth. No. 143, October 1994. *International Journal of Obstetrics and Gynaecology* 1995; 48: 127–129.
11 O'Leary JA. *Shoulder Dystocia and Birth Injury.* McGraw Hill, 1992.
12 Keighley MRB, Radley S, Johannson R. Consensus on prevention and management of post-obstetric bowel incontinence and third degree tear. *Clinical Risk* 2000; 6(6): 231–237.
13 Schofield PF, Grace R. Faecal incontinence after childbirth. *Clinical Risk* 1999; 5: 201–204.
14 Bolam *v* Friern Hospital Management Committee [1957] 2 All ER 118; [1957] 1 WLR 582; 1 BMLR 1.
15 Bolitho *v* City and Hackney HA [1993] 4 Med LR 381; [1993] 13 BMLR 111; [1998] AC 232; [1997] 4 All ER 771; [1997] 3 WLR 1151; 39 BMLR 1; [1998] PNLR 1; [1998] Lloyd's Rep Med 26.
16 Puxon M. The incompetent parturient. *Clinical Risk* 1997; 3: 27.

Part III
Obstetrics

▶10

Prenatal Screening

Nicholas M Fisk

Historically, antenatal care concentrated on improving outcomes for the mother, largely oblivious to problems in the fetus. Over the past two decades, the advent of high-resolution ultrasound and Down syndrome screening programmes, along with ready access to invasive procedures, now renders exclusion of fetal abnormality the focus of the first half of pregnancy. Indeed, with improvements in maternal and perinatal outcomes, it is now arguable that the major risk of serious adverse outcome that parents face is that of having a fetus with a congenital, chromosomal or genetic abnormality. Without prenatal screening, 2% of babies at birth will have a structural anomaly, while 1 in 700–800 will have Down syndrome, and an as yet undetermined, although at least comparable, number will have some other serious genetic disorder. Their prevalence in early pregnancy – when screening takes place – is up to twice as high because abnormal fetuses are more likely to miscarry than normal ones.

Although most parents want screening for reassurance that their baby is normal, the chief impact of screening programmes in reducing adverse outcomes is through identification and termination of abnormal fetuses. The trend to lower family size and older maternal age at child-bearing, together with the rarity of perinatal death (ca. 8/1000), has led to increased parental expectations that every pregnancy will have a normal outcome. Such views are fuelled by technological advances whereby most fetuses are now screened for aneuploidy or structural anomalies. 'Wrongful birth' resulting from failed prenatal diagnosis has become a major source of litigation, at least in terms of quantum, and joins birth asphyxia/cerebral palsy as the two pivotal focuses of any obstetric risk management strategy.

Principles

Prenatal screening differs from other forms of disease screening in two respects. Firstly, a positive screening result may lead to diagnostic tests such as amniocentesis, which entail a small but definite risk of procedure-related fetal loss. Secondly, the downstream implications of a positive result include the option of termination of pregnancy, a sensitive issue on which parents will have differing views depending on their religious and cultural backgrounds, and their own ethical and moral frameworks. Thus, prenatal screening must always be *voluntary*.

Pre-test counselling may be face to face, but should include provision of written information. The voluntary nature of screening is stressed, along with its rationale and limitations, and the implications of a positive screen, including diagnostic tests, their risks, and the option of termination of pregnancy. The detection rate is also important, in particular so that parents appreciate the chance of a false-negative screening result, resulting in a missed antenatal diagnosis. These points may be reiterated in post-test counselling, although the latter largely refers to the more detailed and specific counselling given to women with high-risk or positive results of screening.

Those involved in counselling should appreciate the difference between screening and diagnostic tests. The former are designed to have high sensitivity but may have a high false-positive rate (ie they identify as high a proportion of affected fetuses as possible at the expense of also identifying a number of unaffected fetuses). Their imperfect accuracy contrasts with that of diagnostic tests, which are designed instead to be highly accurate on which further management and decision-making can be based. Screening tests are usually safe and applicable to low-risk populations, whereas diagnostic tests may involve invasive procedures, and are applicable to high-risk groups, including those with positive screening tests. Although Down syndrome screening is the obvious example, ultrasound can also be both a screening and a diagnostic test. A screening scan need only detect a suspicion that an abnormality may be present, whereas high-resolution ultrasound, often in a referral centre, is used to confirm or refute the diagnosis.

Over 90% of structural and chromosomal abnormalities arise in pregnancies without specific risk factors (ie in low-risk pregnancies). For this reason, anomaly and aneuploidy screening is offered universally. In other instances, screening will be selective, confined to certain ethnic groups or those with a family history. Screening programmes may be national, although most operate at a regional and particularly local level. Written protocols have become an important clinical risk strategy for reducing exposure in this area.

Down screening

Down syndrome

Down syndrome babies have three, instead of the normal two, copies of chromosome 21, or at least the critical region of chromosome 21. It is the most common chromosome disorder identified postnatally or at any time after the first 10 weeks of pregnancy, and is the most common genetic cause of mental retardation. The phenotype comprises the following features: upward slanting eyes, prominent epicanthic folds, spots on the iris, a flat nasal bridge, protruding tongue, short neck, flat occiput, short, broad and incurved little fingers, single transverse palmar creases, and a sandal gap between the first and second toes. Babies with Down syndrome are more likely to have structural malformations in other organ systems, in particular the heart, gut and kidneys. Intellectual disability and learning difficulties occur to some degree in all, and are usually moderate to severe. Ninety percent have conductive hearing loss; there is an increased frequency of leukaemia and a very high risk of premature-onset Alzheimer's disease.

Although the exact cause of Down syndrome is not known, most arise due to a non-disjunctive error in the meiosis-I stage of oogenesis in the mother. This risk increases with advancing maternal age, from 1 in 1500 at birth at age 20, to 1 in 900 at 30, one in 450 at 35, 1 in 100 at 40, to more than 1 in 30 at 45 years. These risks are considerably higher at conception, but fall progressively with gestation due to selective loss of aneuploid fetuses.

Diagnosis

Diagnosis is based on demonstrating an extra copy of chromosome 21 in metaphase culture, which allows the full karyotype to be determined. At least 95% have the 47 XY +21 or 47 XX +21 karyotype, denoting the common or full form of trisomy 21 in male and female fetuses, respectively. The remainder arise secondary to an unbalanced translocation in one parent, typically involving chromosomes 14 and 21; in such cases, the karyotype is abnormal when the fetus inherits one, instead of neither or both, the abnormal parental chromosomes.

Newer forms of DNA testing for Down syndrome using molecular methods, such as fluorescent *in situ* hybridization (FISH) or chromosome-specific short tandem repeats (STRs),[1] instead test for only one or more fragments of chromosome 21. They are highly accurate in detecting Down syndrome, but do not distinguish full from translocation cases.

Screening strategies

There is no way of preventing conception with Down syndrome. The only definitive way of diagnosing or excluding Down syndrome prenatally is by invasive testing – ie inserting a needle inside the womb to obtain a sample of fetally derived tissue for karyotype determination in the laboratory. The two most common invasive tests are chorion villus sampling (CVS) at 11–13 weeks, or amniocentesis after 14 weeks. Although highly accurate in diagnosing or excluding Down syndrome, these invasive tests carry a risk of procedure-related complications, in particular a risk of miscarriage in the region of 1%.[2,3] For this reason, women are not offered routinely, nor would most want, amniocentesis or CVS unless they were demonstrated to be at increased risk. Instead, they normally undergo a screening test.

The traditional way of determining whether a woman was at increased risk was her age. In the 1970s and 1980s, the generic age-related risk for Down syndrome was given to women over the age of 35–38 years, who then decided whether or not they wished to undergo an invasive diagnostic test. However, the relationship with age was weak, such that age-based screening strategies detected only around 30% of affected fetuses, and have thus been abandoned.

More recently, obstetric services have used one of two types of screening test together with a woman's age to determine her individual risk of having a baby with Down syndrome. The first strategy was serum screening, developed in the late 1980s and adopted into widespread practice in the early 1990s.[3,4] The second strategy of measuring the thickness of the subcutaneous tissue on the back of the baby's neck on ultrasound, called nuchal translucency screening, was developed in the mid-1990s,[5] and is increasingly replacing mid-trimester serum screening in many centres. A number of newer strategies have emerged in the past few years, but these essentially reflect combinations of serum screening and ultrasound.[6]

It is known that 75–80% of pregnant women wish to avail themselves of an offer of voluntary Down screening. Every obstetric service now has a duty of care to offer some form of screening for Down syndrome. Although there is still no national screening strategy for Down syndrome, it is no longer acceptable to offer age-based screening as the sole strategy for Down syndrome screening. This is because serum and nuchal translucency screening have been demonstrated clearly to have much greater detection rates for the same, or lower, false-positive rates.

These temporal changes in prenatal screening have been highlighted in the UK by data from the National Down Syndrome Cytogenetic Register.[7] Between 1989 and 1997, the proportion of Down syndrome diagnoses made antenatally increased from 30% to 53%; this change was most marked in younger mothers, the proportion diagnosed antenatally in those <35 years increasing from 9% to 45%. Over the same interval, the proportion of cases detected based on advanced maternal age fell from 78% to 16%, while the proportion based on serum screening and ultrasound increased from 6% and 13%, respectively, in 1989, to 37% and 43% in 1997. Note that the figure for ultrasound-based screening is not solely a reflection on the uptake of nuchal translucency screening, as it also includes cases in which an invasive test was performed for any abnormal ultrasound finding, including structural anomalies detected in later pregnancy. Additional information comes from surveys of screening practice for Down syndrome in the UK.[8,9] Between 1994 and 1998, the number of health authorities offering age-related screening alone decreased from 23% to 8%, while those offering serum screening, in one form or another, to all women increased from 60% to 72%. By 1998, however, only 8% of health authorities had introduced nuchal translucency as their primary screening strategy for all women.

Both serum and nuchal translucency screening remain inherently inaccurate, based on risk adjustment rather than accurate prediction. Although they detect around two-thirds to three-quarters of pregnancies with Down syndrome as being in a high-risk group, they also categorize around 5% of women with normal babies as high risk. Under both strategies invasive testing is offered to women whose risk of Down syndrome exceeds 1 in 250 or 1 in 300, albeit still with only a relatively small chance of having a baby with Down syndrome (1 in 50–100). Because of this, risks are expressed numerically, with the terms 'high-risk' and 'low-risk' preferred over 'positive' and 'negative'. Most high-risk results are false positives, while a third to a quarter of babies with Down syndrome will be associated with low-risk results. Such high false-positive rates would be unacceptable in most screening programmes outside pregnancy but, in the absence of alternatives, are tolerated in pregnancy because the diagnostic test involves a risk of fetal loss.

Serum screening

Unconjugated oestriol (uE3) and α-fetoprotein (AFP) levels are slightly lower (0.72 and 0.75 multiples of the median, respectively) and inhibin A and free β human chorionic gonadotrophin (hCG) levels slightly higher (1.92 and 2.2 multiples of the median, respectively) in mothers with a Down syndrome fetus.[3] Although not sufficiently abnormal to be diagnostic, these levels are used in regression analysis to modify the mothers *a priori* age-related risk of trisomy 21. Double test (AFP and hCG), triple test (AFP, hCG, uE3), quadruple test (AFP, hCG, uE3, inhibin A), serum screen and Bart's test are all names for serum screening – the exact name depending on local preference and the particular combination of hormones measured.

Typically, a woman would be offered the serum screen after she had been counselled as to its voluntary and screening nature, its detection and false-positive rate, and the implications of a high-risk result. She consents to a single blood sample, usually at 15–16 weeks but at any time between 14 and 21 weeks, for assay of one of the hormone combinations above. The risk of Down syndrome at birth is calculated based on computer modelling of the hormone results adjusted for maternal weight, and sometimes race, against her age and gestational age in days. Typically, ultrasound dates are used to determine gestational age, as these have proved more accurate than menstrual dating in estimating Down syndrome risk. If the result exceeds a high-risk threshold, usually 1 in 250, she is offered an invasive test, usually amniocentesis, to establish definitively whether or not the baby has Down syndrome.

Screening results can be influenced by prior vaginal bleeding, such that an elevated AFP negates its utility in Down screening. Serum screening is less applicable in diabetic pregnancies, where many of the markers are around 10% lower than in normal mothers. Serum screening is now considered inapplicable in twin pregnancies, because any abnormal hormonal production from one Down's placenta or fetus is likely to be masked by normal hormone production from the normal co-twin. Repeat testing is not recommended, especially where the initial result is high risk.

By convention, the screening performance of the various tests is compared for a fixed 5% false-positive rate. Wald *et al.*[3] recently modelled available data from the published literature and their own Barts/Oxford series and reported that sensitivity improves from 58% with AFP and total hCG to 69% for the optimal three-marker combination of AFP, total hCG and uE3. The best detection rate of 76% was achieved when inhibin A was added for quadruple testing, as shown in Figure 10.1. The 1998 NHS Health Technology Assessment Report on Down screening concluded that serum screening should be the standard method of screening, and be offered to all women regardless of where they live or their age.[3]

Screening services are best organized on a regional or consortium basis, overseen by an overall coordinator responsible for quality control and audit, in particular monitoring sensitivity and false-positive rates.

Nuchal translucency screening

The second and newer strategy is nuchal translucency screening on an ultrasound scan at 10–14 weeks.[5] Here, a measurement is made of the thickness of the subcutaneous tissues on the back of the fetal neck; the degree of nuchal oedema is greater in Down syndrome although, as with serum screening, there is considerable overlap between normal and Down fetuses. Although the mechanism is not entirely understood, it appears related in chromosomally abnormal fetuses to minor cardiac anomalies.[10] Cardiac dysfunction is further supported by a high frequency of abnormal ductus venosus Doppler waveforms in Down fetuses. Nuchal translucency measurements

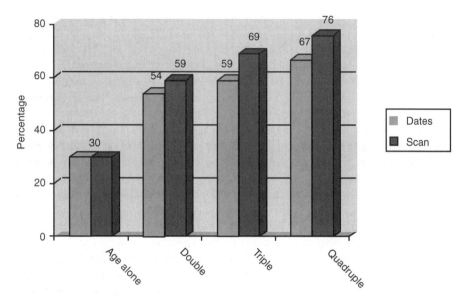

Fig. 10.1. Comparison of detection rates assuming a 5% false-positive rate for various combinations of maternal weight-adjusted serum parameters in the mid-trimester, double testing with AFP and total hCG, triple testing with AFP, unconjugated estriol and total hCG, and quadruple testing with AFP, unconjugated estriol, total hCG and inhibin. The increase in detection rate in the black compared to grey boxes illustrates the improved sensitivity found if ultrasound dating is used. After Wald et al.[3]

increase with gestation, so values are referenced to the crown–rump length. In normal fetuses, the upper reference limit increases from 2.2 to 2.8 mm at crown–rump lengths of 38 to 84 mm, with 5% of fetuses having a value above this, and 1% >4 mm. As with serum screening, the result is combined with maternal age and crown–rump length (ie gestational age) for software calculation of the risk of Down syndrome. Again, results over a predetermined threshold, typically 1 in 300, are considered high risk, and the mother is then offered invasive testing.

The main demonstration project screened over 96,000 women in 22 centres to report an 82% detection rate for Down syndrome for a 8.3% false-positive rate.[5] Correcting this for a 5% false-positive rate yielded a 77% detection rate for trisomy 21. This detection rate has been criticised as a possible overestimate, for two reasons.[3,11] Firstly, it involved a high-risk population, with a median maternal age of 31 years, and there is evidence that screening performance is better in high-risk populations. Indeed, there is as yet a paucity of published information on low-risk pregnancies. Secondly, detection rates were based on the first-trimester incidence of trisomy 21. It is known that around 40% of Down fetuses will miscarry in the interval until birth, and there is some suggestion that the chance of this may be higher among trisomic fetuses with increased nuchal translucency compared to those without.[12] Notwithstanding these reservations, the UK multicentre project screened more than twice as many women as the largest demonstration project for serum screening, including more than three times the number of Down syndrome fetuses. This consortium, through King's College Hospital and the Fetal Medicine Foundation in London, is now evaluating screening performance in large-scale low-risk populations in a number of countries, which it is able to do as a legacy of non-commercial dissemination of its risk estimation software to centres fulfilling its training and audit requirements. Further information on screening performance will come from two large non-intervention studies, one nearing completion in the UK, and one underway in the USA.

As with anomaly scanning, nuchal translucency scanning is a skilled procedure requiring high-resolution equipment and appropriately trained staff. Although these should now be standard in all obstetric ultrasound services, resource implications have been a barrier to the uptake of nuchal translucency scanning in many centres. A particular problem in nuchal translucency scanning is ensuring that the fetus is measured in the correct plane (see Figure 10.2). Although adjusting the angle of the transducer, tapping the mother's abdomen or using a transvaginal approach may help, most of the time this simply involves waiting for the baby to move into the correct position. Some early studies suggested that an adequate nuchal translucency measurement could not be obtained around 20% of the time, but most groups now achieve an appropriately aligned measurement close to 100% of the time. However, to achieve this can take up to 30 minutes, or, rarely, a further visit may be needed.

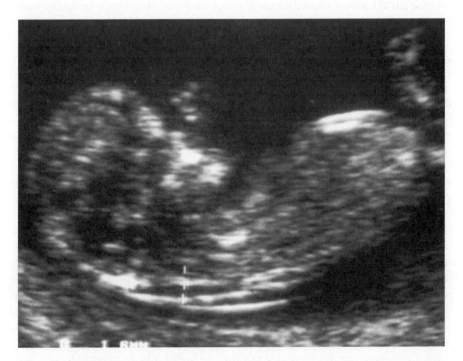

Fig. 10.2. Nuchal translucency measurement. Note the image is magnified, the focal zone is on the fetus, that the fetus is lying longitudinally, the neck is neither unduly flexed or extended, the amnion is resolved separately from the neck, and the calipers are positioned in an 'on and on' fashion to define the borders of the nuchal translucency.

Another disadvantage of nuchal translucency screening, at least in centres where sonographers do the screening, is that a high-risk result is apparent at the time. This can generate considerable anxiety, and here the sonographer may be forced into initiating post-test counselling in the course of a busy scanning session. In contrast, post-test counselling after serum screening can be arranged or initiated by a trained counsellor at an appropriate time after the result is obtained. The immediacy of the result, on the other hand, is an advantage in fetal medicine services where scans are undertaken by doctors able to undertake immediate post-test counselling.

There are several advantages to a first-trimester scan, which increase the justification for nuchal translucency screening. Firstly, it will identify the 2–3% of pregnancies at this stage that are non-viable.[13] Secondly, in multiple pregnancies it allows accurate determination of chorionicity, to distinguish the 80% of twins with separate placentas (dichorionic) from the 20% with a shared monochorionic placenta indicative of a three- to tenfold increased risk of fetal and perinatal loss and morbidity.[14] This is important, as chorionicity cannot always be distinguished reliably in later pregnancy. Also, it means that multiple pregnancies can be screened, as the biochemical strategies are inapplicable in multiple pregnancy. Notwithstanding this, monochorionic twins have a higher than expected false-positive rate,[15] while the incidence of Down syndrome in twin fetuses appears little over half that expected in singletons.[16] Thirdly, a limited anomaly scan can also be done at this time, which may detect many of the more gross structural abnormalities. Lastly, women seem to prefer nuchal screening, in particular the opportunity to observe their baby on a first-trimester scan, as well as the transparency and immediacy of the result.

In chromosomally normal fetuses, a raised nuchal translucency measurement, particularly >3.5 mm, has prognostic implications. The chance of fetal/perinatal loss increases exponentially from 4 to 8, 15 and 53/1000 with measurements ≥3.5, 4.5 and 5.5 mm, respectively.[17] A wide range of genetic and skeletal syndromes has been associated with a raised nuchal translucency. Similarly the chance of the baby having a major congenital heart defect increases from 0.5/1000 to 3, 5 and 23/1000 with measurements of ≥3.5, 4.5 and 5.5 mm, respectively.[18] Nuchal translucency may have a role in screening for congenital heart disease, the sensitivity of which on routine ultrasound is poor, and accordingly most centres now offer referral for fetal echocardiography to those with euploid fetuses with a nuchal translucency measurement ≥3.5 mm.

Raised nuchal translucency has a comparable or better sensitivity for most non-Down syndrome aneuploidies, whereas serum screening has some utility, but only for trisomy 13 and 18. The latter are lethal in late pregnancy or early infancy, and are almost all detected on a routine higher resolution anomaly scan. Sex chromosome abnormalities on the other hand (Turner, Kleinefelter and triple-X syndromes) are associated with a milder phenotype. The rationale for the detection of these aneuploidies is thus less robust than for Down syndrome.

Mid-trimester ultrasound markers

A number of markers, or soft tissue signs, increase the risk of Down syndrome. These can be identified on mid-trimester ultrasound, typically on a scan prior to amniocentesis at 16 weeks, or the routine anomaly scan at 18–20 weeks. Markers include nuchal skin oedema, short femoral or humeral length measurements, choroid plexus cysts, bilateral renal pelvic dilatation, echogenic fetal bowel and hyperechogenic foci ('golf balls') in the fetal heart. Early publications reporting increased prevalence of these markers in Down fetuses compared with euploid fetuses were used to derive increased risks for trisomy 21. Because the relative risk attributable to these markers was usually small in magnitude, a dilemma emerged as to whether women should be informed of such findings is isolation. Many patients in the early to mid-1990s were counselled about their increased risk in the presence of markers, with little regard to their background risk, any previous screening, the sensitivity and specificity of such findings in large-scale studies in low-risk populations, or whether there were other abnormalities present.

There were several problems with this approach. Firstly, the sensitivity of these markers was considerably lower than that for serum screening, or the emergent nuchal translucency screening. For instance, the highest sensitivity for any marker was with nuchal oedema, but this was still only 34–38% in pooled studies.[3,19] Secondly, these markers were also present in a substantial proportion of healthy fetuses (hyperechogenic bowel in 1%, nuchal oedema in 1%, renal pelvic dilatation in 2–3%, short femurs in 6–8%, short humeri in 5%). If invasive testing were offered to all those with one marker, up to 15% of women would be identified as at increased risk. Thirdly, the populations on which these risk estimates were based had not undergone prior Down screening. If earlier nuchal translucency or quadruple serum screening removes around 75% of affected fetuses from the pool undergoing mid-trimester ultrasound, then the utility of mid-trimester markers falls substantially. Finally, their predictive value is heavily influenced by whether they are found in isolation or in association with other markers and structural anomalies. A recent meta-analysis of 56 studies found sensitivities for individual markers in isolation of only 1–16% (Table 10.1), whereas the sensitivity of multiple markers in association with structural anomalies was 69%.[20] Most of the markers in isolation had low relative risks (positive predictive values or likelihood ratios of only 3–7). Indeed, it is now known that choroid plexus cysts in isolation, which are found in 0.65% of normal fetuses, do not increase the risk of Down syndrome at all.[20,21] The highest relative risk for any marker in isolation was for a thickened nuchal fold,[17] but this was found in only 4% of fetuses with Down

Table 10.1. Test performance for mid-trimester ultrasonic markers as isolated findings to predict trisomy 21, based on a meta-analysis of 56 studies.[20]

Marker	Sensitivity (%)	Positive likelihood ratio (%)
Thickened nuchal fold	4	17
Choroid plexus cyst	1	1
Short femur length	16	2.7
Short humeral length	9	7.5
Echogenic bowel	4	6.1
Echogenic intracardiac focus	11	2.8
Renal pyelectasis	2	1.9

syndrome. The finding of two or more markers, however, does need to be discussed with the woman.[22]

For all these reasons, mid-trimester ultrasound is not recommended as a practical or primary screening test for Down syndrome.[3,20] Although absence of markers on a mid-trimester ultrasound in the absence of prior screening has been suggested to reduce the chance of Down syndrome by 50–80%,[23] most health authorities do not advocate ultrasound to modify high-risk serum screening results, as this necessarily reduces the detection rate in any screening programme.

Current status

There has been considerable debate as to whether biochemical or ultrasound screening for Down syndrome is superior. The pro-nuchal translucency camp argues that detection rates are higher, that women prefer earlier diagnosis, and that abnormal results not associated with aneuploidy predict other complications. The pro-biochemical screening camp respond that earlier screening predicts pregnancies destined to miscarry, and that serum screening is simpler to implement.

Accordingly, recent efforts have gone into combining the two strategies. First trimester maternal levels of PAPP-A (pregnancy-associated plasma protein-A) are lower on average (0.38 multiples of the median) and β-hCG higher (1.83 multiples of the median) in pregnancies carrying a Down fetus.[3] Although demonstration projects suggest a higher sensitivity in the first trimester of combined nuchal translucency and serum screening than with either technique alone,[24,25] there is a practical difficulty in avoiding stepwise results and ensuring that a single risk estimate is generated. One way of achieving this is to use an automated serum-testing device in the ultrasound clinic for one-stop on-the-spot risk assessment. Another suggested modification is to integrate both forms of first-trimester screening with mid-trimester serum screening.[26] Theoretical calculations suggest that the principle advantage of integrated screening lies in reducing the false-positive or invasive-procedure rate to 1%, but whether women will accept undergoing first-trimester assessment without being given a risk estimate until 15–16 weeks, remains to be seen.

Given the controversies above, the paucity of large-scale screening studies in low-risk pregnancies, and regional disparities in priorities and resources, a wide range of screening strategies is likely to remain in use for the foreseeable future. Notwithstanding this, a recent NHS report on cost effectiveness and safety concluded that of the four efficient screening strategies, integrated testing would be the most effective and safest option, but the most expensive, costing £51,000 more per baby detected than the cheapest effective option of nuchal translucency screening.[6] Combined first-trimester screening and mid-trimester quadruple testing were both more sensitive than nuchal translucency testing alone in the model, but cost an additional £57,000 and £75,000, respectively, per baby detected, with a total service cost between that of nuchal translucency and integrated screening. The main implication of this report for service providers is that switching from a primary strategy of double or triple serum screening in the mid-trimester to nuchal translucency screening in the first trimester would result in a comparable detection rate, but almost a 30% saving in cost.[6]

Other genetic screening

Although there are many hundreds of inherited single-gene disorders, genetic screening exists currently for only a handful. We each carry about six genes for severely disabling conditions, but fortunately most of us by chance reproduce with someone who carries a different six. Thus, for many diseases with the common autosomal recessive mode of inheritance, a couple only becomes aware that they are at risk after having an affected child. Autosomal dominant inheritance is less prevalent in severely disabling conditions, because the nature of the disease means that affected individuals rarely reproduce. An exception is Huntington disease, which usually manifests only in the post-reproductive age group. Accordingly, dominant conditions, such as thanatophoric dwarfism and achondroplasia, often occur instead as a result of new mutation. X-linked dominant conditions, on the other hand, such as muscular dystrophy and the haemophilias, are inherited vertically via unaffected carrier females.

A family history remains the commonest form of genetic screening, and is a routine and important part of early antenatal care. Simple genetic risks for common diseases can usually be estimated at the time, while rare, complex or multifactorial conditions may require access to databases such as Online Mendelian Inheritance in Man (OMIM; see URL http://www3.ncbi.nlm.nih.gov/Omim/searchomim.html) or consultation with a clinical geneticist.

There are no genetic conditions for which universal antenatal screening is undertaken in the UK. However, universal screening has been recommended for cystic fibrosis, and screening for haemoglobinopathies is currently undertaken in many regions, especially urban ones with sizeable multiethnic populations. Procedure-related miscarriage in couples at risk of these genetic disorders is less an issue than in Down screening because women are typically only offered an invasive test where their genetic risk is ≥ 1 in 4. Antenatal screening is likely to expand in future as a result of the cloning of increasing numbers of disease genes, together with advances in screening technology, particularly the development of DNA microarrays. Indeed, the eventual translation of promising laboratory studies of non-invasive prenatal diagnosis using fetal cells or DNA in maternal blood into clinical practice raises the prospect of every fetus being screened directly, rather than indirectly through screening the parents for carrier status as at present. Notwithstanding this, screening is usually only justified where the condition results in severe morbidity, and its identification *in utero* may alter the outcome, either through parental reproductive choices, or through timely treatment *in utero* or at birth. Reproductive choice predominantly means entertaining the option of termination of pregnancy, but also extends to other options for future pregnancies – such as changing partners, using donor gametes (sperm or oocytes), or pre-implantation diagnosis to select unaffected embryos for implantation.

Cystic fibrosis

Cystic fibrosis is an autosomal recessive condition characterized by thick secretions from exocrine epithelia, resulting in progressive respiratory and gastrointestinal morbidity and infertility. It has a high case fatality ratio, although with advances in treatment, predicted life expectancy now exceeds 40 years. The carrier frequency in the UK is around 1 in 24, making it the commonest recessive gene found in Caucasian populations. Over 800 mutations have been described in the cystic fibrosis transmembrane regulator gene at 7q31, which encodes a protein regulating chloride secretion and sodium absorption. The ΔF_{508} gene accounts for about 75%, although fewer in black people and those of Asian and Ashkenazi backgrounds. Screening for three mutations would cover around 80% of cases, whereas increasing the number of mutations tested to 12 and 56 would increase the detection rate only marginally, to 83 and 86%, respectively.

Historically, screening of immediate family members for carrier status has been indicated once a relative had been diagnosed. However, this cascade-based approach will only detect around 15% of carriers. Accordingly, population-based screening has been attempted but has the disadvantage of denoting up to 1 in 20 individuals as high risk, often when they are single and at a time remote from reproductive intent. This is why the uptake of population screening in demonstration projects is well under 50%, but rises in pregnancy to around 75%, comparable to other forms of prenatal screening.[27–29] Antenatal screening has the advantage of immediacy to the reproductive process, and can either be done sequentially, testing the second partner only where the first is a carrier, or together as a couple. The chance of having a child with cystic fibrosis falls from 1 in 4, where both parents are carriers, to 1 in around 500 where only one is, and to around 1 in 50,000 where neither carries the common cystic fibrosis mutations.

The utility of antenatal screening has been confirmed in 11 demonstration projects in four countries in which over 50,000 couples were screened. Although antenatal screening has been recommended in the UK,[29] this has not translated into widespread clinical practice. One issue is financial, each prevented live birth costing an estimated £46,000–£53,000. This is considerably more than neonatal screening at £5000–£6000 per diagnosed child, but still considerably less than the lifetime medical costs of caring for an affected child. Another is the increasing life expectancy and quality of life of affected individuals with cystic fibrosis, which may improve further with therapies currently under development such as gene replacement. Indeed, it can be argued that an antenatal diagnosis of cystic fibrosis may not necessarily satisfy the requirements of serious mental or physical handicap for termination under section 1 (1)(b) clause E of the Abortion Act 1967 (as amended by the Human Fertilization and Embryology Act 1990).

Haemoglobinopathies

In the UK, it has been estimated that 43 conceptions each year are homozygous for β-thalassaemia (0.07/1000) and 178 (0.28/1000) for sickle cell disease. These autosomal recessive disorders mainly affect black, Asian and Mediterranean ethnic minorities. Universal screening has been recommended in areas where these groups, which average around 10% of UK residents, comprise more than 15% of the local population. Antenatal screening is always stepwise, with mothers identified as carriers then invited to have their partner tested and, if at risk, to consider invasive prenatal diagnosis. As the chief rationale of screening is reproductive choice – that is, termination of unwanted affected fetuses – it is important to distinguish the two commoner forms among the 600 types of haemoglobinopathy. Although both sickle cell anaemia and β-thalassaemia are associated with reduced life expectancy and considerable morbidity, the phenotype of the former is milder, with management aimed at preventing infections and sickling crises, whereas individuals with β-thalassaemia major in the absence of bone marrow transplantation have a lifelong requirement for blood transfusion and iron-chelation therapy. For this reason, unselected women identified as carriers for sickle cell disease by antenatal screening are less likely to avail themselves of partner testing and prenatal diagnosis than those shown to be carriers for β-thalassaemia (16% versus 80%).[30,31] In contrast, α-thalassaemia, which is rare in the UK, being largely confined to East Asians, is usually lethal *in utero*. A recent systematic review estimated that universal haemoglobinopathy screening is cost effective in all populations with 1% or more ethnic minorities, providing that at least 25% of these carry the β-thalassaemia trait.[31]

Screening requires haemoglobin electrophoresis, with further investigation using DNA studies. For the thalassaemias, the distinction between universal and selective screening is somewhat tenuous, in that all women have their mean cell volume estimated as part of the full blood count done with their routine antenatal booking investigations. However, this approach, in addition to failing to detect sickle cell carriers, will also fail to detect couples at risk of variants and combination disorders (ie haemoglobin Sβ-thalassaemia). Whatever the arguments about the necessity for electrophoresis on those with normal red cell indices, there is universal agreement that women with a low mean red-cell volume should be further investigated by haemoglobin electrophoresis.

Tay-Sachs disease

Tay-Sachs disease is a progressive neurodegenerative autosomal recessive disorder resulting from deficiency of the enzyme hexosaminidase A, which leads to accumulation of the lipid GM2 ganglioside in nerve cells. The classic form results in almost undetectable enzyme levels, and death within the first five years, although there is a rarer late onset form with levels around 2–4% of normal. In contrast, carriers have hexosaminidase A levels in the region of 20–50% of normal.

One in around 30 Ashkenazi Jews are carriers, although the incidence is only around a hundredth of this in non-Jews. Accordingly, biochemical carrier testing should be offered in early pregnancy to couples of Ashkenazi background; many will already have been screened either as a couple or individuals because of the high level of awareness in these communities. Further DNA testing may then be indicated to identify which of around 80 different mutations in the *HEX A* gene on chromosome 15 is involved, and thus predict the phenotype. Most centres still screen biochemically, although more recently screening for the three commoner mutations alone has been suggested, given the incomplete sensitivity (93–99%) and specificity (88–98%) of the enzyme assay alone.[32] Experience in susceptible communities in North America suggests that screening has resulted in around a 90% reduction in the incidence of Tay-

Sachs disease.[33] Some centres also offer this group screening for Canavan disease, and the recent cloning of the gene for primary familial dysautonomia, carried by 1 in 30 Askenazim, may lead to it being added to a 'Jewish screen'.

Anomaly scanning

Universal mid-trimester screening

Ninety five percent of structural fetal abnormalities occur in women who are not considered at high risk of fetal abnormality. For this reason, the practice of routine ultrasound screening (ie examining all pregnant women) for fetal abnormality was introduced. Randomized controlled trials and observational studies show that routine is preferable to selective screening for this purpose.[11,34-36] Routine ultrasound screening for fetal abnormality has been shown to reduce perinatal mortality through the selective identification and termination of malformed fetuses.[37] The effect of the uptake of routine anomaly scanning in the 1980s on the prevalence of fetal anomalies is demonstrated in a report from the Northern Region. This showed that half of the decline in perinatal mortality between 1982 and 1990 was accounted for by antenatal recognition of serious abnormalities leading to termination of pregnancy prior to viability.[38] Although routine ultrasound screening for this purpose has been advocated for many years by expert groups[39,40] and a 1994 Royal College of Obstetricians and Gynaecologists (RCOG) guideline felt there was little doubt about the value of ultrasound in excluding many fetal anomalies,[41] the uptake of routine ultrasound in the UK remained incomplete well into the 1990s. A survey of UK obstetric ultrasound services in 1995 with a 65% response rate found that only 82% of units offered a routine scan for fetal anomalies.[42] More recently, the RCOG Working Party on Ultrasound Screening for Fetal Abnormalities concluded in 1997 that, on the basis of current evidence, an ultrasound scan undertaken between 18 and 20 weeks was the most effective available method to detect a wide range of fetal abnormalities.[43] A systematic review in 2000 similarly concluded that a scan undertaken between 18 and 20 weeks was the most effective method available to detect fetal abnormalities at a stage in pregnancy when there was still time to perform invasive diagnostic procedures and/or offer termination of pregnancy if indicated.

Congenital malformations are common, and structural malformations occur in 2.1% of pregnancies.[11] Several large unselected series of fetal anomaly screening in district hospitals in the UK published in the early 1990s had shown that abnormalities were detected in 1.0–1.6% of pregnancies.[44-46] Pregnant women are at far greater risk from structural abnormalities than they are from chromosomal abnormalities such as Down syndrome (live birth incidence: 0.12%), for which there is universal screening.

Not all abnormalities detected by ultrasound will be major or of clinical significance. Some will lead to further investigation during the pregnancy or arrangements for further investigation or special management after delivery; a very few can be treated *in utero*. Some women with a fetus with a non-viable or severely handicapping abnormality will choose to continue with the pregnancy, and may gain value from parental preparation. Notwithstanding this, the principal purpose of fetal anomaly scanning is so that women identified as having a fetus with a severe or handicapping abnormality can be offered termination of pregnancy. Failure to offer a routine ultrasound screening service for fetal abnormality effectively denies mothers of severely anomalous fetuses this option.

The ability to offer a routine service has resource implications and depends on having the requisite skills and number of staff available, and the appropriate ultrasound equipment. It also depends on the legality of termination of pregnancy and its acceptability to women.[11] There is general agreement that adequately trained staff and modern machinery are essential for this task.[40,41] Some have argued that resource issues within the NHS have not allowed every obstetric service to offer such a service on a routine basis, at least in the 1980s and early 1990s.[47] However, an anomaly scan has been estimated to cost only £15–£50 at 1997 prices,[11] while a study from Sheffield in 1993/4 estimated that replacing selective screening with routine screening resulted in a net saving of nearly £1 million per year through reduced care costs for children with long-term handicap.[48] Extrapolating this result to the whole NHS, it was estimated that universal routine anomaly scanning would save £170 million annually.[48] Routine anomaly scanning is now the norm, and any health authority that fails to offer such a service not only exposes its patients to an increased risk of having a child with long-term handicap, but also itself to litigation.

Sensitivity

The sensitivity of ultrasound for fetal anomaly detection varies widely in the published literature from 17% to 96%, depending on the scanning policy, the gestational age, the skill of the operator, the study population and the type of anomaly included. Routine ultrasound screening between 18 and 22 weeks of unselected populations in the UK has achieved consistently high detection rates for major abnormalities of 73%–92%.[34,44–46] Systematic review of the available studies of routine mid-trimester ultrasound, as shown in Table 10.2, reveals that detection rates in studies published since 1990 vary considerably depending on the organ system, from highs of 76% for central nervous system abnormalities and 67% for renal tract anomalies, to 17% and 24% for cardiac and skeletal anomalies, respectively.[11] Within each organ system there are major and minor anomalies with very different prognoses; therefore, the RCOG Working Party proposed a four-tiered classification as follows: lethal anomalies, anomalies associated with possible survival and long-term morbidity with or without surgery, anomalies amenable to intrauterine therapy, and anomalies associated with possible short-term/immediate morbidity. Subcategorization using this classification in the systematic review confirmed the trend towards higher detection rates with increasing severity of the malformation as per Table 10.2.

The detection rates shown in Table 10.2 are likely to underestimate contemporary standards of routine ultrasound, because many of these studies started in the 1980s when standards of equipment and training were lower, and because they were often done in the introductory phases of routine ultrasound screening programmes.

Table 10.2. Prevalence and detection of congenital anomalies at second-trimester routine ultrasound scan according to RCOG classification[43] in 96,633 fetuses in 11 studies published since 1990. Note that the category of anomalies amenable to intrauterine therapy (obstructive uropathy, pleural effusions) has not been included because no data were available to extract in this category. After Bricker et al.[11]

Category	Anomaly	Prevalence per 1000	Detection rate (%)
Lethal		2.0	60/79 (76%)
	Anencephaly	0.6	37/38 (97%)
	Trisomy 13/18	0.7	5/8 (63%)
	Hypoplastic left heart	0.4	9/16 (56%)
	Bilateral renal agenesis	0.4	7/7 (100%)
	Musculoskeletal	0.4	2/10 (20%)
Possible survival with long-term morbidity		8.8	161/409 (39%)
	Spina bifida	0.6	22/33 (67%)
	Hydrocephalus	0.7	18/32 (56%)
	Encephalocele	0.2	7/7 (100%)
	Holoprosencephaly	0.2	4/7 (57%)
	Down syndrome	1.8	11/70 (16%)
	Complex cardiac	1.7	24/103 (23%)
	AVSD	0.5	1/13 (8%)
	Gastroschisis	0.2	11/11 (100%)
	Exomphalos	0.2	7/7 (100%)
	Diaphragmatic hernia	0.3	9/20 (45%)
	Tracheo-oesophageal fistula	0.3	2/15 (13%)
	Bowel obstruction	0.3	2/15 (13%)
	CAML	0.3	6/6 (100%)
	Bilateral renal dysplasia	0.3	3/5 (60%)
	Multiple abnormalities	1.3	30/38 (79%)
Anomalies associated with possible short-term/ immediate morbidity		4.8	66/313 (21%)
	ASD/VSD	1.4	2/87 (2%)
	Isolated valve abnormality	0.3	5/12 (42%)
	Facial clefts	1.0	20/61 (33%)
	Talipes	1.5	30/142 (23%)
	Unilateral renal dysplasia	0.6	9/11 (82%)

AVSD = atrioventricular septal defect; ASD/VSD = atrial or ventricular septal defect.

Detection rates in the Belgian multicentre study doubled in the early 1990s compared with the mid to late 1980s.[49] For instance, the sensitivity of detection of spina bifida in the systematic review was only 67%, well below that achieved in virtually all the studies of ultrasound screening for spina bifida. Of more relevance are sensitivities achieved in the three large studies of routine screening in UK district general hospitals, which, accepting the limitation of small numbers, were 10 out of 10 for spina bifida. A large population-based study in Scotland between 1989 and 1994 showed that a minimum standard 18–20 week anomaly scan detected 92% (80 out of 87) of spina bifidas.[34]

Diagnostic accuracy

After termination of pregnancy for ultrasonically diagnosed congenital anomalies, it is well established that important additional information, usually in the form of other undetected anomalies, is obtained at autopsy in 20–45% of cases.[50-53] This is primarily of relevance to determining the aetiology of malformation complexes and syndromes, and thus the recurrence risk. It also indicates some of the limitations of ultrasound, which fails to reveal anomalies in organ systems not associated with fluid accumulations or detectable alterations in ultrasonic phenotype.

False-negative diagnoses are more likely in the presence of oligohydramnios and maternal obesity. In addition, some malformations may not actually be present/detectable at the time of the mid-trimester scan, such as ventriculomegaly, duodenal atresia or minor renal lesions. Minor or progressive cardiac lesions, especially those involving the outflow tracts, are notoriously difficult to detect. Some anomalies, such as hypospadias, congenital dislocation of the hip, anal atresia, isolated cleft palate, and ear and eye malformations, are unlikely to be detectable at any stage. The reasons for variable detection rates for individual anomalies within each organ system have been reviewed in detail by Chitty.[54]

Any false-positive diagnosis is of concern in that it might lead to termination of a structurally normal fetus. Here, it must be remembered that, unlike other forms of prenatal testing, ultrasound is both a *screening* and a *diagnostic* test. The purpose of a screening examination is only to raise the suspicion that something may be wrong, which should then prompt referral to someone with specialized skills in fetal abnormality scanning. In the first instance, this may be an obstetrician or a radiologist in a district general hospital with responsibility for anomaly scanning. Unless such a scan is normal, or the diagnosis is obvious and the counselling straightforward (eg in anencephaly), women with antenatally diagnosed or suspected fetal abnormalities should then be referred to a fetal medicine specialist and/or tertiary referral fetal medicine centre.

The past decade has seen the establishment in most regions of tertiary referral fetal medicine centres, which offer high-resolution ultrasound by experts in fetal abnormality management, diagnostic and therapeutic invasive procedures, and which have ready access to input from allied specialists in paediatrics, surgery, genetics and the laboratory sciences. Before management decisions are reached, further investigation may be needed to establish the diagnosis and extent of any abnormality. Examples include colour and power Doppler, fetal echocardiography, amnioinfusion, invasive procedures such as amniocentesis, CVS, fetal blood sampling or fluid aspiration, karyotyping, and DNA studies. Consultation with subspecialists in paediatric surgery, cardiology, cardiothoracic surgery, neurology, neurosurgery, craniofacial surgery, urology, orthopaedics and clinical genetics may help in deciding diagnosis and management options, while parents find counselling by specialists directly involved in the care of affected children after birth invaluable in understanding the likely prognosis for their child, and the nature of any surgical or medical treatment entailed.

The term 'temporary false positive' may thus be more appropriate, and rates as low as 0.5% can be achieved.[43] Temporary false positives are in fact a necessary part of ultrasound screening, as high detection rates require referral of cases with equivocal findings, in which abnormalities may then be excluded on a detailed high-resolution scan in a referral centre. The sonographer in the district centre as an expert in routine, and thus predominantly normal scans, cannot be expected to have the extensive diagnostic experience of the fetal medicine specialist who deals with fetal anomalies on a day-to-day basis; the sonographer, however, should be expert in recognizing when findings are atypical. Hub-and-spoke networks of screening and diagnostic centres are now an established part of routine mid-trimester anomaly screening. Fortunately, sustained significant false positives (ie resulting in termination of a normal fetus) are exceedingly rare. The figure is zero in all but one study in the systematic review; the rate of 0.00006% in the Oxford region study[35] was due to two fetuses, one with isolated nuchal translucency and the other with an isolated absent stomach, for which the issue of termination had not been raised with the parents by the prenatal diagnosis team.

Counselling

Screening for fetal anomalies is a sensitive area because it involves the option of termination of affected pregnancies, which is unacceptable to some couples. Like Down syndrome screening, anomaly scanning therefore must be voluntary and consent sought. However, it differs from Down screening in that its purpose is not entirely the detection of fetal abnormalities, for which termination of pregnancy can be offered. Firstly, an ultrasound yields additional benefits such as accurate dating, confirmation of viability, early diagnosis of twins, parental bonding and placental localization. Notwithstanding this, many of these benefits are better achieved through an earlier dating scan while the benefit of routine mid-trimester placental localization remains controversial. Secondly, termination is not a relevant option, or indeed the only option, for many anomalies for which there may be value in parental preparation, fetal treatment, *in-utero* transfer to a specialist centre, or early delivery for postnatal management. Although around 99% of parents want an ultrasound, many do so for reassurance that the baby is normal, but it is still important they appreciate the potential significance of antenatal detection of fetal abnormality.

The RCOG Working Party concluded that while formal written consent before a scan seems unnecessary, women should be positively allowed to opt in for the scan to be performed.[43] There should be an opportunity for discussion both before and after the scan so any relevant concerns can be addressed. It was recommended that written information be provided before a routine anomaly scan, which identified the objectives of screening, and likely detection rates for the more common severe fetal abnormalities (eg spina bifida, cardiac defects, aneuploidy, etc). A proforma information sheet recommended in a supplementary report is shown in Table 10.3.[22]

Standards for the routine anomaly scan

The main risk from ultrasound comes from its use by inadequately trained staff working in relative isolation using poor equipment.

Table 10.3. Suggested information sheet for women undergoing a two-stage scanning protocol.[22] Reproduced with permission of the Royal College of Obstetricians and Gynaecologists.

Your ultrasound scan
Please read this carefully.

As part of your antenatal care we are offering to do a scan of your pregnancy.

The first scan will be done at your antenatal visit. It is to check how many weeks pregnant you are, that there are not twins, and that the baby is doing well. Usually, the scan will be through your abdomen and you should have a full bladder. Sometimes the scan will be done through the front passage (vagina) but the ultrasonographer will talk to you about this if it proves necessary.

A second scan, done at about 20 weeks, is to check that your baby is normal. Mostly babies are healthy, but sadly some have problems which could be serious. If you really do not wish to know if the baby has an abnormality, it may be best to decide not to have this scan. If you do decide to have a scan, we will assume that you wish to know about anything that we find.

The scan will involve you lying down on a couch, and a trained scan operator putting scan gel and then the scan head onto your abdomen. This will give images on the screen which allow measurements of the baby and give moving pictures. These can be quite difficult to see clearly, but the scan operator will try to ensure that all is well.

About half of the major abnormalities that cause serious difficulties will be seen on a scan and half will not be seen. This means that even if your scan is normal there is a small chance that your baby will still have a problem.

Below is a list of different types of congenital abnormality, and how likely scanning is to identify each problem.

Problem	What the problem is	Chance of being seen
Spina bifida	Open spinal cord	90%
Anencephaly	Absence of the top of the head	99%
Hydrocephalus*	Excess fluid within the brain	60%
Major congenital heart problems		25%
Diaphragmatic hernia	A defect in the muscle which separates the chest and abdomen	60%
Exomphalos/Gastroschisis	Defects of the abdominal wall	90%
Major kidney problems	Missing or abnormal kidneys	85%
Cerebral palsy	Spasticity	Never seen
Autism		Never seen
Down syndrome	May be associated with heart and bowel problems	About 40%

Many cases present late in pregnancy or even after birth.

The scan can sometimes tell what sex the baby appears to be, but not always, and we would usually not do extra scans just to identify the sex of the baby. If the scan does predict the sex of the baby this is right about 95% of the time. The scan operator will only tell you the sex of the baby if you, and all the people in the scan room with you, want to know that information.

If the scan finds a problem you will be told at the time of the scan that there is a problem, but a full discussion of the problem may require you to come back to the hospital for a further scan and discussion with a specialist. Most problems that need repeat scanning are not serious and approximately 15% of scans will need to be repeated for one reason or another.

Although ultrasound may be done by obstetricians, midwives, technicians or radiographers, the best ultrasonographers are those with specific training, such as radiographers. Detection rates rise substantially with training and increasing experience,[46,49] with rates of 40% in district centres rising to 90% in referral centres.[55] Thus midwives wishing to be involved in ultrasound screening should have undertaken professional training with certification. Ultrasound training programmes leading to diplomas and masters degrees are now well established for professions supplementary to medicine, and are accredited through the Consortium for the Accreditation of Sonographic Education (CASE), whose members include the British Medical Ultrasound Society, the College of Radiographers, the Royal College of Midwives and the UK Association of Sonographers. Doctors may gain appropriate training through the combined RCOG/Royal College of Radiologists' joint Diploma in Obstetric and Gynaecological Ultrasound, the Fetal Medicine Foundation, or through subspecialty training in maternal and fetal medicine. The RCOG Working Party felt that scanning should be undertaken by qualified sonographers who would devote a substantial proportion of their time to obstetric scanning, while medical practitioners would be expected to perform the equivalent of two obstetric scanning sessions per week to maintain expertise.[43] District centres should have a medical practitioner, typically an obstetrician or radiologist with particular interest in obstetric ultrasound, with overall responsibility for the service, including invasive procedures, giving consultant opinions, referrals, developing protocols in conjunction with the sonographers, and overseeing audit and continuing medical and professional development. A superintendent sonographer would have responsibility for day-to-day management of the ultrasound unit, including scanning protocols, and maintenance of professional and equipment standards.

The recommendation from the RCOG Working Party, which is having the biggest impact, was that ultrasound examinations for fetal anomaly detection should be carried out on equipment no older than five years. The only exception was where relevant electronic software and hardware upgrades had been installed, in which case this should have been done not more than five years previously. Visualization is significantly impaired by the use of older or inferior equipment. This is both because ultrasound transducers decay with time, and because there have been rapid advances in transducer design and image processing, analogous to advances in other computational technology over the past five to ten years. Obstetric ultrasound historically has been underfunded by comparison with other imaging equipment, and this recommendation is proving a powerful argument when obstetric ultrasound services negotiate with their managers for equipment.

Although hard-copy images of routine ultrasound examinations are normal practice in the USA and Australasia, this has not been the case in the UK for cost reasons. The recent supplement to the RCOG Working Party report notes that the use of hard copy for routine normal scans has major cost implications, and reaffirms current minimum practice in relation to image archiving. When abnormalities are detected, or when there are suspicious findings, hard copy or – preferably – video recordings are recommended.[22] There are problems with the longevity of thermal paper records, however; and video will soon become an obsolete technology, now that most new high-resolution machines come fitted with DICOM digital storage capability.

Protocols

The RCOG working group recommended minimum standards for a 20-week anomaly scan. Twenty minutes should be allocated to the examination. This should be conducted using a checklist approach. As shown in Table 10.4, and Figure 10.3, the optimal scan will include extended views of the cardiac outflow tracts, the fetal face and lips, and the position of the hands and feet.

Table 10.4. Minimum standards for a 20-week anomaly scan as recommended by the RCOG Working Group.[22]

Head: shape and internal structures	Cavum septum pellucidum
	Cerebellum
	Ventricular atrial width (<10 mm)
Spine:	Longitudinal and transverse
Abdomen: shape and content	At level of stomach
	At level of kidneys and umbilicus
Renal pelves :	<5 mm AP measurement
Longitudinal axis:	Abdominothoracic appearance
	Diaphragm
	Bladder
Thorax:	At level of four-chamber cardiac view
Arms:	Three bones
	Hand (not counting fingers)
Legs:	Three bones
	Foot (not counting toes)

The anatomical features of the various structural anomalies are detailed in numerous textbooks and reports and will not be repeated here. However, a few examples of diagnoses/organ systems will be considered, in which missed diagnoses not infrequently give rise to risk management and litigation.

Spina bifida

Spina bifida is the most common form of neural tube defect (NTD), a group of disorders comprising spina bifida, anencephaly and encephalocele, which results from failure of closure of the neural tube in the first months of pregnancy. The birth prevalence has declined four- to fivefold over the past two to three decades, in large part as a result of prenatal diagnosis and termination of affected pregnancies. It is now rare for a baby to be born with an unsuspected spina bifida defect.

The older screening strategy comprised maternal serum AFP testing at 16 weeks gestation; a level >2.5 MOM (multiples of the median) may reflect leakage of fetal cerebrospinal fluid through the open neural tube, although there were many other non-NTD causes of high AFP, including wrong dates, fetal death, multiple pregnancy and fetal abdominal-wall defects. Maternal serum AFP testing detected 79% of open spina

Baseline fetal anomaly scan

Extended views

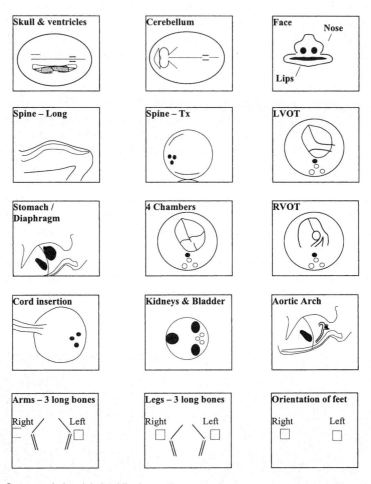

Fig. 10.3. Suggested pictorial checklist for routine anomaly scan at 20 weeks including minimum views in the first two columns, and optional extended views in the right hand column.[22] Reproduced with permission from the Royal College of Obstetricians and Gynaecologists.

bifidas, but was then abandoned in many centres undertaking routine ultrasound screening at 18–20 weeks because of a number of reasons: (i) the superior detection rate of ultrasound alone (ca. 90%) for open spina bifida; (ii) the large number of inaccurate results with AFP testing; and (iii) the need to investigate positive AFP results by amniocentesis. Notwithstanding this, it has been retained in some centres, as the AFP test forms part of maternal serum screening for Down syndrome.

In the latter part of the 1980s, it became widely recognized that almost all fetuses with open spina bifida also have abnormal cranial appearances on ultrasound.[56–58] These comprised ventriculomegaly in 71%, a lemon-shaped head or frontal bossing in

97%, and a banana-shaped or non-visualized ('absent') cerebellum in 97% (see Figure 10.4).[59] This means that even if the sonographer failed to detect a lesion in the skin over the back, or an abnormality in the bony part of the spine, these intracranial findings would still suggest the presence of a spina bifida lesion, and prompt referral for a high-resolution diagnostic scan. Inspection of the shape of the fetal head and cerebellum thus became an integral part of NTD screening by ultrasound. Cerebellar shape is the most accurate predictor of all these as, when it is found, 100% of studied fetuses have spina bifida.[57,58]

Ultrasound alone is thus the optimal screening policy for NTDs. It is very unlikely that a district general hospital obstetric ultrasound service acting with due care and attention would fail to diagnose an open spina bifida lesion on a routine anomaly scan, in the absence of extenuating factors which impede the quality of ultrasonic visualization (eg maternal obesity, previous abdominal surgery or scarring, or reduced amniotic fluid volume). However, it is still rarely possible for a district general hospital ultrasound service acting with due care and attention to miss a spina bifida lesion on a routine anomaly scan, especially if the lesion is small or unassociated with ventriculomegaly or intracranial signs, and the spinal anatomy is difficult to assess when not delineated by surrounding amniotic fluid, such as when the back is up against the uterine wall. Nevertheless, even if some or most of the above features were missed, detection of any one of the several abnormal ultrasound findings on a screening scan normally will prompt referral for a more detailed diagnostic scan, thus avoiding a false negative antenatal diagnosis.

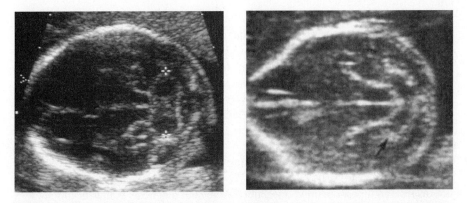

Fig. 10.4. Cranial signs of spina bifida at 18–20 weeks. The left-hand picture shows the normal shape of the cranial bones and the normal dumbbell shape of the cerebellum between the calipers, which contrast with the lemon-shaped head, and the banana-shaped cerebellum (arrow), found in almost all fetuses with open spina bifida.

Congenital heart disease

Congenital heart disease is the commonest type of structural abnormality found in fetal life or at birth, with an overall frequency of eight per 1000. Around half of these will be life threatening or associated with severe morbidity. The components of the fetal heart are the most complex and difficult to visualize of all the fetal organs usually examined, and it is the only one for which fetal medicine specialists may need to refer on for fetal echocardiography by a paediatric cardiologist.

The four-chamber view is the minimum standard screening plane, comprising a cross-sectional view of the fetal chest, in which the four separate chambers of the fetal heart are seen in a single plane. The intraventricular septum is inspected for its integrity to exclude major atrial or ventricular septal defects, and the mitral and tricuspid valves to exclude major valvular defects; the four chambers of right and left atrium, and right and left ventricle, are inspected to check that they are roughly of equal size. The offset junction of the valves with the atrioventricular septum helps exclude atrioventricular septal defects.

Because published studies indicate that only 15–63% of major heart defects are normally detected antenatally using the four-chamber view,[60–62] a missed diagnosis of complex congenital heart disease is unlikely to indicate a breach of acceptable standards for a screening examination. Indeed, a large study of 7500 pregnancies screened using the four-chamber view showed that only 26% of major heart defects (defined as lethal or requiring surgical correction) were detected on a routine examination at 16–22 weeks in a low-risk population.[63] Extracardiac abnormalities increase the likelihood of detection, isolated cardiac anomalies being detected in only 7% of cases in one study, compared with 36% with multiple problems.[64] The RCOG Working Party, in reviewing the wide range of detection rates reported in the literature, estimated that around 60% of severe cardiac conditions would be detected using four-chamber view screening alone.[43]

The majority of district obstetric units only screen for congenital heart disease by examining the four-chamber view. Increasingly, the outflow tracts are also inspected, which is now recommended as part of an optimal screening examination.[22] This involves following the origin of the aorta from the left ventricle, inspecting its calibre and continuity with the left ventricular outflow, and similarly the origin of the pulmonary artery from the right ventricular outflow tract, and confirming the normal cross-over relationship between the two. Addition of the latter views in teaching centres has been associated with improved detection rates of up to 86%.[61,65]

Although some cardiac lesions continue to carry a very poor prognosis, such as hypoplastic left heart, many are now survivable with corrective surgery, albeit with a not insubstantial peri-operative morbidity. Antenatal diagnosis is thus becoming less about the option of termination, and more about delivery in a centre with ready access to paediatric cardiology and cardiothoracic surgery. Antenatal diagnosis usually prompts an offer of antenatal karyotyping, as 16% of isolated defects, and more than half in the presence of other anomalies, are associated with fetal aneuploidy. Atrioventricular septal defects in particular are associated with trisomy 21 in about half of cases. In addition it has been recognized that around 10% of conotruncal defects are associated with diGeorge syndrome or the CATCH phenotype; this can be diagnosed by showing a microdeletion in 22q, which, if present, alters the prognosis.[66,67]

Limb reduction

Limb reduction deformities occur with a frequency of around 1 in 2000 live births. Some are the result of genetic or syndromal conditions, but these are usually of lesser severity, predominantly involve the forearms, and are associated with other abnormalities. The cause of many limb reduction deformities is not known, but a vascular aetiology at a crucial early stage of development has been implicated in some, particularly those with unilateral forelimb defects, either as a spontaneous event, or secondary to CVS or maternal cocaine or solvent ingestion. Limb amputations have been implicated in a condition called amniotic band or amniotic disruption and mutilation syndrome.

There are several reasons for examining the limbs at a routine anomaly scan: (i) detection of gross limb shortening, which could be evident in either the limb or the forelimb; (ii) detection, as in other long bones, of fractures and deficient mineralization; (iii) detection of limb reduction deformities, both of the isolated and syndromal type; (iv) detection of major deformity in the hands, feet or digits; and (v) detection of positional defects which would indicate an increased risk of aneuploidy. As the last three of these would only be detectable if the lower portion of the limb were examined, it would seem logical for any routine policy to examine the limb in its entirety.

Bilateral limb reduction deformities are usually a straightforward and technically simple diagnosis on a routine anomaly scan. However, it is possible for a minor or partial limb abnormality to be missed on obstetric ultrasound, especially if unilateral. On occasion, it may be difficult to visualize both limbs adequately, especially when the lower-most limb, usually an arm, is obscured beneath the fetal trunk or head, or both, where its visualization would be impaired by acoustic shadowing. This occurs not infrequently when the baby is lying with the shoulder girdle in a direct antero-posterior position. It is good practice to examine all four limbs in their entirety, which may require manipulating the transducer angle or waiting for the baby to move. However, the minimum standards set for routine anomaly scan refer only to examining all three bones in one upper and one lower limb.[22]

First-trimester anomaly scanning

A limited anomaly scan can be performed at the time of a nuchal translucency scan.[68,69] In expert hands, using transvaginal scanning where necessary, up to 65% of major anomalies can be detected at this time, or 79% of the total diagnosed antenatally.[70] Many of the anomalies are towards the more gross end of the spectrum, such as anencephaly or holoprosencephaly. A number of organ systems, however, are not well seen at this gestation, including the heart and the renal tract. First trimester anomaly scanning is technically and diagnostically challenging,[71] and has yet to be subject to large-scale audit in a routine setting.[72]

Although first-trimester anomaly scanning cannot be recommended as a primary screening strategy in low-risk populations at this time,[11] it is acknowledged that more structural anomalies are potentially detectable as a result of a nuchal translucency scanning programme than are chromosomal abnormalities. Further research is needed into detection rates in low-risk populations and the natural history of anomalies diagnosed in the first trimester.

In the interim, there are good arguments in centres not offering routine nuchal translucency scans for a booking scan before 15 weeks in addition to the routine anomaly scan at 18–20 weeks. The RCOG working party recommends that this two-stage policy is ideal,[43] and that the purpose of the first scan is to determine gestational age accurately, to demonstrate fetal viability, to establish fetal number, and in multiple pregnancies amnionicity and chorionicity, and to detect gross fetal abnormalities.[22] There is some evidence from a randomized trial that a booking scan in a two-stage policy leads to more accurate dating, which can facilitate optimal timing of the morphology scan, and less anxiety in women compared with a one-stage anomaly scan at 18–20 weeks.[73]

Invasive procedures

Current methods of prenatal diagnosis for aneuploidy and monogenic disorders involve fetal tissue sampling. Invasive procedures (CVS, amniocentesis and fetal blood sampling) carry a risk of fetal loss and morbidity. This leads to incomplete uptake, and thus missed diagnoses, of handicapping congenital diseases. For this reason, research is focusing on the alternative of non-invasive fetal diagnosis by harvesting the 1 in 10^5–10^7 fetal cells found in the mother's blood stream; although no technique is yet near clinical application.

An obstetrician would normally counsel a woman contemplating an invasive procedure about her risk of the condition being tested for, the voluntary nature of the test, the option of another test or of not testing, the nature of the procedure proposed, the risk of procedure-related miscarriage, and any other relatively common risks specific to the procedure. Because of the possibility of fetal loss as a result of the procedure, it is important the woman balances potential impact of fetal loss on the one hand against that of having an affected child on the other. Her views are likely to be influenced by her age, fertility, reproductive history, and social circumstances, as well as her cultural background and personal beliefs. In particular, the decision as to whether or not to undergo an invasive test can be traumatic for many parents, so it is important that they not be rushed into premature decisions.

The similarities between the different types of invasive procedures are greater than their differences. All are done under continuous ultrasound visualization of the needle tip. Usually, the operator introduces the needle with one hand while using the other hand on the scan transducer for ultrasound guidance. Each has a small procedure-related miscarriage risk of between 1% and 2%, with higher rates in the presence of multiple needle insertions, or where carried out by less skilled operators. Each has a small chance of laboratory failure or inaccuracy. A few operators use a needle guide, but this has the disadvantage of being less flexible if the needle position needs to be realigned. A few centres, particularly in the USA or on the Continent, have a Sonographer do the scanning while the operator introduces the needle. This has for the operator the advantage of not needing to be trained in ultrasound, but the disadvantage of poorer hand/eye coordination.

Amniocentesis

The miscarriage rate after amniocentesis is 1%, based on the only randomized controlled trial, which was done in Denmark at 16–18 weeks in the mid-1980s.[2] A 22 G needle is recommended, and transplacental insertions are best avoided. Continuous ultrasound guidance was shown in the 1980s to reduce the number of dry and bloody taps,[74,75] compared with the older semi-blind technique of preprocedural ultrasound localization of a target pool. There is also a 1 in 200 risk of cytogenetic culture failure, about which patients should be warned, as it may lead to the need for a repeat procedure. This is less of an issue in centres offering rapid DNA testing for aneuploidy, as failure to obtain a full karyotype once the major aneuploidies have been excluded may not necessarily warrant further invasive testing.

In general, only two needle insertions should be attempted, and where there is difficulty obtaining a sample, the woman should instead be referred to a tertiary centre. A number of studies have highlighted the significance of operator experience in terms of reduced needle insertions and fewer bloody taps.[75,76] In one series, doctors undertaking fewer than 50 procedures in three years had a single pass success rate of 82% compared with those with greater than 50 procedures of 93%.[77] Because of this, amniocentesis is no longer a routine procedure considered within the remit of every obstetrician and obstetric registrar, but is instead restricted to those who have been trained in the procedure, and maintain skills through a regular caseload. The RCOG guideline on amniocentesis (http://www.rcog.org.uk/index.html) recommends that 30 supervised procedures are required before a trainee be deemed competent, and thereafter 30 procedures annually to maintain skills.

Amniocentesis is usually done at 15–16 weeks, but can be done for various indications right up until term. Because of the potential advantages of first, as opposed to second, trimester diagnosis, early amniocentesis has been evaluated, but associated with clear increased risks of miscarriage compared with both first-trimester CVS and mid-trimester amniocentesis,[78–80] as shown in Figure 10.5. This is consistent with gestational age being a more important determinant of miscarriage rates than the type of procedure itself. Early amniocentesis in randomized trials was also associated with a 1.5% risk of talipes.[78,81] Amniocentesis should not be undertaken before 14 weeks.

There is now a considerable number of published case reports in which significant brain or eye damage detected after birth has been attributed to amniocentesis based on the pattern of damage together with lack of obvious other cause for injury. In several cases, subcutaneous nodules or skin scars were considered to indicate the site of passage of the needle into the baby. The asymmetric neuropathology of such injury has been described recently.[82] Notwithstanding the above, damage from needle trauma at amniocentesis would seem very rare. Direct trauma to the fetus from an amniocentesis needle has been reported almost exclusively in cases where the procedure was not performed under ultrasound guidance and continuous visualization of the needle tip. There are no cases reported in large recent series where amniocentesis was done by experienced operators predominantly under continuous ultrasound guidance.[2,74,83] In litigation terms, this should now be a historical issue, the risk management lesson being that the needle tip should be visualized at all times. Even if a needle were

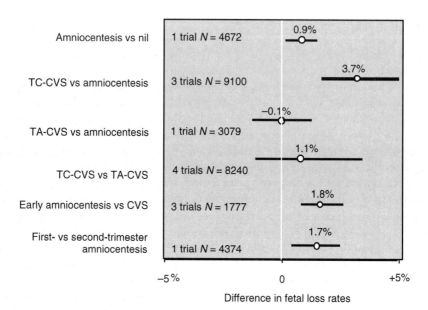

Fig. 10.5. Mean and 95% confidence intervals for the difference in fetal loss rates in randomized trials of invasive procedures, with a value to the right of the midline indicating an increased loss rate for the index compared with the comparator procedure. For instance, amniocentesis is associated with a 0.9% increase in loss rate compared with no procedure. After Wald *et al.*[3]

inadvertently to penetrate a fetal skull, it seems likely that the damage is largely done by aspiration; fluid should only be aspirated at amniocentesis where the needle tip is observed clearly within the amniotic cavity.

Chorion villus sampling

CVS at 10–13 weeks is generally accepted as a slightly more risky procedure than conventional amniocentesis at 15–16 weeks, with a procedure-related miscarriage rate more in the region of 2% compared with 1% after amniocentesis (Figure 10.5). There are two approaches. The first is the conventional transcervical approach developed in the early 1980s where a cannula or biopsy forceps is inserted through the cervix into the placental substance. Meta analysis of the randomized trials (Figure 10.5) of transcervical CVS yield an excess loss rate in the CVS group of 3.7% compared with mid-trimester amniocentesis, although there were some issues relating to operator inexperience in the largest study which may render this an overestimate.[83] The second, and newer, procedure developed in the late 1980s and early 1990s is transabdominal CVS, whereby in a technique similar to that used for amniocentesis, a needle is inserted through the mother's abdomen into the placenta. There is a non-significant trend in the meta analysis of the randomized trials of transcervical versus transabdominal CVS for the transabdominal approach to be associated with a lower risk of miscarriage, which is then comparable to that after amniocentesis.[3] The transabdominal approach is preferred, not just because it may be associated with a lower miscarriage risk, but also because it avoids for women what has been termed the ignominy of the lithotomy position. In addition, the similarities of transabdominal CVS to other ultrasound-guided invasive procedures make it easier to learn than transcervical CVS.

Parents undergoing elective invasive procedures for karyotyping are usually offered the choice of either amniocentesis or CVS. The difference in miscarriage rates forms an important part of this counselling, and the greater safety of amniocentesis results in some couples choosing to delay testing until 15–16 weeks. This choice does not apply at the gestation at which serum screening results are available, but it does for high-risk nuchal translucency results.

Unlike amniocentesis, which tests fetal skin and urinary cells, CVS tests the placental cells which do not always have exactly the same karyotype as the fetus, especially if there has been a post-zygotic non-disjunctive event after cells destined to become the placenta have separated off from those giving rise to the fetus. Extensive cytogenetic experience now shows that this phenomenon of confined placental mosaicism occurs in around 1% of chorion villus samples.[84] This is unlikely to lead to diagnostic error in that such samples usually show bizarre polyloidies or mosaicism for monosomic or trisomic chromosomes not usually compatible with a live fetus on ultrasound. Parents should be counselled in advance about this risk, because, if found, it is likely that further investigation by amniocentesis will be indicated.

Care must be taken in processing the sample to exclude maternal contamination by decidual tissue. This is done by careful microscopic dissection of the villus sample. For DNA studies, where the extreme sensitivity of the polymerase chain reaction means that amplification of only a few maternal cells in error could lead to a false-negative diagnosis, it is now routine to exclude this by demonstrating non-maternal (ie paternal) minisatellite repeats in the sample.

Concern was raised in 1991 that CVS might damage the fetus. Among a series of 289 patients undergoing transabdominal CVS between 56 and 66 days gestation, five had anomalies (1.7%), four with abnormalities consistent with oromandibular limb hypogenesis syndromes (missing segment[s] of the lower limb associated with facial abnormalities) and one with an isolated transverse limb reduction defect.[85] A few publications subsequently appeared to support this association, but most found few, if any, cases of oromandibular limb hypogenesis syndrome, and an incidence of limb reduction defects no higher than the usual background incidence of 1 in 2000. In the largest series of 138,000 babies who underwent CVS *in utero*, the incidence of limb reduction defects was 1 in 1878, similar to the incidence of 1 in 1692 found in the largest population registry of >1.2 million unexposed babies in British Columbia.[86] Thus, there is no firm evidence that CVS does cause limb reduction or other deformities. Notwithstanding this, most units stopped doing CVS before nine or 10 weeks gestation as a result of the original report,[85] and thus most procedures analysed in the literature are of those done after nine weeks.[87,88] It remains possible, even probable, that early CVS before nine weeks might cause limb and other defects. The postulated mechanism is vascular disruption to the placental circulation leading to vasospastic phenomenon in the limbs and elsewhere. In keeping with this, animal experiments show that disrupting uteroplacental blood supply leads to limb haemorrhages,[89] while observation, using minitelescopes, of human fetuses undergoing CVS has shown facial haemorrhages appearing during the procedure.[90,91] CVS should not be done till 10 and, arguably on safety grounds, 11 weeks gestation.

Multiple pregnancy

Invasive testing in multiple pregnancy requires attention to chorionicity and zygosity, the need to sample each fetus separately, and the applicability of selective fetocide if the results are discordant. Invasive procedures in twins require a high degree of ultrasound and invasive procedure skills, and for these reasons it has been recommended that they only be done in fetal medicine referral centres.[92] Parents should be counselled beforehand about the chance of a discordant result and the option of selective fetocide. The topography is mapped in terms of location within the uterus, placental site, and plane of the dividing septum in three dimensions. This is a prerequisite for interpretation of discordant results and for selective fetocide.

For monochorionic twins, only one needs sampling for prenatal diagnostic indications, but the operator should be certain of this on first-trimester scanning. With this exception, it is important to ensure that both fetuses are sampled separately. With amniocentesis, this is best achieved by two separate ultrasound-guided procedures, as far away as possible from the dividing septum. Dye instillation techniques are not only no longer necessary but contraindicated, as methylene blue causes fetal intestinal atresia. Some groups use a single needle insertion technique with septal puncture, but there remain, at least theoretical, concerns about both contamination and septal rupture leading to functional monoamnionicity.[93,94] Despite the use of separate cannula insertions and combined transabdominal and transvaginal approaches, CVS in twins remains associated with a 2–6% risk of contamination, so that many operators opt instead for amniocentesis. Otherwise, DNA fingerprinting and/or confirmatory amniocentesis may be necessary in dichorionic twins with concordant sex karyotypes at CVS.

There are no randomized trials to indicate procedure-related loss rates in twins. Background loss rates, however, are appreciably higher. Recent series suggest that total fetal loss rates in twins after amniocentesis (ca. 3.5–4.0%) or CVS (2–4%) may not be much higher than background rates. A case control study of 202 twins undergoing mid-trimester amniocentesis reported a loss rate only 0.3% higher than in control twins.[95]

Another important technical consideration in performing invasive sampling in twin pregnancies is to ensure that the procedure is documented adequately and the specimens labelled meticulously, such that, if the results prove discordant, there is no doubt which twin is the abnormal one. An error in this respect might result in termination of a normal baby and survival of a baby with Down syndrome. Ideally, the operator doing the diagnostic procedure should also undertake any selective fetocide to minimize uncertainty, and obviate any need for confirmatory invasive testing. Selective fetocide in dichorionic twins discordant for fetal abnormality by injection of intracardiac potassium chloride is associated with a 7% loss rate in the international registry, with lower rates if the procedure is done before rather than after 12 weeks

(5% versus 9%).[96] The same technique in monochorionic twins leads to death of the healthy twin due to sharing of their circulation along vascular anastomoses, and as a result selective fetocide generally has been considered contraindicated. Recently, however, ultrasound-guided cord occlusion using bipolar diathermy forceps has been developed to render selective termination in monochorionic twins now feasible.[97]

Termination of pregnancy

Management options

Following a diagnosis of fetal abnormality, the pregnant woman should be seen within 24 hours by the relevant consultant and, if appropriate, within two to three working days by a fetal medicine specialist.[22] Apart from further investigations where indicated, the chief purpose of the consultation is to allow the woman (and usually her partner) to understand the nature of the abnormality, the possibility of therapy, and the probable outcome for the child. Further consultation with the relevant paediatric specialist may be indicated, especially where postnatal interventions are contemplated or where there is a major risk of serious handicap. Counselling should be non-directive, and not hurried; it should address the certainty of the diagnosis, the possibility of additional anomalies, the likelihood that anomalies are part of a more serious undiagnosed genetic syndrome, the difficulties prognosticating based solely on findings *in utero*, the chance of intrauterine or early neonatal death, the range of prognoses for the child with and without surgery, the risk of peri-operative morbidity and mortality, life expectancy, and the seriousness of any handicap, including its modification by aids and prostheses. Pregnant women should be offered a further or follow-up consultation, and access should be given to written or web-based information, such as those now provided by various professional organizations and parental support groups.

Although some conditions are amenable to fetal treatment, neonatal correction or surgery in infancy, there is no treatment for chromosomal anomalies and many structural abnormalities, and the management issues are essentially limited to termination versus continuation of pregnancy. Unless the abnormality is trivial, termination of pregnancy is a mainstream management option to be discussed in parental counselling.[98] The RCOG report on termination of pregnancy for fetal abnormality[99] advises that where abortion falls within the grounds specified in the Abortion Act, doctors 'must advise the woman that she has this option. They must ensure she understands the nature of the fetal abnormality, and the probable outcome of the pregnancy, whether it continues to term or is aborted. The woman is then able to decide whether she wishes to have an abortion and to give her informed consent. Practised obstetricians are often able to mention the option of abortion at an early stage in the consultation process, which is then largely concerned with providing the woman with the information on which she can base her decision'.

It is emphasized that the specialist's decision here is whether or not termination should be *offered*, not whether or not it should be *recommended*. Failure to mention the option of termination of pregnancy is a predictable source of litigation, especially from parents who later find themselves faced with life-long care for a child with a major handicap. On the other hand, it is inappropriate to offer the option of termination early in a consultation, only later to withdraw such offer after deciding that the fetal abnormality falls outside the requirements of the Abortion Act. Borderline or controversial cases are best decided by a fetal medicine specialist in consultation with colleagues, ideally reaching consensus in a multidisciplinary meeting with the relevant paediatric subspecialists.

The decision as to whether to continue the pregnancy or accept an offer of termination of pregnancy is one for the parents. Such decisions are made against a complex background of the parents' own moral, ethical and religious perspectives, in addition to their life circumstances, perception of risk and reproductive intent. It is axiomatic that specialists must not presuppose parental responses to an offer of termination, based on their views prior to antenatal diagnosis, or their stated religious beliefs. Stating that the woman/parents did not request termination is no defence to an allegation of failure to offer termination, as parents may not appreciate the legality or availability of termination, particularly if from abroad, or at later gestations. Ten percent of obstetricians have conscientious objections to abortion. Where a doctor has a particular personal or moral objection to termination, however, it remains standard of care to advise patients of this situation and the availability of termination elsewhere. The RCOG Ethics Committee advises that obstetricians who are unable to comply with a request for termination of a pregnancy for fetal abnormality should be prepared to refer the pregnant woman to a colleague for another opinion.[100]

The Abortion Act 1967 as amended by the Human Fertilization and Embryology Act 1990

In England and Wales, termination of pregnancy is allowed where two medical practitioners acting in good faith certify that '. . . there is a substantial risk that if the child were born it would suffer from such physical or mental abnormalities as to be seriously handicapped' (s1[1][(b] clause E of the 1967 Abortion Act). A respectable body of medical opinion would support many common fetal abnormalities, such as spina bifida, Down syndrome, severe ventriculomegaly, complex congenital heart disease, severe skeletal dysplasia, bilateral limb reductions, as satisfying this requirement. Indeed, this is implicit in the various screening programmes for spina bifida and Down syndrome that have been in operation in recent decades.

Termination can also be offered under clause C of the Act (1[a]) where 'the pregnancy has not exceeded its 24th week and the continuance of the pregnancy would involve risk, greater than if the pregnancy were terminated, of injury to the physical or mental health of the pregnant woman or any existing children of her family'. This is the clause which, rightly or wrongly, has been widely interpreted as sanctioning 'social grounds', and the one under which more than 90% of terminations in England and Wales are performed. Where practitioners have difficulty justifying termination prior to 24 weeks for fetal abnormality which they do not necessarily consider 'severe' (clause E), termination is instead then frequently offered under clause C. There is, however, no duty of care imposed on an obstetrician or fetal medicine specialist to offer a woman termination of pregnancy for a fetal abnormality considered minor.

Late termination

In England and Wales, the modifications to the Abortion Act under the Human Fertilization and Embryology Act 1990 removed any gestational limit from termination of pregnancy under clause E (section 37[1][d]). A previous case (*Rance v Mid-Downs Health Authority and Storr*, Mr Justice Brooke, 1990) of failed diagnosis of spina bifida on a scan at 27 weeks foundered on the fact that termination at this late stage of pregnancy would have been in contravention of the Infant Life Preservation Act 1929. In contrast, the modifications to this clause under the Human Fertilization and Embryology Act 1990, which came into effect on 1 April 1991, also repealed the offence created by the Infant Life Preservation Act insofar as it related to terminations of pregnancy performed by medical practitioners.

Thus termination has been allowable for severely handicapping conditions at any stage of gestation since 1991, and is a standard management option in most fetal medicine centres,[100,101] although fewer than a hundred are done each year. Legally, it may be argued that gestational age becomes irrelevant to the offer of termination under clause E in that gestation is not mentioned. Paintin, for instance, argues, 'An important reason for termination when the fetus has abnormalities is to enable the woman to avoid the considerable long-term burden of providing care for a severely handicapped child. If such an abortion is ethical at 22 weeks, it can be argued that it remains ethical whenever in pregnancy the diagnosis is made'.[102] Notwithstanding this, there is anecdotal evidence that obstetricians' thresholds for termination increase with advancing gestation. The RCOG Ethics Committee report acknowledges that 'reasons for termination, at no stage trivial, must be more pressing the longer pregnancy has progressed'. Indeed, in a 1993 survey only 21% of consultant obstetricians indicated that beyond 24 weeks, they would 'recommend' (note, not '*offer*') termination for spina bifida, while only 13% would for Down syndrome.[103] However, a major failing of this study was the exclusion of academics. These clinical problems after 24 weeks would not normally be dealt with by general obstetric and gynaecological consultants, but instead by fetal medicine specialists, the majority of whom at least then were academics. The small number of late terminations under clause E (94 or 0.05% of terminations in 1994) has been interpreted as indicating that British obstetricians have a cautious attitude to late termination; although alternatively this could represent the high sensitivity of diagnosis earlier in pregnancy.[102]

Because termination under clause C is not available in late pregnancy, arguments about whether various fetal anomalies satisfy clause E ('substantial risk ... seriously handicapped') are particularly poignant after 24 weeks. Down syndrome and spina bifida clearly do, as clause E is listed as the relevant clause under which the vast majority of terminations are done for these conditions before 24 weeks. Anecdotal experience is that many fetal medicine specialists would now not offer termination under clause E for the following conditions in isolation: cleft lip and palate, unilateral limb reduction, mild ventriculomegaly, achondroplasia, and cystic fibrosis.

'Substantial' is not defined in the Abortion Act. The 1996 RCOG Report on Termination of Pregnancy for Fetal Abnormality[99] advises that 'a risk may be substantial without satisfying the test of being more likely than not; equally, the risk must be more than a mere possibility. In the context of this Act, obstetricians would be wise to err on the side of caution, bearing in mind that a decision to perform an abortion because there is a substantial risk rather than a certainty of abnormality may result in a loss of a normal fetus'. The same report provides guidance on the scaling of severity (i.e. seriousness of handicap) from the World Health Organization, arguing that only individuals at the third or higher points of the WHO disability scale would be considered by most people to be seriously handicapped. Point 3 on the scale requires support for everyday living classified as 'assisted performance', which includes the need for a helping hand (ie the individual can perform the activity or sustain the behaviour, whether augmented by aids or not, only with some assistance from another person). Point 4 requires support for everyday living classified as 'dependent performance', which includes complete dependence on the presence of another person (ie the individual can perform the activity or sustain the behaviour, but only when someone is with him most of the time).

Late termination for fetal abnormality has become a controversial topic. There are those that disapprove in circumstances of non-lethal malformation, arguing that aborting the third-trimester fetal patient violates beneficence-based obligations to it and is therefore unethical, no matter what the law permits.[104,105] Others argue that gestation is irrelevant when faced with a seriously abnormal fetus.[102] Indeed, the availability of late termination may actually prevent some terminations, in that the prognosis may become clearer with advancing gestation.[106] For instance, anomalies such as mild-to-moderate ventriculomegaly, where there is a substantial chance of a normal outcome, as well as substantial chance of severe handicap, may be observed expectantly with serial scans to determine whether the lesion is progressive, rather than the parents being faced with a yes or no decision on termination earlier in pregnancy. Forty percent of 305 third trimester terminations in one French series had the diagnosis made earlier in pregnancy, but the poor prognosis only became clear in the third trimester.[106]

Termination in later pregnancy is largely confined to referral centres both because of the need for an expert opinion on fetal diagnosis and prognosis, and because of the need to stop the baby's heart beat before it is born (otherwise it would not be a termination). This is usually achieved by ultrasound-guided intracardiac injection of potassium chloride, which is recommended for all terminations after 21 weeks and 6 days' gestation.[99] These are skilled procedures, usually restricted to fetal medicine specialists, who take care to ensure that fetal asystole is sustained, both by monitoring the absence of a fetal heart beat for at least five minutes post-asystole, and then checking again on ultrasound half an hour later.

Conclusion

It is hardly surprising that prenatal diagnosis is a frequent source of litigation, given the imprecision of the methods used, the variation in screening techniques employed and the costs of a 'wrongful birth' following a false-negative diagnosis. Risk management strategies need to focus on counselling women as to the limitations of prenatal diagnosis, and on ensuring uniform standards through protocols, appropriate staff training and modern equipment.

References

1 Verma L, Macdonald F, Leedham P, McConachie M, Dhanjal S, Hulten M. Rapid and simple prenatal DNA diagnosis of Down's syndrome. *Lancet* 1998; 352: 9–12.
2 Tabor A, Philip J, Madsen M, Bang J, Obel EB, Norgaard-Pedersen B. Randomised controlled trial of genetic amniocentesis in 4606 low-risk women. *Lancet* 1986; 1: 1287–1293.
3 Wald N, Kennard A, Hackshaw A, McGuire A (eds.) Antenatal Screening for Down's Syndrome. Southampton: Health Technology Assessment, 1998; 2(1).
4 Wald NJ, Cuckle HS, Densem JW *et al.* Maternal serum screening for Down's syndrome in early pregnancy. *BMJ* 1988; 297: 883–887.
5 Snijders RJM, Noble P, Sebire N, Souka A, Nicolaides KH. UK multicentre project on assessment of risk of trisomy 21 by maternal age and fetal nuchal-translucency thickness at 10–14 weeks of gestation. *Lancet* 1998; 352: 343–346.
6 Gilbert R, Augood C, Gupta R *et al.* Cost effectiveness and safety effectiveness of first and second trimester screening strategies for Down syndrome. London: Systematic Reviews Training Unit, Department of Epidemiology and Public Health, Institute of Child Health, University College London, 2000.
7 Mutton D, Ide RG, Alberman E. Trends in prenatal screening for and diagnosis of Down's syndrome: England and Wales, 1989–97. *BMJ* 1998; 317: 922–923.
8 Wald NJ, Huttly W, Wald K, Kennard A. Downs syndrome screening in the UK. *Lancet* 1996; 347: 330.
9 Wald NJ, Huttly WJ, Hennessy CF. Downs syndrome screening in the UK in 1998. *Lancet* 1999; 354: 1264.
10 Hyett J, Perdu M, Sharland G, Snijders R, Nicolaides KH. Using fetal nuchal translucency to screen for major congenital cardiac defects at 10–14 weeks of gestation: population-based cohort study. *BMJ* 1999; 318: 81–85.
11 Bricker L, Garcia J, Henderson J, Mugford M, Neilson J, Roberts T. Ultrasound screening in pregnancy: a systematic review of the clinical effectiveness, cost effectiveness and women's views. *Health Technology Assessment* 2000; 4(16).
12 Hyett JA, Sebire NJ, Snijders RJM, Nicolaides KH. Intrauterine lethality of trisomy 21 fetuses with increased nuchal translucency thickness. *Ultrasound in Obstetrics and Gynecology* 1996; 7: 101–103.
13 Pandya PP, Snijders RJ, Psara N, Hilbert L, Nicolaides KH. The prevalence of non-viable pregnancy at 10–13 weeks of gestation. *Ultrasound in Obstetrics and Gynecology* 1996; 7: 170–173.
14 Fisk N, Bennett P. Prenatal determination of chorionicity and zygosity. In: Ward R, Whittle M (eds.) *Multiple Pregnancy*. London: RCOG Press, 1995: 56–67.
15 Sebire NJ, Snijders RJM, Hughes K, Sepulveda W, Nicolaides KH. Screening for trisomy 21 in twin pregnancies by maternal age and fetal nuchal translucency thickness at 10–14 weeks of gestation. *British Journal of Obstetrics and Gynaecology* 1996; 103: 999–1003.
16 Cuckle H. Down's syndrome screening in twins. *Journal of Medical Screening* 1998; 5: 3–4.
17 Souka AP, Snijders RJM, Novakov A, Soares W, Nicolaides KH. Defects and syndromes in chromosomally normal fetuses with increased nuchal translucency thickness at 10–14 weeks of gestation. *Ultrasound in Obstetrics and Gynecology* 1998; 11: 391–400.
18 Hyett JA, Perdu M, Sharland GK, Snijders RS, Nicolaides KH. Increased nuchal translucency at 10–14 weeks of gestation as a marker for major cardiac defects. *Ultrasound in Obstetrics and Gynecology* 1997; 10: 242–246.
19 Vintzileos AM, Egan JF. Adjusting the risk for trisomy 21 on the basis of second-trimester ultrasonography. *American Journal of Obstetrics and Gynecology* 1995; 172: 837–844.
20 Smith-Bindman R, Hosmer W, Feldstein VA, Deeks JJ, Goldberg JD. Second-trimester ultrasound to detect fetuses with Down syndrome: a meta-analysis. *JAMA* 2001; 285: 1044–1055.
21 Chitty LS, Chudleigh P, Wright E, Campbell S, Pembrey M. The significance of choroid plexus cysts in an unselected population: results of a multicenter study. *Ultrasound in Obstetrics and Gynecology* 1998; 12: 391–397.

22 *Routine Ultrasound Screening in Pregnancy: Protocol, Standards and Training.* Supplement to *Ultrasound Screening for Fetal Abnormalities.* London: Royal College of Obstetricians and Gynaecologists, 2000.

23 Vintzileos AM, Guzman ER, Smulian JC, Day-Salvatore DL, Knuppel RA. Indication-specific accuracy of second-trimester genetic ultrasonography for the detection of trisomy 21. *American Journal of Obstetrics and Gynecology* 1999; 181: 1045–1048.

24 Spencer K, Souter V, Tul N, Snijders R, Nicolaides KH. A screening program for trisomy 21 at 10–14 weeks using fetal nuchal translucency, maternal serum free beta-human chorionic gonadotropin and pregnancy-associated plasma protein-A. *Ultrasound in Obstetrics and Gynecology* 1999; 13: 231–237.

25 Spencer K, Spencer CE, Power M, Moakes A, Nicolaides KH. One-stop clinic for assessment of risk for fetal anomalies: a report of the first year of prospective screening for chromosomal anomalies in the first trimester. *British Journal of Obstetrics and Gynaecology 2000*; 107: 1271–1275.

26 Wald NJ, Watt HC, Hackshaw AK. Integrated screening for Down's syndrome based on tests performed during the first and second trimesters. *New England Journal of Medicine* 1999; 341: 461–467.

27 Cuckle H, Quirke P, Sehmi I *et al.* Antenatal screening for cystic fibrosis. *British Journal of Obstetrics and Gynaecology* 1996; 103: 795–799.

28 Livingstone J, Axton RA, Gilfillan A *et al.* Antenatal screening for cystic fibrosis: a trial of the couple model. *BMJ* 1994; 308: 1459–1462.

29 Murray J, Cuckle H, Taylor G, Littlewood J, Hewison J. Screenng for cystic fibrosis. *Health Technology Assessment* 1999; 3(8).

30 Modell B, Petrou M, Layton M *et al.* Audit of prenatal diagnosis for haemoglobin disorders in the United Kingdom: the first 20 years. *BMJ* 1997; 315: 779–784.

31 Davies SC, Cronin E, Gill M, Greengross P, Hickman M, Normand C. Screening for sickle cell disease and thalassaemia: a systematic review with supplementary research. *Health Technology Assessment* 2000; 4(3).

32 Bach G, Tomczak J, Risch N, Ekstein J. Tay-Sachs screening in the Jewish Ashkenazi population: DNA testing is the preferred procedure. *American Journal of Medical Genetics* 2001; 99: 70–75.

33 Kaback MM. Population-based genetic screening for reproductive counselling: the Tay-Sachs disease model. *European Journal of Paediatrics* 2000; 159(Suppl 3): S192–S195.

34 Smith NC, Hau C. A six-year study of the antenatal detection of fetal abnormality in six Scottish health boards. *British Journal of Obstetrics and Gynaecology* 1999; 106: 206–212.

35 Boyd PA, Chamberlain P, Hicks NR. 6-year experience of prenatal diagnosis in an unselected population in Oxford, UK. *Lancet* 1998; 352: 1577–1581.

36 Bucher HC, Schmidt JG. Does routine ultrasound scanning improve outcome in pregnancy? Meta-analysis of various outcome measures. *BMJ* 1993; 307:13–17.

37 Saari-Kemppainen A, Karjalainen O, Ylostalo P, Heinonen OP. Ultrasound screening and perinatal mortality: controlled trial of systematic one-stage screening in pregnancy. The Helsinki Ultrasound Trial. *Lancet* 1990; 336: 387–391.

38 Northern Regional Survey Steering Group. Fetal abnormality: an audit of its recognition and management. *Archives of Diseases in Childhood* 1992; 67: 7704.

39 Royal College of Obstetricians and Gynaecologists. *Report of the Working Party on Routine Ultrasound Examination in Pregnancy.* London: RCOG, 1984.

40 Drife J, Donnai D (eds.) *Antenatal Diagnosis of Fetal Abnormalities. Proceedings of the 23rd Study Group of the Royal College of Obstetricians and Gynaecologists.* London: Springer–Verlag, 1991.

41 Royal College of Obstetricians and Gynaecologists. *The Value of Ultrasound in Pregnancy.* London: RCOG, 1994.

42 Royal College of Obstetricians and Gynaecologists / Royal College of Radiologists. *Recommendations from the Survey of the use of Obstetric Ultrasound in the UK.* London, 1995.

43 Royal College of Obstetricians and Gynaecologists. *Ultrasound Screening for Fetal Abnormalities: Report of the RCOG Working Party.* London: RCOG, 1997.

44 Luck CA. Value of routine ultrasound scanning at 19 weeks: a four year study of 8849 deliveries. *BMJ* 1992; 304: 1474–1478.

45 Chitty LS, Hunt GH, Moore J, Lobb MO. Effectiveness of routine ultrasonography in detecting fetal structural abnormalities in a low risk population. *BMJ* 1991; 303: 1165–1169.

46 Shirley IM, Bottomley F, Robinson VP. Routine radiographer screening for fetal abnormalities by ultrasound in an unselected low risk population. *British Journal of Radiology* 1992; 65: 564–569.

47 Chamberlain G. Antenatal care and the identification of high-risk women. In: Clements RV (ed.) *Safe Practice in Obstetrics and Gynaecology: a Medico-Legal Handbook.* Edinburgh: Churchill Livingstone, 1994: 169–190.

48 Long G, Sprigg A. A comparative study of routine versus selective fetal anomaly ultrasound scanning. *Journal of Medical Screening* 1998; 5: 6–10.

49 Levi S, Schaaps JP, De Havay P, Coulon R, Defoort P. End-result of routine ultrasound screening for congenital anomalies: the Belgian Multicentric Study 1984–92. *Ultrasound in Obstetrics and Gynecology* 1995; 5: 366–371.

50 Clayton-Smith J, Farndon PA, McKeown C, Donnai D. Examination of fetuses after induced abortion for fetal abnormality. *BMJ* 1990; 300: 295–297.

51 Weston MJ, Porter HJ, Andrews HS, Berry PJ. Correlation of antenatal ultrasonography and pathological examinations in 153 malformed fetuses. *Journal of Clinical Ultrasound* 1993; 21: 387–392.

52 Medeira A, Norman A, Haslam J, Clayton-Smith J, Donnai D. Examination of fetuses after induced abortion for fetal abnormality – a follow-up study. *Prenatal Diagnosis* 1994; 14: 381–385.

53 Faye-Petersen OM, Guinn DA, Wenstrom KD. Value of perinatal autopsy. *Obstetrics and Gynecology* 1999; 94: 915–920.

54 Chitty LS. Ultrasound screening for fetal abnormalities. *Prenatal Diagnosis* 1995; 15: 1241–1257.

55 Bernaschek G, Stuempflen I, Deutinger J. The influence of the experience of the investigator on the rate of sonographic diagnosis of fetal malformations in Vienna. *Prenatal Diagnosis* 1996; 16: 807–811.

56 Nicolaides K, Campbell S, Gabbe S, Guidetti R. Ultrasound screening for spina bifida: cranial and cerebellar signs. *Lancet* 1986; 2: 72–74.

57 Campbell J, Gilbert WM, Nicolaides KH, Campbell S. Ultrasound screening for spina bifida: cranial and cerebellar signs in a high-risk population. *Obstetrics and Gynecology* 1987; 70: 247–250.

58 Van-den-Hof MC, Nicolaides KH, Campbell J, Campbell S. Evaluation of the lemon and banana signs in one hundred thirty fetuses with open spina bifida. *American Journal of Obstetrics and Gynecology* 1990; 162: 322–327.

59 Sturgiss S, Robson S. Prognosis for fetuses with antenatally detected myelomeningocele. *Fetal and Maternal Medical Review* 1995; 7: 235–249.

60 Achiron R, Glaser J, Gelernter I, Hegesh J, Yagel S. Extended fetal echocardiographic examination for detecting cardiac malformations in low risk pregnancies. *BMJ* 1992; 304: 671–674.

61 Bromley B, Estroff JA, Sanders SP *et al.* Fetal echocardiography: accuracy and limitations in a population at high and low risk for heart defects. *American Journal of Obstetrics and Gynecology* 1992; 166: 1473–1481.

62 Ott WJ. The accuracy of antenatal fetal echocardiography screening in high- and low-risk patients. *American Journal of Obstetrics and Gynecology* 1995; 172: 1741–1747.

63 Tegnander E, Eik Nes SH, Johansen OJ, Linker DT. Prenatal detection of heart defects at the routine fetal examination at 18 weeks in a non-selected population. *Ultrasound in Obstetrics and Gynecology* 1995; 5: 372–380.

64 Stoll C, Dott B, Alembik Y, Roth MP. Evaluation of routine prenatal diagnosis by a registry of congenital anomalies. *Prenatal Diagnosis* 1995; 15: 791–800.

65 Stumpflen I, Stumpflen A, Wimmer M, Bernaschek G. Effect of detailed fetal echocardiography as part of routine prenatal ultrasonographic screening on detection of congenital heart disease. *Lancet* 1996; 348: 854–857.

66 Raymond FL, Simpson JM, Sharland GK, Ogilvie Mackie CM. Fetal echocardiography as a predictor of chromosomal abnormality. *Lancet* 1997; 350: 930.

67 Raymond FL, Simpson JM, Mackie CM, Sharland GK. Prenatal diagnosis of 22q11 deletions: a series of five cases with congenital heart defects. *Journal of Medical Genetics* 1997; 34: 679–682.

68 Souka AP, Nicolaides KH. Diagnosis of fetal abnormalities at the 10–14-week scan. *Ultrasound in Obstetrics and Gynecology* 1997; 10: 429–442.

69 Chitty LS, Pandya PP. Ultrasound screening for fetal abnormalities in the first trimester. *Prenatal Diagnosis* 1997; 17: 1269–1281.

70 Economides DL, Braithwaite JM. First trimester ultrasonographic diagnosis of fetal structural abnormalities in a low risk population. *British Journal of Obstetrics and Gynaecology* 1998; 105: 53–57.

71 Whitlow BJ, Economides DL. The optimal gestational age to examine fetal anatomy and measure nuchal translucency in the first trimester. *Ultrasound in Obstetrics and Gynecology* 1998; 11(4): 258–261.

72 Whitlow BJ, Chatzipapas IK, Lazanakis ML, Kadir RA, Economides DL. The value of sonography in early pregnancy for the detection of fetal abnormalities in an unselected population. *British Journal of Obstetrics and Gynaecology* 1999; 106: 929–936.

73 Crowther CA, Kornman L, O'Callaghan S, George K, Furness M, Willson K. Is an ultrasound assessment of gestational age at the first antenatal visit of value? A randomised clinical trial. *British Journal of Obstetrics and Gynaecology* 1999; 106: 1273–1279.

74 Anandakumar C, Wong YC, Annapoorna V *et al.* Amniocentesis and its complications. *Australian and New Zealand Journal of Obstetrics and Gynaecology* 1992; 32: 97–99.

75 Romero R, Jeanty P, Reece EA *et al.* Sonographically monitored amniocentesis to decrease intra-operative complications. *Obstetrics and Gynaecology* 1985; 65: 426–430.

76 Wiener JJ, Farrow A, Farrow SC. Audit of amniocentesis from a district general hospital: is it worth it? *BMJ* 1990; 300: 1243–1245.

77 Silver RK, Russell TL, Kambich MP, Leeth EA, MacGregor SN, Sholl JS. Mid-trimester amniocentesis. Influence of operator caseload on sampling efficiency. *Journal of Reproductive Medicine* 1998; 43: 191–195.

78 Sundberg K, Bang J, Smidtjensen S *et al.* Randomised study of risk of fetal loss related to early amniocentesis versus chorionic villus sampling. *Lancet* 1997; 350: 697–703.

79 CEMAT: Randomised trial to assess safety and fetal outcome of early and midtrimester amniocentesis. The Canadian Early and Mid-trimester Amniocentesis Trial Group. *Lancet* 1998; 351: 242–247.

80 Nicolaides K, Brizot MdL, Patel F, Snijders R. Comparison of chorion villus sampling and early amniocentesis for karyotyping in 1,492 singleton pregnancies. *Fetal Diagnosis and Therapy* 1996; 11: 9–15.

81 Farrell SA, Summers AM, Dallaire L, Singer J, Johnson JA, Wilson RD. Club foot, an adverse outcome of early amniocentesis: disruption or deformation? CEMAT (Canadian Early and Mid-Trimester Amniocentesis Trial). *Journal of Medical Genetics* 1999; 36: 843–846.

82 Squier M, Chamberlain P, Zaiwalla Z *et al.* Five cases of brain injury following amniocentesis in mid-term pregnancy. *Developmental Medicine and Childhood Neurology* 2000; 42: 554–560.

83 MRC. Medical Research Council European trial of chorion villus sampling. MRC working party on the evaluation of chorion villus sampling. *Lancet* 1991; 337: 1491–1499.

84 Hahnemann JM, Vejerslev LO. Accuracy of cytogenetic findings on chorionic villus sampling (CVS): diagnostic consequences of CVS mosaicism and non-mosaic discrepancy in centres contributing to eucromic 1986 1992. *Prenatal Diagnosis* 1997; 17: 801–820.

85 Firth HV, Boyd PA, Chamberlain P, MacKenzie IZ, Lindenbaum RH, Huson SM. Severe limb abnormalities after chorion villus sampling at 56–66 days gestation. *Lancet* 1991; 337: 762–763.

86 Froster UG, Jackson L. Limb defects and chorionic villus sampling: results from an international registry, 1992–94. *Lancet* 1996; 347: 489–494.

87 Johnson J. Chorionic villus sampling: introduction and techniques. In: Harman C (ed.) *Invasive Fetal Testing and Treatment.* Oxford: Blackwell Scientific Publications, 1995: 21–46.

88 Holzgreve W, Tercanli S, Surbeck D, Miny P. Invasive diagnostic methods. In: Rodeck C, Whittle M (eds.) *Fetal Medicine: Basic Science and Clinical Practice.* Edinburgh: Churchill Livingstone, 1999: 417–434.

89 Webster WS, Lipson AH, Brown-Woodman PD. Uterine trauma and limb defects. *Teratology* 1987; 35: 253–260.

90 Quintero RA, Romero R, Mahoney MJ, Vecchio M, Holden J, Hobbins JC. Fetal haemorrhagic lesions after chorionic villous sampling. *Lancet* 1992; 339: 193.

91 Quintero RA, Romero R, Mahoney MJ *et al.* Embryoscopic demonstration of hemorrhagic lesions on the human embryo after placental trauma. *American Journal of Obstetrics and Gynecology* 1993; 168: 756–759.

92 Royal College of Obstetricians and Gynaecologists. Recommendations arising from the Royal College of Obstetricians and Gynaecologists' 30th study group: multiple pregnancy. In: Ward H, Whittle M (eds.) *Proceedings of the RCOG Study Group on Multiple Pregnancy.* London: RCOG Press, 1995: 349–352.

93 Sebire NJ, Noble PL, Odibo A, Malligiannis P, Nicolaides KH. Single uterine entry for genetic amniocentesis in twin pregnancies. *Ultrasound in Obstetrics and Gynecology* 1996; 7: 26–31.

94 Buscaglia M, Ghisoni L, Bellotti M *et al.* Genetic amniocentesis in bi-amniotic twin pregnancies by a single transabdominal insertion of the needle. *Prenatal Diagnosis* 1995; 15: 17–19.

95 Ghidini A, Lynch L, Hicks C, Alvarez M, Lockwood CJ. The risk of second-trimester amniocentesis in twin gestations: a case-control study. *American Journal of Obstetrics and Gynecology* 1993; 169: 1013–1016.

96 Evans MI, Goldberg JD, Horenstein J *et al.* Selective termination for structural, chromosomal, and Mendelian anomalies: international experience. *American Journal of Obstetrics and Gynecology* 1999; 181: 893–897.

97 Deprest JA, Audibert F, Van Schoubroeck D, Hecher K, Mahieu-Caputo D. Bipolar coagulation of the umbilical cord in complicated monochorionic twin pregnancy. *American Journal of Obstetrics and Gynecology* 2000; 182: 340–345.

98 Joint Working Party of the Royal College of Obstetricians and Gynaecologists and of the Royal College of Paediatrics and Child Health. *Fetal Abnormalities: Guidelines for Screening Diagnosis and Management.* London: RCOG and RCPCh, 1997.

99 Royal College of Obstetricians and Gynaecologists. *Termination of Pregnancy for Fetal Abnormality in England, Wales and Scotland.* London: RCOG, 1996.

100 Royal College of Obstetricians and Gynaecologists. A *Consideration of the Law and Ethics in Relation to Late Termination of Pregnancy for Fetal Abnormality.* London: RCOG, 1998.

101 Fisk NM, Fordham K, Abramsky L. Elective late fetal karyotyping. *British Journal of Obstetrics and Gynaecology* 1996; 103: 468–470.

102 Paintin D. Abortion after 24 weeks. *British Journal of Obstetrics and Gynaecology* 1997; 104: 398–400.

103 Green JM. Obstetricians' views on prenatal diagnosis and termination of pregnancy: 1980 compared with 1993. *British Journal of Obstetrics and Gynaecology* 1995; 102: 228–232.

104 Chervenak FA, McCullough LB, Campbell S. Is third trimester abortion justified? *British Journal of Obstetrics and Gynaecology* 1995; 102: 434–435.

105 Chervenak FA, McCullough LB, Campbell S. Third trimester abortion: is compassion enough? *British Journal of Obstetrics and Gynaecology* 1999; 106: 293–296.

106 Dommergues M, Benachi A, Benifla JL, des Noettes R, Dumez Y. The reasons for termination of pregnancy in the third trimester. *British Journal of Obstetrics and Gynaecology* 1999; 106: 297–303.

▶11 ⁄

Antenatal Care

Julian Woolfson

Introduction

When the first antenatal outpatient clinic was opened by JW Ballantyne in Edinburgh in 1915, most women in the United Kingdom had no routine antenatal care from midwives or doctors. Before this time, their first contact with either of these professionals was usually when things were going wrong, by which time it was often too late to do anything to improve the outcome for the woman or her fetus. Maternal mortality and morbidity were high, and most families could tell of a relative who had died or become permanently handicapped as a result of what would today be considered avoidable factors. Fetal mortality and morbidity were even higher. Stillbirth was common and babies who were born alive prematurely, or handicapped as a result of what would now be avoidable pregnancy-related problems, rarely survived.

The availability of antenatal care spread quickly, partly as a result of the efforts of Janet Campbell, who as a senior civil servant in the 1920s was responsible for starting the National System of Antenatal Clinics.[1] By 1935, 80% of women in the United Kingdom were receiving some antenatal care and this figure had risen to 91% by 1946.[2] It would be unrealistic to say that the increasing availability of antenatal care was the sole reason for the progressive reduction since then in maternal and perinatal mortality and morbidity, but its importance should not be underestimated. It cannot be a coincidence that outcomes were improved when as much attention was paid to the 40 weeks of pregnancy as to the 12 hours or so of labour.[3]

The aims of the first antenatal clinics were modest but even today those aims still form the basis for antenatal care: to maintain maternal health; to recognise potential problems at an early stage; and to educate the mother in the duties of motherhood and dispel the ignorance and fears of pregnancy and labour.

If the aims of antenatal care have not changed over the past 80 years, its scope and complexity have, largely as a result of two principal and inter-related driving forces: namely, the advances in medical knowledge and technology and the changing nature of society.

For example, pregnancy-related conditions such as *pre-eclampsia* and *antepartum haemorrhage* were well known long before the introduction of the first antenatal clinics. There was, however, little that could be done about them. There were no effective drugs to treat high blood pressure and although it was known that delivery of the baby was the only cure for pre-eclampsia or eclampsia, there were no safe methods of inducing labour. Nor was it likely that a baby delivered prematurely in order to avoid the maternal complications of these conditions would survive. Caesarean section carried such high risks to the woman herself that it was very rarely performed.

Similarly, the management of antepartum haemorrhage as a result of a placental abruption amounted to little more than hope and prayer. The risks of haemorrhage from a *placenta praevia* were overcome by inserting a hand or instrument through the cervix and placenta and pulling the fetus down in order to stop the bleeding. Both were usually fatal for the fetus and often for the mother as well. Blood transfusion was very rare and where it was used the danger of a transfusion reaction was high. It was only the advances in medical knowledge and technology that changed the management of these conditions and improved their outcomes.

As important as these advances have been, the effect of the changing nature of society has been at least as great. Over the past fifty years, there has been a *socialization of nature*[4] in that phenomena that used to be regarded as 'natural', or given in nature, have now become 'social': they depend on our own social and political decisions. The most notable of these has been the will and the ability to control fertility, which has on its own probably been the most significant factor in the reduction of maternal and fetal morbidity and mortality.

Until the early part of the 20th century, *grand multiparity*, traditionally defined as having had five or more children, was common. Its associated risks, which include maternal anaemia, malpositions of the fetus and a greatly increased risk of postpartum haemorrhage, were also well known but, again, there was little that could be done about any of them other than advise delivery in a hospital and counsel against further pregnancies. The former did not guarantee a better outcome and the latter was, of course, more easily said than done, partly because contraception was regarded by many as sinful or even criminal, and partly because there were simply no suitable or safe methods available. Nevertheless, the early antenatal clinics provided an opportunity at least to explain the risks of further pregnancies and thereby provided the basis for the widespread acceptance and implementation of contraception as the methods became available.

Social change has, however, also had other wider and more subtle effects. By the late 20th century, maternal and perinatal morbidity and mortality had fallen to the point where maternal deaths were counted individually rather than expressed as a rate, and perinatal deaths accounted for less than 1% of all births. Few families today have suffered the devastation and grief of a maternal death and few have had experience of stillbirth or neonatal death. As a result, such occurrences are now less likely to be regarded as vagaries of life than as failure on the part of others, usually the medical and midwifery professions. Many will result in litigation.

There have been other highly significant changes over the past few decades. Parents once had to wait until the day of birth to learn the sex of their newborn child and whether it would be healthy. Today, a wide range of prenatal diagnostic techniques will not only determine the sex of the fetus but identify structural or chromosomal abnormalities sufficiently early to allow termination of the pregnancy (see Chapter 10). The availability of such tests and their ability to influence the outcome of the pregnancy inevitably raises the expectations of prospective parents but at the same time presents them – and society – with new and complex ethical and legal decisions. The healthcare system, whether as part of the National Health Service or the private sector, is increasingly relied upon to make the technology and expertise available, often at disproportionate cost and with the prospect of rationing in other, less emotive, areas of healthcare. Once again, both individuals and society may regard failures in any of these areas as a failure on the part of those charged with their care.

And yet despite these changes in knowledge, technology and the nature of society, the underlying principles of antenatal care still remain the same: maintenance of maternal health, recognition of potential problems, and education. In this respect, antenatal care is a prime example of risk management in its widest sense: identifying potential problems, analysing and evaluating them and then taking steps to avoid or minimize adverse outcomes.

This chapter is not intended to be a detailed guide to the provision of antenatal care; nor should it be taken as a guide to every possible intervention, for these are ever-changing and are covered in other chapters in this book. Rather, it is a contextualized and risk-management-oriented look at antenatal care and the duties and responsibilities it places on both the pregnant woman and those responsible for her care. It starts with a general overview of the purpose and structure of antenatal care and then goes on to consider some of those clinical situations which pose the greatest clinical and ethical difficulties – and therefore risks.

The infrastructure of antenatal care

Most pregnant women in the United Kingdom now book for confinement in a consultant unit with their antenatal care arranged under the *shared-care* system, in which their care is shared between their GP, community and hospital-based midwives and doctors. Women who are considered to be low risk may not attend a hospital antenatal clinic at all, whereas a few, particularly those who are considered to be high risk, will be booked for full care and will attend a hospital antenatal clinic at every visit. The rest – probably the majority – will attend a variable number of hospital antenatal clinics. In all cases, the midwife has a key role in the provision of care that is 'flexible, sensible and responsive to the needs of women and fully involves them as partners in care'.[5,6]

The midwife will, however, still be expected to recognise those clinical situations where a pregnancy may not be progressing normally and to refer the woman accordingly. The referral may be to the woman's GP or to one of the hospital obstetric staff, the seniority of that hospital doctor being decided by the midwife on the basis of her perceived assessment of the nature of the situation and the protocols for that hospital. In general terms, however, a senior house officer (SHO) in obstetrics would be expected to deal with basic obstetric problems such as a urinary infection or mildly raised blood pressure. A *specialist registrar*, a more senior speciality trainee known as an 'SpR', would be expected to see more complex problems – such as a moderately raised blood pressure together with protein in the woman's urine (collectively signifying pre-eclampsia) – or to decide whether induction of labour was required. A *consultant* would be expected to see any woman whose clinical situation was deemed to require a more experienced assessment or where difficult decisions might have to be made.

It is important to stress that these are not in any way intended to be hard and fast rules. Much depends on the level of experience of each doctor. For example, an experienced SHO would be expected to have at least the experience of a junior SpR. An experienced SpR in his/her fourth or fifth year and having already passed the specialist examination (Membership of the Royal College of Obstetricians and Gynaecologists [MRCOG]) and having been accredited as a specialist by that College would be as experienced as a (relatively) new consultant. It is for this reason that the term 'experienced obstetrician' is used in this chapter to denote a doctor who is sufficiently capable of making the kind of decisions that a senior SpR or a consultant would be expected to make. Where the term 'consultant' is used with regard to the seniority required, it is an expression of the author's opinion and should not be regarded as prescriptive or setting the standard of care. In many respects, it is as much political as it is medical and it applies to those situations where the most senior person should not only be involved but also be *seen* to be involved.

Wherever the setting of the antenatal clinic and whatever the arrangements with regard to the level of staff available, certain basic principles apply. There should be adequate facilities provided and there should be reasonable access to basic services and investigations such as routine blood testing and ultrasound scan. There are also guidelines with regard to the healthcare professional's behaviour. These are set out in the guideline on ethical considerations relating to good practice in obstetrics and gynaecology issued by the Royal College of Obstetricians and Gynaecologists:[7]

> Patients should be treated with courtesy and respect at all times. Medical staff should take as a model either how they themselves would like to be treated, or those they care about such as their mother, partner or daughter. The relationship between clinician and patient should be characterised by symmetry of status and the presumption of formal address should be used as a reflection of professional attitude.

> In situations where history taking and examination are carried out adequate privacy should be ensured. Intimate examinations should be carried out in accordance with the GMC guidance[8] which includes the use of a chaperone wherever possible. Any third person present, such as another doctor or medical student, should be introduced, and any objections to that presence should be respected. In communicating with patients, language should not be pitched so high as to be unintelligible, nor so low as to be patronising.

It could be argued that guidance such as this should never have been necessary but the truth is that the combination of poor antenatal clinic facilities and over-booked clinics in many obstetric units resulted, in a few of them, in a diminution of attention to these important non-clinical details. Coupled with the changing nature of the doctor–patient relationship and the increasingly widely spoken 'language of human rights',[9] it is perhaps not surprising that women who feel belittled or demeaned by the manner in which they were treated are much less kindly disposed to actual or perceived errors of judgement on the part of the medical and midwifery staff. The woman who is treated in accordance with the Royal College of Obstetricians and Gynaecologists guidelines is probably less likely to resort to official complaint or litigation when, for example, a breech presentation is missed, resulting in an unexpected and unplanned emergency Caesarean section, than her counterpart who – perhaps only in her view – has not been treated in the way she expected or was entitled to. Courtesy, patience, respect and kindness are arguably the easiest and most important constituents of effective risk management.

The booking visit

This is the most important antenatal visit. It starts with a full and detailed history, usually taken by an experienced midwife, and is followed by a careful general physical examination which includes height, weight, blood pressure, abdominal palpation and, if appropriate, a vaginal examination. The woman's urine is checked for the presence of glucose, protein and bacteria. There will then be a number of blood tests, including haemoglobin estimation, blood group and antibodies, immunity to rubella and screening for haemoglobinopathies and syphilis. More recently, screening for HIV, hepatitis and other infections has become part of the normal range of investigations. Given the sensitive nature of some of these tests, it is essential that the pregnant woman be informed of the need for the test and the significance of a potentially devastating positive result. She should be able to decline a particular test if she wishes.

Many hospitals now offer an early first-trimester ultrasound scan at around 12–13 weeks gestation. This will confirm that the fetus is alive and, by then measuring it, it will provide a more accurate assessment of the duration of the pregnancy and the estimated date of delivery (EDD) than could otherwise be derived. Multiple pregnancy can be confirmed or excluded and, in some units, the *nuchal translucency* (the thickness of the pad of tissue at the back of the fetus' neck) can be measured and used as a basis for calculating the risks of Down syndrome. A second scan should be performed at around the 20th to 24th week of pregnancy. The main purpose of this scan is to exclude major fetal anomalies and assess fetal growth and placental position. It follows that if facilities or the woman's wishes allow only one scan, this should be it.

The range of invasive and non-invasive ultrasound-based tests for fetal anomalies has grown dramatically over the past few years, so much so that prenatal screening has become an obstetric subspecialty in its own right. Thus, many women will be advised to undergo other scans or tests as well. The reader is referred to Chapter 10 for a fuller discussion of this important area.

The information gathered at the booking visit is now often recorded on a computer system but it should also always be recorded in the woman's notes. Many hospitals encourage women to carry their own antenatal records, although there will usually be a 'backup' copy in their main files. The principal benefit of the woman carrying her own notes is that information about the pregnancy is available immediately if she has to be admitted to another hospital in an emergency. However, the notes also provide an opportunity to inform the woman (and her partner) about the progress of the pregnancy and involve her in any decisions that may have to be made.

Evaluating the information gained at the booking visit is probably the most important part of antenatal care. Fit, healthy women who have delivered healthy children successfully in the past are least likely to develop problems in pregnancy and labour, whereas those who have had previous difficult pregnancies and labours are more likely to have problems again. Women who have never had a child before* are in effect 'unknown quantities' in that there is no past 'form' to guide the obstetrician or midwife.

A considerable amount of time must therefore be taken with the *past obstetric history*. Details should include any problems during the pregnancy, the mode of onset of labour and the gestation at which the baby was born. The nature of the labour, the type of delivery and the baby's condition at birth are very important, as is the baby's weight and subsequent health. Where there has been an operative delivery, the indication should be clearly recorded and additional details sought, such as whether there were any problems as a result of the delivery. Wherever possible, the woman's account of the delivery should be checked against the records of that pregnancy and any relevant details noted. If the woman has previously delivered at another hospital, it may be necessary to write to that hospital to obtain more information.

The implications of the outcomes of previous pregnancies will be discussed in more detail later in this chapter but an example of the importance and value of the previous obstetric history would be a woman who has already had one Caesarean. There are several options open to her with regard to the route of the delivery and so she should be seen at about 34 weeks gestation in the current pregnancy by someone who is sufficiently experienced to assess her particular situation and discuss the route of delivery. If it is decided that an *elective* Caesarean section is required, a reasonably competent specialist registrar can then do it. In short, the decision requires more skill and experience than the subsequent action.

In contrast, a woman who has had two previous Caesarean sections would usually be advised to have a third. Making the decision to perform another Caesarean section requires little skill and can therefore be made antenatally by a midwife or junior doctor. However, a third Caesarean section can be quite difficult to perform and so it should be performed by a more senior obstetrician. Thus, knowledge of the past obstetric history is of considerable assistance in planning both the nature of the antenatal visits and the level of seniority of the medical staff at the delivery.

The *history of the present pregnancy* is particularly important, especially if it is the woman's first pregnancy. Thanks to accurate ultrasound dating, estimating the due

---

* The nomenclature in general use can be very confusing. A woman who has had children before is called a *multipara*. A woman who has never had a child before is said to be *nulliparous*. Women who are in their first pregnancy are known as *primigravidas*, those who have been pregnant more than once are *multigravidas*. Miscarriages or abortions are traditionally – and wrongly – not included and so a woman who has had one or more miscarriages or abortions but who is now in an ongoing 'first' pregnancy is still commonly referred to as a primigravida. The recommended nomenclature is the *para/gravida* system, where every pregnancy over 28 weeks gestation is counted as a 'para' and every pregnancy, whatever the outcome, is counted as a 'gravida'. Thus, a woman who is pregnant for the fourth time having had one miscarriage and two children is a *para two, gravida four*. A woman who has only been pregnant once but who has had twins is a *para two, gravida one*. One of the greatest of advantages of women carrying their own notes is that they quickly deal with any confusion by simply telling anyone who asks that they have been pregnant 'x' times and have had 'y' children.

date is now relatively easy and so the problems of both *iatrogenic prematurity* (inducing labour too early in the mistaken belief that the woman is overdue) and postmaturity (waiting too long) can be avoided. Many of the problems reported by women in their first pregnancy may be relatively trivial, at least to the medical and midwifery staff, but they offer an invaluable opportunity to discuss the problems of pregnancy in general and to begin a dialogue with regard to her wishes, anxieties and expectations.

If the woman is a smoker, she can be advised to give up or at least cut down. The same applies to alcohol consumption and the use of recreational drugs. Most women who smoke or drink alcohol or use drugs in pregnancy are distressed by the thought that they might be harming their unborn child but are nevertheless unable to stop. They need help and support, not a lecture on the evils of smoking, drinking or taking drugs, and if sensitively counselled these women will usually respond favourably. The worst case scenario is when a woman is so distressed by the things said to her by a (well-meaning) midwife or doctor that she defaults from the rest of her antenatal clinic visits.

The booking examination not only provides a baseline height, weight, blood pressure and urine analysis but can also provide an opportunity to discuss things arising from it. Weight gain (or loss) can lead to advice about the importance of a balanced diet and such basics as care of the nipples can provide an opportunity to discuss breast-feeding. Examination of the abdomen – *palpation* – provides an estimate of the size of the uterus and establishes physical contact in what may be an embarrassing situation for some women. Again, gentleness, sensitivity and non-patronizing explanation facilitates the establishment of a trust between the patient and her carers.

Subsequent antenatal visits

Advances such as ultrasound scan have changed many of the traditional intentions and content of antenatal care. For example, palpation of the uterine size on a regular basis in order to assess fetal presentation and growth may offer the reassurance of 'hands-on care' but it is less accurate in assessing fetal presentation and growth than ultrasound scan. In this respect, one might justifiably question whether palpation now serves a useful purpose, or whether additional routine scans should either replace palpation or else be performed routinely in the third trimester of the pregnancy to eliminate any doubts about fetal presentation or growth.

This is not to say that regular antenatal clinic visits will no longer be needed. There are other purposes, such as the detection of raised blood pressure or pregnancy-induced hypertension, and to allow women the opportunity to receive advice and support from the midwives or doctors. The advantages and reassurance given by hands-on contact also cannot be underestimated; nor, for that matter, should one disregard the benefits of giving the woman and her partner or family an opportunity to have regular meetings with her healthcare professionals.

A consensus is gradually emerging with regard to the balance between the needs of pregnant women, the use of technology and a respect for the traditional roles of the midwife and doctor. Women are now encouraged to book early and to undergo a first-trimester scan, usually around the 12th–13th week. Having confirmed fetal viability, excluded multiple pregnancy and having provided a baseline for accurately dating the pregnancy, the woman can then be seen at monthly intervals by her midwife or GP in an appropriate and more convenient setting. This is, in effect, a *triage* system starting with the midwife, progressing to the GP and ultimately involving a consultant obstetrician if required.

Providing that the second scan, at around 22–24 weeks gestation, excludes fetal or placental position anomalies and confirms normal growth, the woman can continue seeing her midwife or GP at monthly intervals. Her blood pressure and urine can be checked at each visit and her haemoglobin level and blood group antibodies checked routinely. Advice can be given on diet, skin care and other areas of concern. Parentcraft classes can be held for the convenience of the women and their partners.

It is still traditional for the pregnant woman to be seen by a doctor – whether trained or in training – at around 34–36 weeks, although in many obstetric units this is no longer considered necessary for those women who have already delivered one or more children uneventfully and whose current pregnancy is progressing normally. In medical terms, the value of a hospital visit at this gestation is questionable but to the pregnant woman herself it may be of enormous value in terms of reassurance and an opportunity to ask questions about the pregnancy and labour.

Providing that the pregnancy is continuing normally, the woman can again continue to be seen by her midwife or GP at fortnightly intervals to about 36 weeks and then weekly intervals thereafter. If any abnormality is detected, the midwife or GP should refer the woman to the consultant unit and the hospital system should ensure that a specialist or consultant opinion can be obtained with the appropriate degree of urgency.

Finally, the woman should be seen in the hospital antenatal clinic at or just after her due date, depending on her parity and any other factors, such as her age. If it is decided that no intervention is required, the woman needs to be seen at least weekly in a consultant clinic and preferably in a day-assessment unit or similar setting every few days.

Where the past obstetric history and/or the nature of the current pregnancy warrant it, the woman should be able to attend a consultant clinic more frequently. An outline of such visits will be discussed later in this chapter but the key principle should be that the frequency of visits and seniority of the person attending the woman are specifically tailored to the individual woman and her needs.

For example, a woman known to be diabetic needs to be seen by a diabetic physician or nurse specialist at regular and frequent intervals throughout the pregnancy and then by a specialist obstetric registrar or consultant at each obstetric visit. A woman who has previously had a small for gestational age baby generally needs more intensive assessment in the last trimester of pregnancy, as does the woman who has previously had a very large baby (but is not diabetic). A woman who has had a stillbirth or neonatal death in the past should be seen as often as she wishes to be seen, irrespective of the cause of the previous stillbirth or the likelihood of its recurrence.

Antenatal admission to hospital

The routine admission of pregnant women to hospital as part of their antenatal care is as recent as antenatal care itself and has undergone as many changes. The earliest uses of this form of medical intervention were intended to avoid maternal death or morbidity. Women with pre-eclampsia (also known as *toxaemia*, as it was thought to be due to a toxin or poison in the blood) were admitted into quiet darkened rooms in order to avoid any stimulation that might lead to *eclampsia* and were kept there until labour started. Women with antepartum haemorrhage thought to be due to a placenta praevia were admitted to minimize the risk of provoking further bleeding.

As medical technology and knowledge advanced, the indications for admission widened and began to include those solely intended for the benefit of the fetus. Not unsurprisingly, this caused a significant increase in the need for resources and was not popular with the women themselves, especially those with other children. The most recent trend has therefore been towards admission to 'day wards' – often nothing more than a part of an existing ward set aside for the purpose. Here, the woman can be observed closely over the course of a day and the fetus monitored by means of cardiotocograph and scan.

Formal admission to hospital, however, is still required occasionally. Whatever the reason for the admission, it represents a 'step change' in the concern about the pregnancy, particularly to the woman and her family. The nature of the care required may therefore also need to change, with a greater degree of maternal and fetal surveillance and regular review by a senior obstetrician. This is particularly so when the admission has been for such things as pain, concern about fetal movements or suspected pre-term labour. In most such cases, there is actually very little that can be done other than to exclude the more obvious conditions, confirm fetal viability or administer a corticosteroid to help the fetal lungs mature. Nevertheless, in those cases where problems subsequently arise weeks or even months later, the conduct and outcome of the admission will feature prominently in the woman and her family's minds. They may come to believe that labour could or should have been prevented or induced, that a particular treatment should or should not have been given or that a fetal problem could or should have been detected or treated.

Every practising obstetrician will be familiar with situations such as these and few will fail to recognise that a complaint or attempt at litigation is understandable when seen through the patient's eyes. Good communication and careful explanation after the event is obviously necessary but in some cases it is too late. It should have begun during the antenatal admission and it should have extended to a careful explanation of the situation and the possible outcomes. The reality, however, is that many admissions occur at night, or over a weekend, or have been too short for the woman to have been seen by an obstetrician senior enough to assess the situation and explain it to the woman and her family. This is not to say that it is necessary for a consultant to see the woman every day during the admission but she should be seen by a doctor – preferably of SpR status – each day.

If she remains in hospital for more than a few days, she should be seen by a consultant, and if she is discharged before being seen by a consultant she should attend a hospital antenatal clinic within a week or so for further assessment and discussion. This may not affect the eventual clinical outcome but it will at least confirm that the woman's concerns and health are being taken seriously and that good communication is part of her care.

Evaluating specific risks

A pregnancy can only be called 'normal' in retrospect, and so if antenatal care is to be risk management in its truest sense it must start with the identification of those women whose own health, or the health of their fetus, may be at greater risk than would normally be expected. The spectrum is naturally wide and does not always follow the traditional teaching that 'healthy women have healthy babies'.

In all cases, a sense of perspective and balance is essential. Not all maternal and fetal risks are of the same magnitude or severity; nor can there be a balance between the risks of death or injury to the fetus and those to the woman. However much a woman might be prepared to suffer in the interests of her unborn child, it would be both unethical and a breach of duty for an obstetrician or midwife not to put the life and well-being of the mother before those of the fetus.

Some risks can be predicted or avoided before pregnancy; others only emerge or can be evaluated during the pregnancy or even labour. Of these, some will do no more than identify the woman as being of 'higher risk', or someone that should be seen by a senior obstetrician antenatally. Examples include the woman with diabetes or a growth-restricted fetus, both of whom require senior obstetric opinions with regard to the timing and nature of the delivery. In others, the risks can be evaluated and acted upon by any member of the team, although that action may require the experience and skills of a more experienced obstetrician.

Risks that can be predicted or avoided before pregnancy

Maternal conditions such as hypertension, diabetes, cardiac disease (congenital or acquired) and liver disease can all adversely affect the outcome of pregnancy if steps are not taken to bring them under control before the start of the pregnancy. The same applies to more subtle indicators such as the mother's general health, her nutritional state, her alcohol consumption and her smoking or drug habits. With the exception of low folic acid levels, which are associated with fetal neural-tube defects such as spina bifida and anencephaly and which are only amenable to treatment with folic acid *before* conception occurs, the other factors can at least be remedied and their effects on the fetus minimized if steps are taken to overcome them early enough in pregnancy.

The essence of good antenatal care therefore starts with pre-pregnancy education and counselling. All women should be encouraged to take folic acid supplements *before* they embark on a pregnancy and those with medical conditions such as those above should be seen by their GP or the appropriate specialist well beforehand. General advice with regard to nutrition, smoking and alcohol or drug usage are (or should be) components of general public education programmes but health professionals in socio-economically deprived areas should, wherever possible, also undertake specific health education promotion.

This advice should be reinforced in the antenatal clinic, although by that stage it is, of course, too late to reduce the chances of neural-tube defect by giving folic acid supplements. Nevertheless, a reduction in alcohol consumption will reduce the incidence of Fetal Alcohol Syndrome and stopping smoking will reduce the incidence of intrauterine growth restriction and premature delivery. Breast feeding can be discussed and encouraged.

Risk factors that only emerge or can only be assessed during pregnancy

Where the woman has a medical condition such as those described above, and irrespective of the severity and the medical management up to that time, she should be seen in a consultant antenatal clinic early in the pregnancy and a further risk evaluation conducted. Where necessary, other specialists should be involved, particularly when the woman is diabetic or has pre-existing hypertension or heart disease.

A plan of management should be agreed and recorded in both the main hospital records and the woman's own self-carried records, along with the names of the professionals involved. The GP should be informed and his/her involvement in the woman's care should be set out. Most importantly, however, the woman herself must be involved in the discussions and must be clearly advised about the nature and purpose of any investigations and interventions. The opportunity for health education at this time should not be underestimated and good communication between all concerned will optimize the chances of a successful outcome.

Particular problems that require a consultant or senior obstetric opinion as part of the antenatal care

Certain conditions or situations will always arise and each will require a more senior opinion if the risks are to be properly identified, analysed and acted upon. The following list is neither exhaustive nor intended to be prescriptive but outlines some of the problems that have to be dealt with on a regular basis.

Women having babies at the extremes of their reproductive life

Pregnancy at the extremes of reproductive life is associated with a higher incidence of spontaneous miscarriage and early failure of the fetus to develop, now usually diagnosed at routine scan by the appearance of an empty gestation sac. In addition to this greater early pregnancy loss, the very young (by and large those women aged 16 or younger) are more likely to develop pre-eclampsia. They are also more likely to have cephalo-pelvic disproportion (the fetal head is too big to engage in the mother's pelvis) because their pelvic growth may lag behind their increase in height.[10] The very young are also much more likely to come from a socio-economically deprived background, with all its additional social and medical morbidity.

The older woman is probably less likely to come from a deprived socio-economic background and her pelvis is fully grown, making cephalo-pelvic disproportion unlikely. Nevertheless, she has her own specific age-related problems. She is more likely to have a chromosomally abnormal fetus and her baseline blood pressure is likely to be higher. She may have smoked for many years and as a result is more likely to have a growth-restricted fetus. The general ageing process may result in an increase in joint pain and backache and any underlying disease such as diabetes will have become more established.

A good basic rule is that any pregnant woman under the age of 17 or older than 40 should attend a hospital antenatal clinic more frequently than others and should be seen at least once by a consultant, preferably in the early part of the third trimester. Her blood pressure should be carefully assessed at each visit and sufficient time set aside to discuss the particular problems if and when they arise. Additional home support may be required for the very young and the maternity department and community social workers may need to be involved at an early stage. The decision to allow a *trial of labour* – that is to say allowing labour to proceed under careful observation to make sure that the fetal head can and does engage in the mother's pelvis – in the young woman should be made in the last week or so of the pregnancy by a senior obstetrician. An entry should be made in the labour records to watch out for any labour disorder that may be a sign of cephalo-pelvic disproportion.

The grand multipara

Like all women, grand multipara fall broadly into two categories: those who intended to be pregnant and those who did not. There are differences, however. While grand multipara who intended to be pregnant bring with them a unique confidence and realism which usually makes them easy to care for, those who did not intend to be pregnant may be distressed at the thought of having to cope with the prospect of an additional child. The confidence may be less and the realisation of the difficulties ahead may be depressing. Some may be lucky enough not to have financial or social problems but others may not be so fortunate. Once again, the involvement of the social worker may be advisable.

The obstetric risks include both the problems of the older woman, outlined in the previous section, and those problems specific to multiparity, namely an increased risk of fetal malpresentation and *unstable lie*. These women should therefore be seen and assessed by an experienced obstetrician at around 36 weeks. If the lie of the fetus is abnormal or unstable, it should not be assumed that it is due to the woman's grand multiparity. The size of the fetus should be estimated, preferably by scan, and placenta praevia excluded before concluding that the unstable lie is due to the lax uterus of the multiparous woman.

Grand multiparity is not *per se* an indication to induce labour earlier but as the risk of *precipitate labour* increases significantly, it may be prudent to consider induction, especially if the woman lives some distance from the hospital. It may also be necessary to perform a *stabilizing induction* if the lie is unstable. (This procedure involves correcting the lie and holding it in this position while the membranes are ruptured and an intravenous infusion of oxytocic is administered. Once the contractions have begun, the head can be released and hopefully will not return to its former position.) For obvious reasons, the decision to perform an induction of this sort must be made by an experienced obstetrician and conducted by one of equal seniority, traditionally assisted by a medical student or midwife to hold the head in place until the contractions commence. It must be done in a well-equipped labour ward setting with facilities for immediate Caesarean section if the umbilical cord should prolapse.

Previous Caesarean section

With Caesarean section rates in the United Kingdom now approaching 30% in some areas, the antenatal assessment of the pregnant woman who has already had a previous Caesarean section is a common and routine occurrence. The question that must be asked in each case is straightforward: by which route should the baby be delivered?

There are always two options. The first is to resolve any doubts about the route of delivery by advising the woman to have an elective Caesarean section at around 39 weeks gestation. The advantages are that a date can be given well in advance, the choice of anaesthesia and analgesia can be discussed at leisure, and preparations made for the care of the other members of the family. The disadvantages of this approach are that the woman will then have had two Caesarean sections and few obstetricians would advise a subsequent attempt at vaginal delivery. If the woman has not yet delivered a child vaginally, she may regret not having an opportunity to do so.

The second option is to advise a *trial of scar* with a view to achieving a vaginal delivery. In this situation – referred to in the American literature as 'vaginal birth after Caesarean' (VBAC) – the ideal management is to aim for spontaneous labour or to induce labour under carefully controlled conditions and then to allow nature to take its course, albeit under careful supervision (including continuous fetal monitoring).

Apart from failure to progress, which usually results in another Caesarean section, the most serious risk of labour following a Caesarean section is *dehiscence* or rupture of the previous Caesarean section scar. While this is not common – estimates are that it will occur unpredictably in around 0.5–2.0% of cases allowed a trial of labour[11] – it *can* and *does* occur. Providing that there is ready recourse to emergency Caesarean section, these dehiscences are seldom associated with serious sequelae for mother or baby. Even so, a small number of babies will be exposed to sufficient hypoxia to cause cerebral palsy or even stillbirth. In the worst case scenario, both mother[12] and baby may die.

Advising the pregnant woman who has had one previous Caesarean section on how she should deliver the subsequent baby or babies is now arguably one of the most difficult situations facing the obstetrician. On the one hand, advising elective Caesarean section in every case – the old doctrine of 'once a Caesarean, always a

Caesarean' – will virtually eliminate any fetal and maternal morbidity or mortality as a result of scar dehiscence, even allowing for the usual surgical and anaesthetic risks to the mother. On the other hand, many studies have shown good outcomes to trial of labour after Caesarean section, with up to 80% of those opting for a trial of labour giving birth vaginally.[13] Many women will still want to attempt at vaginal delivery after Caesarean section even though there is up to a 25% risk of needing an emergency Caesarean section in labour and a three to four times greater risk of complications when Caesarean section is performed as an emergency rather than electively.[14]

In certain situations, the decision to advise a woman to undergo a repeat Caesarean section is easy to make. More than one previous Caesarean section, or a woman with a single previous Caesarean section who then has a breech presentation, or twins, or a larger than average fetus or a medical conditions such as diabetes are all widely considered to be contraindications to a trial of labour. For the rest, however, it is not so straightforward and all the obstetrician can do is counsel the pregnant woman about the pros and cons of each decision and allow her to make a choice.

The problem with counselling along these lines is that the 'standard' rules do not always apply. To the vast majority of women, even the smallest risk of damage to the baby is unacceptable and they would far rather undergo what might in medical eyes be regarded as an 'unnecessary' Caesarean section than put their fetus at risk by attempting a vaginal delivery. The traditional risk/benefit analysis is therefore likely to result in a very different decision when it is the woman herself who makes it. The frequently quoted study by Al-Mufti *et al.*[15] revealed that 31% of female obstetricians would want an elective Caesarean section for the delivery of their first baby, albeit for concerns about incontinence and sexual problems following a vaginal delivery. This confirms that women's choices are not always dictated by statistical considerations.

Conversely, some women may for a variety of reasons feel that a repeat Caesarean section would imply a failure on their part, and they may insist on a trial of labour however great the risks. When the attempt is successful, there is great satisfaction. However, where it fails, or where it ends in fetal or maternal damage as opposed to 'just' another Caesarean section, there is likely to be recrimination and a significant chance of litigation based on a failure to 'properly advise' about the risks entailed.

Every experienced obstetrician will have evolved his or her own strategy for counselling women who have had a previous Caesarean section but certain key risk management principles still apply. First, the counselling should be given at an appropriate time or times during the third trimester, and the gist of the discussion clearly set out in the woman's records on each occasion. Second, the counselling should be comprehensive and include mention of both the likely success rates for a vaginal birth and the risks of scar dehiscence. It should be non-confrontational and non-directional, with no pressure put on the woman to decide one way or the other, at least at the initial discussion. That is not to say that the obstetrician cannot say what he or she considers to be the right decision. Since the majority of women form good relationships with their doctors and midwives, looking to them for guidance and advice, they would be disappointed if that advice was not forthcoming. Third, the woman should know both that the obstetric situation can change and that she can change her mind if she wishes. On occasion, the 'wrong' decision will be made but this will invariably be accepted if the woman genuinely feels that she has been able to play a part in deciding about her care. Fourth, not all pregnant women will be able to understand and appreciate the variables that must be taken into account. Time, a non-patronizing attitude, a clear explanation, and encouraging the woman to bring along her partner, a member of her family or a friend will usually result in an acceptable conclusion.

The author tries to see every woman who has had a previous Caesarean section at about 34 weeks gestation in her subsequent pregnancy to begin a discussion about the route of delivery. In many cases, the woman has a fairly clear idea of what she would like to do, but whether she has or not, the pros and cons of each approach are discussed in detail. Even if an agreed decision can be made at that visit, the woman is asked to return two or three weeks later for further discussion. If she cannot make a decision, or if the obstetric aspect has not yet become clear – for example, the size of the fetus cannot be properly estimated – then she is also asked to return a few weeks later for further discussion. In all cases, and on every occasion, a record is made in the woman's hand-held records as an *aide memoire*. If she has chosen an elective Caesarean section, this is booked for around 39 weeks gestation. If she has decided to aim for a vaginal delivery then she is seen at weekly intervals from 38 weeks onwards and the decision reviewed on each occasion. Whatever her decision, and whether or not it changes during the last few weeks of the pregnancy, every effort is made to introduce her to the other members of the medical staff who, even if not likely to be present during labour or to perform the elective Caesarean section, will be seeing her postnatally.

In those cases where the woman decides to attempt a trial of scar after a Caesarean section, the fact of the previous Caesarean section should be clearly recorded in the labour section of the woman's notes so that all concerned are aware of her situation. Every labour ward in the UK should have a protocol for the management of trial of scar but it is also useful to set out a management plan in the patient's notes as well.

More than one previous Caesarean section and/or placenta praevia

Where a woman has had two or more Caesarean sections, or where there is a known placenta praevia (ie the placenta is so low-lying that safe vaginal delivery is not possible), the route of delivery is clear: a Caesarean section is required.

It does not matter who makes the decision but it is very important who does the operation. Previous Caesarean sections result in considerable tissue scarring and placenta praevia results in increased vascularity of the *lower segment* of the uterus through which the baby has to be delivered. Both can make the Caesarean section difficult to perform and so an experienced obstetrician should either do the operation or directly assist the trainee.

Where there has been more than one Caesarean section *and* there is a placenta praevia, the operation is even more likely to be difficult because the placenta may be abnormally adherent to the scar of the previous Caesarean sections. In such cases, it is essential that the operation be performed by an experienced consultant obstetrician who is capable of performing a Caesarean hysterectomy, if required. It follows that a senior anaesthetist also should be present. The woman should be advised of the possible need for hysterectomy in advance and, ideally, should sign an appropriately worded consent form.

Before leaving this subject, it would be worth remembering that any operation can become complicated and that emergency hysterectomy may become the only way of saving the woman's life. In such circumstances, the consultant (or consultants, because by now a second consultant obstetrician should have been called if at all possible) must act in the patient's best interests even without her specific consent. If her partner or family are immediately available, they should be informed that hysterectomy is necessary but their consent is neither required nor valid in law.

The big fetus

The big or *macrosomic* fetus is associated with two principal risks: *cephalo-pelvic disproportion* and *shoulder dystocia*. In the first, the fetal head is simply too large to pass through the mother's pelvis. Labour becomes obstructed and unless the disproportion is overcome, either by means of enhancing the contractions in order to cause the fetal head to *flex* into a smaller diameter, or by opting for emergency Caesarean section, fetal and maternal damage are likely to ensue. Fortunately, the universal adoption of the Partogram,[16] which provides an easily recognisable graphic record of progress in labour, has meant that disproportion can generally be detected and emergency Caesarean section performed well before the fetus comes to any harm.

In cases of shoulder dystocia, however, the fetus' head has already passed through the mother's pelvis and delivered but its shoulders fail to do so. By the time that this has happened, it is too late to do a Caesarean section. Shoulder dystocia can therefore justifiably be called an obstetric nightmare. The baby is stuck with its shoulders wedged in the birth canal, its chest and umbilical cord are compressed and if fetal asphyxia is to be avoided, the obstetrician must expedite delivery. In doing so, however, physical injury to the baby, in particular the brachial plexus of nerves, may be unavoidable, resulting in a permanent Erb's palsy of the affected arm.

If shoulder dystocia could be predicted antenatally, it could be prevented by performing a Caesarean section either electively, before the onset of labour, or alternatively, during labour itself. The problem is that while there are certain associations with shoulder dystocia, there are no reliable predictors for it, either antenatally or in labour, and without them there is a very high risk of dramatically increasing the number of Caesarean sections performed, with no evidence that any benefits that might theoretically accrue will not be outweighed by complications of the Caesarean sections themselves. Furthermore, while it would seem logical to assume that shoulder dystocia will only occur when the fetus is macrosomic, almost half the reported cases occur in infants weighing less than 4 kg.[17]

Having said this, however, the *pro rata* incidence of shoulder dystocia is greater when the fetus weighs more than 4 kg in diabetic women and 4.5 kg in non-diabetic women.[18] Thus, if nothing else an accurate estimate of fetal weight may guide the obstetrician either towards advising elective Caesarean section or, if not, to at least put the labour ward staff on notice of the possibility of shoulder dystocia so that the appropriate level of midwifery and medical staff can be present in case it occurs. Unfortunately, however, clinical estimates of fetal weight before delivery are notoriously inaccurate and even ultrasound measurement, which is more accurate than clinical estimation, has an unavoidable error even with the most up-to date machines and expert ultrasonographers. Nevertheless, and because scan is more reliable, good clinical practice (and risk management) dictates that if the woman is diabetic, or gains an excessive amount of weight during pregnancy, or if there is an excess of liquor making accurate palpation of the fetus difficult, or if the fetus feels large, any or all of which are associations with fetal macrosomia, the fetal weight should be estimated by ultrasound scan at around 38 weeks gestation.

Wherever possible, a woman with a fetus estimated to weigh more than 4 kg at around this gestation should then be seen by an experienced obstetrician for further assessment. The situation should be discussed with her in detail and her views taken into account. If the delivery is to be by elective Caesarean section, the operation should be done by an experienced surgeon because a big fetus can be difficult to deliver even by Caesarean section. If a vaginal delivery is intended, the risk of shoulder dystocia should be recorded clearly in the notes.

Shoulder dystocia in a previous pregnancy

There was little written about the risks of shoulder dystocia in a previous pregnancy until Smith *et al.*[19] reviewed the outcomes of pregnancies in women who had had a shoulder dystocia before and found that there was a recurrence rate of 9.8% in the next pregnancy – 17 times the background rate amongst all deliveries.

This does not mean that a woman who has had a problem with shoulder dystocia in a previous pregnancy should automatically be advised to have an elective Caesarean section. What should happen is that the woman should have an ultrasound scan at around 36 weeks in order to estimate fetal weight and then be seen by an experienced obstetrician to discuss route of delivery. Provided that the fetus is not unduly large, the chances of avoiding shoulder dystocia are still good – around 90%.

Finally, and before leaving the subject of shoulder dystocia, it is worth remembering that brachial plexus injury and Erb's palsy have been reported in the absence of traction and even when the baby is delivered by Caesarean section.[20]

The small fetus

The abnormally small fetus, which in this context means one that is growth-restricted as opposed to premature, presents significant antenatal problems. The first is making the diagnosis, which is more difficult than it would seem. It is possible to suspect from palpation of the woman's abdomen that the fetus is small but this gives no indication as to whether the fetus is simply genetically small or that the woman's dates are incorrect. The only way that intrauterine growth restriction can be diagnosed reliably is by demonstrating a fall in *growth velocity* (that is to say that the fetus has not grown as much as would normally be expected) by means of two consecutive ultrasound scans at about a two-week interval. Since it is not considered either necessary or indeed possible to scan every woman in this way at present, it is essential that the woman's abdomen be palpated carefully at every antenatal visit and the height of the fundus of the uterus measured with a tape measure. This may be relatively crude when compared with ultrasound scan but it provides the basis for a simple screening test to decide which women should then have a scan to estimate fetal size and growth.

The second problem is deciding when to deliver. Deliver too soon, and the baby may develop respiratory distress syndrome as a result of its prematurity. Deliver too late and the baby may have already sustained permanent brain damage or will be unable to withstand the stress of labour. The decision to deliver should therefore be made by an experienced obstetrician and only on the basis of ultrasound scan and, where appropriate, antenatal cardiotocograph (CTG) monitoring.

The third problem concerns the route of delivery. Where the fetus is already showing signs of chronic hypoxia, Caesarean section should be performed. Where it is not, it is acceptable to aim for a vaginal delivery but it is essential that the fetal heart rate be monitored continuously and that the facilities for recourse to urgent Caesarean section be available.

Previous stillbirths and neonatal deaths

Whatever the possibility of a recurrence of stillbirth or neonatal death in a subsequent pregnancy, the woman who has been unfortunate enough to have experienced either should be seen by a senior obstetrician, preferably a consultant, at frequent intervals throughout the pregnancy and as often as she wishes, irrespective of the likelihood of a recurrence.

In those case where a second stillbirth or neonatal death are possibilities, and even if the woman was counselled at length about the causes of that previous stillbirth or neonatal death, she should still be seen early in the pregnancy by a consultant obstetrician. The risks of it occurring again should be assessed, particularly if the neonatal death occurred as a result of prematurity, and the woman counselled accordingly. A management plan should be recorded clearly in the notes so that in the event of an unplanned admission to hospital all concerned will be aware of the particular problems. If such an admission occurs, the consultant might also want to be notified and come even if not on call. This may not alter the outcome but the presence of the consultant and any explanation given by him or her is always greatly appreciated by the woman and her family. One would not wish to be unduly cynical, but from a risk management point of view, if something does go wrong they are at least less likely to make a formal complaint or initiate litigation simply 'in order to find out what happened'.

Breech presentation

Breech presentation is a relatively frequent finding during the late second and early third trimester but becomes progressively less frequent as the pregnancy advances and the fetus becomes larger. The two principal risks of breech presentation are prolapse of the umbilical cord when the membranes rupture and difficulty delivering the after-coming fetal head.

Since both are likely to occur in or around the time of labour, it could be argued that all women with breech presentations should be delivered by elective Caesarean section as soon as the fetus is sufficiently mature or, at the latest, as soon as labour begins. It should not, however, be regarded as a sure way of avoiding fetal problems. The fetus which presents by the breech has, among other things, a higher background rate of congenital anomaly and intrauterine growth restriction, although the diameter of its head may be increased.[21] Furthermore, while breech presentation is a predictor for cerebral palsy, breech delivery *per se* is not.[22] It is, of course, ultimately up to the woman to decide whether she would prefer to undergo an elective Caesarean section but she should at least be made aware of the increased risks whichever way the baby is delivered.

When counselling the woman with a breech presentation, it is also essential that the obstetrician takes into account the level of staffing on the labour ward, both in terms of numbers and experience. Many of the stillbirths and neonatal deaths associated with attempted vaginal breech delivery occur as a result of failure to detect or act on an abnormal fetal heart rate pattern on the CTG, and this may be exacerbated by inexperience at the time of delivery.[23] It follows that staffing levels should not only be adequate but that sufficiently senior staff are present on the labour ward and supervise or conduct the actual delivery. If either are lacking, or cannot be safely relied on, this should be explained to the woman before she makes up her mind whether to undergo a Caesarean section or attempt a vaginal breech delivery.

The risks of vaginal breech delivery, including a lack of experienced staff, are now so widely recognised by pregnant women and their carers alike that an increasing number are opting for elective Caesarean section. This has simplified antenatal care in that many consultants now advise elective Caesarean section at 38 weeks or so in every case and insist that their junior staff do the same. If a woman known to have a breech presentation labours before her elective Caesarean section can be done, she simply undergoes an emergency Caesarean section.

It is in some ways ideal risk management but it fails to take five things into account. The first is knowing for certain that no breech presentations will be missed. The only sure way of diagnosing a breech presentation is by ultrasound scan, but many obstetric units do not have sufficient resources to scan every woman in the last weeks of pregnancy. The second is that from time to time a woman known to have a breech presentation will arrive on the labour ward with her cervix fully dilated and the breech about to deliver. There is not sufficient time to perform a Caesarean section and so there must be someone present who is capable of delivering a breech vaginally. The third problem is that second twins are often delivered by breech. One therefore either has to say that all twins should be delivered by Caesarean section or make sure that experienced staff are available, even if the general policy is to deliver breeches by Caesarean section. The fourth problem is that an increased rate of Caesarean section for singleton (and twin) breech delivery will inevitably result in there being no one left capable of delivering a breech vaginally. The fifth is that there are some women who want a vaginal breech delivery and who will not agree to a Caesarean section.

It is therefore both likely, and in the author's opinion advisable, that vaginal breech deliveries will continue to be performed. To this end, the safest way forward is for any woman suspected of having a breech to be advised to undergo a scan to confirm the presentation, the approximate size of the fetus and the *attitude* of its head. Some obstetricians would also recommend *pelvimetry* – that is to say, measurement of the size of the maternal pelvis by means of X-ray or, preferably, magnetic resonance imaging (MRI). There is still some doubt, however, as to whether pelvimetry selects cases accurately for vaginal delivery or whether knowledge of pelvic adequacy gives the obstetrician confidence in allowing women a trial of vaginal breech delivery.[24] Armed with this and all the other factors which must be taken into account, including the level of experience available on the labour ward, the senior obstetrician (preferably the consultant) who sees the woman will be able to advise her of the risks in her particular case and help her decide on a course of action that is acceptable to all concerned.

This may include an external cephalic version (ECV), in which the fetus is physically turned from breech to cephalic presentation. Where suitable, the possibility should be raised and its risks and benefits carefully explained. Apart from occasionally being unsuccessful, ECV carries significant risks, including causing fetal distress and precipitating premature labour. Its advantage, however, is that it eliminates any need for discussion about the route of delivery of the breech. If it is carried out successfully, there is no need to worry further, providing that the fetus does not turn back into breech presentation. If the woman declines ECV, or if it is unsuccessful, the decision about route of delivery still has to be made and further counselling is required.

The risks of delivery by both routes should again be carefully explained, bearing in mind that while the counselling should be non-directional, it is both right and proper that the obstetrician makes his or her views clear. Thus, if a woman chooses in favour of a vaginal breech delivery when the consultant believes that the risks of that course of action in that particular case are unacceptably high (even if only because of a shortage of skilled staff), the consultant should make this clear and, if necessary, offer a second opinion elsewhere. The same applies if the consultant believes that an attempt at vaginal delivery is the correct way forward but the woman does not.

It also follows that senior obstetric staff should personally supervise every vaginal breech delivery.

Twins and higher multiples

All the symptoms and complications of pregnancy are more pronounced in multiple pregnancy. Malpresentation is more common, the placenta is larger and therefore more likely to be low-lying, and conditions such as pre-eclampsia are likely to arise earlier and be more severe. For these reasons, it is considered good practice to ask a woman with a multiple pregnancy to attend the antenatal clinic more frequently and to undergo regular ultrasound scans to monitor fetal growth. An experienced obstetrician should see her at around 34 weeks both to assess the progress of the pregnancy and to begin a dialogue with the woman regarding the nature of the labour. Many women with multiple pregnancies are now being advised to undergo elective Caesarean section (especially with three or more fetuses) but many still attempt – and succeed – with vaginal delivery. Once again, the labour ward management of twins is well recognised but any particular concerns should still be recorded in the woman's labour records well in advance.

Medical conditions in pregnancy

There are too many conditions to discuss them all in this chapter, but in essence the management of each is essentially the same, dependent on the nature and extent of the medical problem. The woman should be assessed by the appropriate specialist (for example, a cardiologist or a specialist in diabetes) and she should also be seen by an experienced obstetrician who can both assess the fetal growth *and* decide on the timing and route of delivery.

The most common medical disorder in pregnancy is pre-eclampsia. Its nature, symptoms and signs are well known and, as a result, the associated morbidity and mortality have fallen dramatically. Nevertheless, it is still a potentially dangerous disease and once again input from a senior obstetrician is essential. This is particularly the case with regard to the decision when to deliver. To a large extent, this decision is based on experience (and learned texts); but regrettably, the decision to deliver is made occasionally by a relatively junior doctor and may result in an unnecessary induction or Caesarean section and a premature baby, or a woman who suffers an eclamptic fit because she was not delivered soon enough. For this reason, no woman should be deemed to have pre-eclampsia without protein in her urine and every woman with pre-eclampsia – that is to say, a raised blood pressure and protein in her urine – should be seen by a senior obstetrician as soon as the condition is diagnosed.

Another area of growing concern is the management of *haemoglobinopathies* – genetic disorders that include sickle cell disease and thalassaemia which, because of the increasingly multiethnic mix of most British communities, are being seen with increasing frequency. In most cases, the mother is not at risk but her children may be, particularly when her partner may have an abnormal haemoglobin as well. For this reason, all women at risk should be screened for haemoglobinopathies in early pregnancy by means of haemoglobin electrophoresis. Those that have a haemoglobinopathy should have their partners tested as well and every effort must be made to review the results of both as soon as possible. There are specialist centres familiar with the problem and so if there is any doubt about the management, the obstetrician can seek help.

Fear of vaginal birth and the woman who requests Caesarean section

It is becoming common for women to ask for an elective Caesarean section. The reasons are numerous and range from fear of a vaginal delivery to extreme concern that something may go wrong in labour. Many obstetricians and midwives are uncomfortable with such 'non-obstetric' indications for Caesarean section and are reluctant even to consider them, although many more are now coming to terms with the fact that such requests are being made by an increasingly educated and aware population who have considered the matter very carefully indeed. So how should the obstetrician or midwife approach these situations?

The obvious starting point is to ask the woman why she wants an elective Caesarean section and then to discuss these reasons. Because it is not an emergency situation, the discussion should include all the potential complications and risks of each option, the level of disclosure being that which the prudent patient would be expect to know in order to make an informed choice, not that which the reasonable doctor would be expected to give. That is not to say that the doctor should not also offer his or her opinion and advice. It is both reasonable and expected that this should happen, although not to the point of confrontation. If the obstetrician is unhappy about the woman's decision, or she is unhappy with the obstetrician's advice, it is perfectly reasonable to suggest a second opinion. Ultimately, however, the woman herself will have to make the risk/benefit analysis and decide one way or another.

The increased awareness of the potential problems and complications of pregnancy, especially in labour, is likely to continue to push women towards requesting elective Caesarean section. In those cases where events in labour have resulted in a less than optimal outcome for mother or baby, there will inevitably be concern that a Caesarean section should have been offered and performed. And where media attention and political opportunism have highlighted problems in the healthcare sector, pregnant women and their carers may feel it safer to avoid them by avoiding labour altogether. There is no doubt that adopting this approach this may result in a further increase in the rate of Caesarean section but this seems inevitable in the context of the current ethical, legal and sociological trends. Obstetricians should not assume that they are totally responsible for the rising Caesarean section rates; nor should society or pressure groups lay the blame for it at their feet.

Conclusion

Few can argue that the advances in antenatal care over the second half of the twentieth century have had at least as great an impact on the outcome of pregnancy as have the advances in the management of labour itself. Much has changed and in all probability will continue to do so over the next 50 years. Advances in prenatal diagnosis and fetal medicine will add to the complexity of antenatal care, and advances in the medical management of conditions such as hypertension and diabetes will mean that there will be more high-risk pregnancies to manage. Changes in the ethical, political and legal framework will affect many aspects of obstetric care and women's expectations of a satisfactory outcome for every pregnancy are unlikely to diminish.

Whatever the changes yet to come, there can be no doubt that good antenatal care will continue to be the foundation for the successful outcome of pregnancy. The way in which antenatal care is delivered undoubtedly will evolve in line with advances in knowledge and technology and the recognition that there must be a partnership between the pregnant woman and her carers. The essential risk-management functions of antenatal care – namely maintenance of maternal and fetal health, recognition of potential problems, and education – are, however, unlikely to change.

References

1 O'Dowd MJ, Philipp EE. *The History of Obstetrics and Gynaecology*. London: The Parthenon Publishing Group, 1994: 83–85.

2 Charles J. Pregnant pause. *Nursing Times* 1992; 88(34): 30–32.

3 Llewellyn-Jones D. *Fundamentals of Obstetrics and Gynaecology*. London: Faber & Faber, 1973: 59.

4 Giddens A. *Sociology*, 3rd edition. Oxford: Polity Press, 1997: 121.

5 Department of Health. *Changing Childbirth*. Report of the Expert Maternity Group. London: HMSO, 1993.

6 Sweet ER. Antenatal care. In: ER Sweet, D Tiran (eds.) *Mayes' Midwifery*, 12th Edition. London: Bailliere–Tindall, 1997: 211.

7 Ethical considerations relating to good practice in obstetrics and gynaecology. http://www.rcog.org.uk/guidelines/ethics/ethical.html.

8 General Medical Council. *Intimate examinations*. A statement by the General Medical Council, 1996.

9 Kennedy I. *Treat Me Right: Essays in Medical Law and Ethics*. Oxford: Clarendon Press, 1988.

10 Moerman ML. Growth of the birth canal in adolescent girls. *American Journal of Obstetrics and Gynaecology* 1982; 143: 528–532.

11 Hofmeyr GJ. *Turnbull's Obstetrics*. London: Churchill Livingstone, 1994.

12 The Report on Confidential Enquiries into Maternal Deaths in the United Kingdom between 1994 and 1996 (published by HMSO, London, in 1998) lists one such occurrence in that triennium.

13 Enkin M, Keirse MJNC, Rebfrew M, Neilson J. *A Guide to Effective Care in Pregnancy and Childbirth*, 2nd edn. Oxford: Oxford University Press, 1995: 285.

14 Thornton JG, Lilford RJ. The Caesarean section decision: patient's choices are not determined by immediate emotional reactions. *Journal of Obstetrics and Gynaecology* 1989; 9: 283–288.

15 Al-Mufti R, McCarthy A, Fisk N. Obstetricians' personal choice and mode of delivery. *Lancet* 1996; 347: 544.

16 World Health Organisation. *The Partograph*, sections I, II, III and IV. WHO/MCH/88.4 Geneva: WHO/Maternal and Child Health Unit, Division of Family Health, 1998.

17 Enkin M, Keirse MJNC, Renfrew M, Neilson J. *A Guide to Effective Care in Pregnancy and Childbirth*, 2nd edn. Oxford: Oxford University Press, 1995: 142.

18 Acker DB, Sachs BP, Friedman EA. Risk factors for shoulder dystocia. *Obstetrics and Gynaecology* 1985; 66: 762–768; Gross TL, Sokol RJ, Williams T, Thompson K. Shoulder dystocia: a fetal-physician risk *American Journal of Obstetrics and Gynaecology* 1987; 156: 1408–1419; Langer O, Berkus M, Huff RW, Samueloff A. Shoulder dystocia: should the fetus weighing ≥4000 grams be delivered by Caesarean section? *American Journal of Obstetrics and Gynaecology* 1991; 165: 831–837.

19 Smith RB, Lane C, Pearson JF. Shoulder dystocia: what happens at the next delivery? *British Journal of Obstetrics and Gynaecology* 1994; 101: 713–715.

20 Johnstone FD, Myerscough PR. Shoulder dystocia. *British Journal of Obstetrics and Gynaecology* 1998; 105: 811–815.

21 Penn ZJ, Steer PJ. In: DK James, PJ Steer, CP Weiner, B Gonik (eds.) *High Risk Pregnancy Management Options*. London: WB Saunders, 1994: 173–174.

22 Nelson KB, Ellenberg JH. Antecedents of cerebral palsy: multivariate analysis of risks. *New England Journal of Medicine* 1986; 315: 81–86.

23 Maternal and Child Health Research Consortium. *Confidential Enquiries into Stillbirths and Deaths in Infancy*, 7th Annual Report.

24 Walkinshaw S. Pelvimetry and breech delivery at term. *Lancet* 1997; 350: 191–192.

▶12

Intrapartum Care

Donald M F Gibb

Introduction

The process of labour and delivery has been described as the most hazardous journey any individual has to face. Until the past 100 years, the risks to mother and baby were substantial and they still are in countries with less developed systems of healthcare. The Taj Mahal is testament to the memory of Mumtaz Mahal who died in her fifteenth pregnancy of postpartum haemorrhage. Advances in fertility control, improving social circumstances, modern anaesthetic techniques, Caesarean section and blood transfusion have been the main factors involved in the huge reductions in maternal mortality over the past 100 years.

The issues of maternal mortality were addressed at the Safe Motherhood Conference in Nairobi 1987, and guidelines were formulated in response.[1] The tragedy of the death of the mother has become rare in this country. Public expectations are high and an adverse result of this nature is likely to result in threatened litigation. The medical profession and the media have presented an idealized picture of perfect reproduction. Sadly the Confidential Enquiries into Maternal Death (*Why Mothers Die*)[2] and the Confidential Enquiry into Stillbirth and Deaths in Infancy (CESDI)[3] reports have highlighted serious deficiencies in care resulting in potentially avoidable deaths and possible injuries. There is much basic work to be done in creating a safer environment. These issues are addressed in the Royal College of Obstetricians and Gynaecologists/Royal College of Midwives document *Towards Safer Childbirth.*[4]

The context of care has to embrace evidence-based medicine and the principles enunciated in the government report *Changing Childbirth.*[5] Evidence-based medicine is widely considered as providing templates which should guide our practice.[6] The Guidelines and Audit Committee of the Royal College of Obstetricians and Gynaecologists makes three grades of recommendations. A Grade-A recommendation requires at least one randomized controlled trial as part of a body of literature of overall good quality, and consistency addressing the specific recommendation. A Grade-B recommendation requires the availability of well-controlled clinical studies but no randomized controlled trials of the topic of recommendations. A Grade-C recommendation requires evidence obtained from expert committee reports or opinions and/or clinical experiences of respected authorities. Grade C indicates an absence of directly applicable clinical studies of good quality.

Grade-A and -B evidence relevant to decisions in intrapartum care is hard to find. The most obvious available Grade-A evidence is the use of steroids in threatened premature birth and the use of prophylactic antibiotics at Caesarean section. Failure to implement such treatments, when the opportunity presents itself, would now be considered an unacceptable standard of care amounting to negligent treatment. However, such evidence is not available to help us to make decisions in most clinical situations. The most common decisions with respect to induction of labour, augmentation of labour, mode of delivery and electronic fetal monitoring continue to be based of grade-C evidence and will continue to be so for the foreseeable future. There has been much debate about whether obstetrics is an art or a science; although many would wish it to be more of a science, largely it continues to be an art.

We are also encouraged to embrace the principles of *Changing Childbirth*[5] in our daily practice. This essentially means that women are at the centre of care and should be offered choice in readily accessible care. The concept of active birth or natural birth has become popular in recent years. This has partly been a reaction to the over-medicalization of birth manifest in one respect as the 'epidemic' of Caesarean birth. Women with birth plans are expressing an intelligent interest in there own biological processes. This should not be discouraged and the professionals should aim to assist in the birth experience that women are seeking. Home birth should be seen as an available option and doctors should not adopt a critical or defensive position about it. Alternative delivery positions, water birth and complementary methods of care should all be included in strategies for safe care.

The organization of care

Care is delivered by midwives and doctors together. Each group of professionals should respect the skills and practices of the other in effective collaboration. All should have a motivation and desire in this important task. Continuing education of both groups should have common elements in problematic areas of care. Clinical risk management is a component of clinical governance. It is an approach to improving the quality of care that places special emphasis on care episodes with unexpected outcomes. It draws from the Department of Health report entitled *An Organisation with a Memory*,[7] an important publication emphasizing that lessons can be learned from medical mistakes.

Midwives are at the frontline of care. Although in principle staff should work where they are happy to work, it is important that they should maintain varied skills. Home birth midwives should also have gained valuable experience with high-risk cases in the labour ward. They should be up to date on emergency procedures, fetal monitoring and practical skills. A home-birth midwife should be trained to do a cardiotocograph (CTG) without a CTG machine. Midwives should be able to depend upon the support of sympathetic doctors; and these doctors should be available and accessible. There should be at least one consultant in each unit who is able to support the midwives providing the home-birth service. Doctors in training have a limited amount of experience and should be well supported by experienced senior colleagues. There are now several practical courses available to teach skills in the labour ward.

In each delivery unit, there should be morning review including midwifery and medical staff. All cases should be considered as team cases. The concept of midwives' cases and doctor's cases is divisive. A low-risk case will be at least 99% midwife care. By the same token, a high-risk woman with numerous problems should receive skilled midwifery input as well as a clear involvement of the doctor. There should be a review of each case and a decision made jointly as to whether it is necessary for the medical staff to see the woman. If the experienced midwife is happy with the situation and the risk assessment, she might not require direct medical input. This should also be dependent on the view of the woman and her partner. In turn, the doctor should not adopt a dominating position denying the midwife her due status as the primary carer. In a busy labour ward there should also be focused systematic reviews at intervals during the day and late in the evening. The Royal College of Obstetricians and Gynaecologists, in a joint report with the Royal College of Midwives, has recommended that the consultant on-call for the labour ward should conduct labour-ward rounds at least twice during the day, with a telephone or physical round during the evening. It is right that doctors and midwives should not work prolonged hours but several shift changes will fragment care. The integrated overview must be retained.

The continuum of pregnancy is from conception to the cot. The journey of late pregnancy and labour is the subject of this discussion.

Late pregnancy

Consideration of the events in labour cannot be considered without setting the clinical scenario in late pregnancy. As outlined in the previous chapter, antenatal care is essentially screening for risk factors. Risk is only of value as a screening concept. When we say there is risk, we must elaborate a risk 'of what? ' The consequential risk of having high blood pressure is different from the consequential risk of placenta praevia or a previous Caesarean section, for example.

At each antenatal visit, a standard assessment is undertaken. It is important to listen to the fetal heart in the antenatal clinic, preferably with a Doptone. There is no grade-A or -B evidence to show that this should be done – especially in a normal pregnancy; however, rarely an arrhythmia may be detected – and women like to hear their baby's heart beat. This alone is enough justification by grade-C evidence. A plan should be discussed and laid out for labour and delivery, bearing in mind the risk factors involved in, for example, multiple pregnancy, breech presentation and previous caesarean section. Full use should be made of the 'special features' box which appears in the case notes and is designed to pass on concern about abnormal features of the pregnancy, especially to the carers in labour. Warning about a small or a large baby is especially important. The fact that there have been serial scans because of intra-uterine growth restriction (IUGR) should be highlighted, for example. A history of good fetal movements is reassuring. Extensive medico-legal experience suggests that this flagging tool is not used properly – forewarned is forearmed.

A minority of women write a birth plan that is usually non-controversial. It should be read, discussed and acknowledged in the late antenatal period; any unusual aspect of it should be flagged for review after admission to the delivery unit.

Types of labour

Labour may be spontaneous or induced. Most women present to the labour ward with a spontaneous event. This is most often contractions, a show, leaking fluid or a combination of these. Many women complain of backache in late pregnancy. Admission to the labour ward is the time for careful review.[8]

Pre-labour rupture of the membranes (PROM)

Leaking of amniotic fluid without the immediate onset of contractions should be considered abnormal, although it occurs remarkably frequently. In natural labour, the membranes tend to rupture late – even remaining intact until the baby has been delivered. Dickens referred to David Copperfield as having been born in a 'caul' – that is, in the bag of intact membranes. Such a phenomenon is still seen in countries where there is a minimum of medical interference in the delivery process. The purpose of the membranes and the contained amniotic fluid is to cushion the fetus and the umbilical cord from outside pressure and to protect the fetus from infection. Absence of this protective mechanism is important. The membrane at term is quite tough and hence sometimes is difficult to rupture. It may be that prior damage to the membrane, whether by infection or previous bleeding, has destabilized it. The woman with membrane rupture presents with a complaint of losing fluid from her vagina. Initial assessment requires a confirmation that amniotic fluid is draining, which can sometimes be difficult. In some cases, leakage of fluid is obvious but in others a speculum examination with or without the use of an amnistix is necessary. Digital examination of the cervix should be avoided unless a decision has already been made to proceed to delivery. A low vaginal swab should be taken for microbiological assessment; and the presence of β-haemolytic streptococcus requires a decision to move towards delivery. If a woman is known to be a carrier of β-haemolytic streptococcus, consideration should be given to induction of labour with the concurrent use of intravenous antibiotics. A hind-water leak is probably relatively common and less threatening to the fetus, although it may be difficult to substantiate. What is important is not how *much* fluid has leaked out but rather how much fluid *remains inside*. This is only determined reliably by an ultrasound scan. Ideally, such an assessment should be available on the labour ward. A CTG is important in this situation.

Pregnancies with reduced amniotic fluid are more prone to umbilical-cord compression, which may be manifest as variable decelerations on the CTG. It must be remembered that fetuses in breech presentation require special consideration – they are even more likely to compress their cord, particularly when active labour commences. It is prudent to monitor continuously and move towards delivery by Caesarean section in these cases.

When the presentation is cephalic, watchful expectancy is appropriate. The woman should be instructed to take her temperature daily and report any change in the nature of the vaginal discharge. A CTG should be performed at least every other day. Most cases will commence labour within three days, but after that it may be wiser to induce labour – especially if there is a maternal pyrexia. Infection may manifest as the onset of labour. Infection does not seem to be a major threat to the term fetus; however, appropriate precautions should be taken to detect and treat it in the baby after birth.

Preterm pre-labour rupture of the membranes (PPROM)

Loss of fluid before maturity presents a greater challenge to the fetus but this is largely due to the threat of premature birth rather than that of infection. In modern practice, with neonatal intensive-care facilities, prematurity is not a significant threat after 34 weeks gestation. Before 26 weeks gestation, however, the couple should be warned of the poor prognosis. Currently, there is debate about the role of antibiotic treatment in this situation, but steroid therapy certainly should be given from 26 weeks gestation. Tocolytic therapy is contra-indicated because the active contractions may be the result of an infective process, and prolongation of the pregnancy may exacerbate the infection. Watchful expectancy is appropriate; however, the added risks of umbilical-cord prolapse with a breech presentation must be considered. Delivery should be considered if there is a breech presentation with membrane rupture in women having reached a gestational age of 32 weeks.

Preterm labour

Premature birth makes a major contribution to perinatal mortality and morbidity. Extensive research has not led to any significant reduction in the rate of premature birth. There are multiple causes such as multiple pregnancy, bleeding, infection, uterine malformation, cervical weakness and elective preterm delivery. There is limited evidence of the value of reduced physical activity, longer-term tocolytic therapy, antibiotic therapy, hormonal therapy or cervical cerclage, except in specific situations. If active contractions are present before 26 weeks, without an obvious treatable precipitant factor, then it is unlikely that short-term tocolytic therapy will lead to a significant prolongation of pregnancy. Between 26 and 34 weeks, there is value in using dexamethasone (12 mg twice daily for two doses) and to inhibit uterine contractions using tocolytic therapy (for 24–48 hours). The most commonly used tocolytics are beta-mimetics such as ritodrine, but these drugs must be used with extreme caution – they cause a maternal tachycardia with the possibility of cardio-respiratory embarrassment. Most of the modern fetal monitors are capable of recording the maternal pulse rate continuously, and this facility is useful in this situation when frequent assessment of maternal pulse is necessary. A guideline with supervision and review by a senior doctor is important. Other tocolytics are becoming more commonly used and should be considered.

If premature labour is well established with a cephalic presentation, vaginal birth with continuous electronic fetal monitoring is reasonable. Preterm labour is usually rapid. If there is a breech presentation or a twin pregnancy, an experienced doctor should consider whether Caesarean section is preferable. Beyond 34 weeks gestation, the decision-making process is based on principles applied to a term pregnancy. There is no grade-A evidence to guide us in this situation.

Spontaneous labour

Most women present to the labour ward with spontaneous contractions. This is the time for an admission review consisting of history, examination and admission CTG.[8] This is the final and most hazardous part of the journey to birth. There is an interplay between the powers of the uterus, the passages of the birth canal, the placenta and the passenger (single or multiple). Each contraction presents a challenge to oxygenation through the feto-placental unit. As uterine pressure rises, blood flow into the placental bed is reduced. Each contraction necessary to promote dilatation of the uterine cervix and descent of the fetus transiently deprives the placenta of blood flow and consequently the fetus of oxygen. In some cases, there is a deficiency in the utero-placental vasculature, which restricts the flow of blood into the intervillous space. The intervillous space itself may be restricted in volume proportionate to a restriction in the size of the placenta. This reduction of feto-placental reserve manifests as progressive CTG abnormalities.

Our access in assessing the health of the fetus is limited to indirect evidence from fetal movement, fetal growth and the fetal heart rate.

Admission assessment

Risk factors in a medical history are well recognized. Some have a condition-specific chance of recurrence (eg premature labour) but others, such as postpartum haemorrhage, are less consistent. The most important factors are those already present in the current pregnancy. There is a continuum from the antenatal period through to labour and delivery. The immediate carer – the bedside midwife – should have a clear grasp of any issues and be able to communicate them to colleagues participating in the care. A very recent history of good fetal movements is very reassuring. Brief general examination is undertaken after admission but the most important examination is that of the abdomen and pelvis. General examination should note the height and weight of the woman, which will already be recorded in the notes. Maternal height bears a direct relationship to maternal pelvic size – it is useful to have some impression of this in women of short stature and women with previous caesarean section.

Examination should focus initially on the maternal abdomen. Large or small fetuses have different implications: a *large* fetus may face the hazard of prolonged labour with the possibility of cephalo-pelvic disproportion or shoulder dystocia; and a *small* fetus may have impaired placental function with IUGR. Attention should be directed to both these features. What is the presentation? In units where there is no routine late ultrasound scan, breech presentation may be missed. The maintenance of clinical skills is important in these 'technology-dependent' days. Consider every pregnancy to be a breech until you are certain it is cephalic. Is the 'deeply engaged' head a breech? A deeply engaged head causes symptoms of pelvic pressure on her bladder and her bowel. Does the woman feel a hard lump under her ribs? When a breech has been missed, the woman often says that she knew it felt unusual and was not right. In a debriefing consultation with a couple after an undiagnosed breech, it is difficult to explain (excuse?) why it has been missed on several examinations. After palpating the abdomen, the fetal heart should be auscultated, ensuring it is at a different rate from the maternal pulse. The maternal pulse should be documented at the start of a CTG and at intervals, to verify that fetal and maternal pulse are different. This will avoid the dreadful mistake of believing the fetus is alive when it is dead.

Vaginal examination provides information about the process, especially by observing the dilation of the cervix and the descent of the presenting part. In abnormal labour, the application of the presenting part to the cervix is important – a thickening cervix or a persisting anterior lip of cervix are adverse signs. The colour and volume of the amniotic fluid should be observed. Absence of amniotic fluid with ruptured membranes is a potentially adverse sign suggesting oligohydramnios. In a woman who has had a previous Caesarean section or who is of short stature, the opportunity should not be lost to gain some impression of pelvic size. This has become a disappearing art in the past 30 years.

The third part of assessment on admission is the CTG. A well grown, moving, healthy fetus is likely to have a normal CTG. However, sometimes there is an unexpected abnormality. There may have been some antenatal adverse event or a risk factor may have been missed. Using a CTG provides additional information that is not available on auscultation concerning baseline variability. This CTG can be limited by starting it when the baby has started moving. Fetuses have quiescent periods when the CTG will not show accelerations for 20–50 minutes. It is important that the CTG is discontinued when it is normal. There is a valid criticism that such a CTG leads to continuing monitoring especially in units where there is a shortage of midwives. This should not be the reason for using CTGs inappropriately. There is no grade-A recommendation for the use of an admission CTG but neither is there for taking a history or performing an examination. There is logic and sense in undertaking such a test. The woman's opinion may also be sought. Most women find an admission CTG reassuring, providing positive support for them at the start of labour.

Strategy of surveillance

Every unit should have its guideline as to how the fetus should be monitored. The word 'monitoring' implies clinical, as well as electronic, techniques. If the admission assessment is normal in all respects, the chance of severe fetal asphyxia supervening in the following four hours is minimal. This could only be because of an acute event such as placental abruption or cord prolapse. A major abruption sufficient to threaten the fetus would also cause signs or symptoms, although these would not necessarily include revealed bleeding. A major concealed abruption would cause pain of a persistent nature. It would also cause the woman to feel distressed and agitated. Pain and agitation are relatively common in the labour ward and busy staff may not be alert to a possible abruption – it should always be born in mind as one of the most threatening pathologies that we see. Umbilical-cord prolapse can also threaten the baby with little warning. We must be aware of the necessity to check for signs of cord prolapse after membrane rupture and always to bear it in mind with breech presentation. It is an eminently treatable condition when it occurs in hospital. If there is significant umbilical-cord compression with or without cord prolapse it will be seen on the CTG as variable decelerations.

After the admission assessment, intermittent auscultation, with the woman mobilizing, should be performed for the following three to four hours or until a risk factor appears. This may be with whatever instrument is suitable; however, it also should be remembered that the woman also likes to hear the heart beat of her baby. There is no national recommendation about the frequency of intermittent auscultation but the Royal College of Obstetricians and Gynaecologists has a Guideline Development Group currently working on fetal monitoring, including this issue. Intermittent auscultation should be carried out around every 15–30 minutes in the first stage of labour, immediately after a contraction, for 30–60 seconds. If there is an audible abnormality of the fetal heart, meconium appears or there is another complication, electronic monitoring should be re-instituted. In a nulliparous woman who may not be delivered in the following four hours, a further strip of CTG is appropriate with the four-hour review.

The late first stage and the second stage of labour are times of the strongest and most frequent contractions. The frequency of auscultation should then be increased to every 5–15 minutes and finally after every contraction when pushing in the second stage of labour. This is a reasonable plan for the low-risk woman with no risk factors. There is high risk and low risk but there is no such thing as *no risk*. High-risk pregnancies merit closer surveillance. This is absolutely essential in pregnancies already recognized to have utero-placental insufficiency, which can only be exacerbated in labour. Continuous electronic fetal heart rate monitoring should also be considered in hypertension, diabetes, twin pregnancy, breech presentation and with other high-risk factors. Amniotic fluid may be noticed to be reduced or discoloured. Failure to see much fluid at artificial rupture of the membranes, referred to as 'scanty', or discoloration of the fluid are risk factors. If no fluid is seen, a gentle attempt should be made to push the fetal head upwards. If this fails to release fluid then the risk of oligohydramnios and possible occult meconium staining should be considered; careful analysis of the CTG is essential. If meconium is present it may be physiological or pathological. The key to this assessment is its volume; just as we are reassured by a good volume of fluid seen on late scan, so we are assured by a good volume of fluid draining. Meconium is not visible on ultrasound scan. There are many ways to describe meconium but this can be simplified into whether it is in a good volume of fluid with the draw sheet widely stained or whether it is scanty meconium only staining the vulval pad. Mature fetuses pass meconium for physiological reasons of maturity into a good volume of amniotic fluid. Fetuses suffering a degree of compromise pass meconium pathologically into a reduced volume of amniotic fluid; this will be 'thick' meconium. Most units recommend continuous electronic fetal heart rate monitoring in the presence of meconium. If it is meconium in a good volume of amniotic fluid, this may not be necessary. Similarly, if a home-birth midwife is convinced that the fetal heart has a normal rate and no decelerations in the presence of meconium, then, after consultation with an obstetrician, the labour may continue at home.

Electronic fetal monitoring

This was introduced in the late 1960s with the hope and expectation that it would reduce intrapartum death and morbidity; unfortunately, however, this has not proved to be the case. Our understanding of the CTG has lagged behind the technological developments. Cerebral palsy (CP) is a non-progressive neurological condition that evolves in the early years of life with development of the nervous system (see Chapter 14 for a detailed discussion). The incidence does not appear to have changed in recent years. Perinatal events may only be implicated in about 15% of cases of CP. and these are usually cases of the dyskinetic (abnormal movement) and spastic quadriplegic types. Other factors – such as the increasing survival of very low birthweight babies – may have contributed to the rate of CP, which could have hidden any improvement from changing standards of intrapartum care.

This static rate of CP cases is not evidence of the lack of effect of intrapartum surveillance. Nonetheless, it is apparent that even when electronic monitoring is undertaken errors are still made by staff. Ennis and Vincent[9] studied 64 cases that had come to litigation in respect of a perinatal death. In 11 cases, continuous fetal heart rate monitoring was omitted although in the event it would clearly have been valuable. In 34 of the remaining 53 cases, the tracing was abnormal but in 11 cases this was not identified by the attending doctor, most of whom were junior (being of senior house officer or registrar grade). Gaffney et al.[10] reported that although most cases of CP are not associated with preventable factors during labour, these are present clinically and medico-legally in a significant number of cases. From a total birth cohort of 132,743 during 1984 to 1987, 339 cases of CP and 63 perinatal deaths (PND) were compared with babies born immediately before and after the index case. Thirty-six percent of the CP cases were associated with preterm birth, 12% with congenital abnormality and 8% a definite postnatal event. Of the 145 singleton term births without congenital abnormalities, 141 could be matched with 257 controls. Only 6% of cases of CP had a five-minute Apgar score of less than two, compared with 65% in cases of PND (controls: zero in both groups). However, in 26% of cases of CP, there were signs of 'fetal distress' in labour which were not responded to, compared with only 7% in controls. The corresponding figures for PND were 50% and 7%. This means that one CP case in every 4023 births possibly were preventable; the corresponding figure for PND was one in 4425 births. Extrapolation to a UK birth rate of 700,000 per annum, this implies that there are around 200 potentially preventable cases of CP per year in this country and another 160 potentially preventable PNDs. More recent data from the CESDI[3] surveys suggest that errors in CTG interpretation are all too frequent.

There is a lack of good evidence from randomized controlled trials concerning the effectiveness of electronic fetal heart rate monitoring (EFM). The only large-scale study looking at the value of intermittent auscultation compared with (the currently more usual) EFM was carried out in Dublin in the early 1980s.[11] In this study, they randomized almost 14,000 women into two groups, and compared those managed with intermittent auscultation and fetal-scalp blood sampling with those managed with EFM. The methodology did not include specification on standards of training in EFM. Moreover, they only included relatively low-risk labours, as demonstrated by the fact that there were only *five* intrapartum stillbirths in the study, a rate of one per 2800 births. This compares with an intrapartum stillbirth rate of about one to two per 1000 births in most UK labour wards during the 1980s. There were only two stillbirths in the intermittent auscultation group compared with three in the EFM group. It is notable that the practice of EFM in the National Maternity Hospital, Dublin, has grown steadily in recent years.

There has been a notable lack of education and understanding of CTGs. In a programme of education over the past 12 years, midwives showed a much greater interest in attending educational seminars than doctors. The role of the midwife is to detect any deviation from normal and then ask a doctor to review (Rule 40, Midwives Rules, United Kingdom Central Council for Nursing and Midwifery). The decision then rests in the hands of the doctors. In medico-legal practice, it is unusual to find cases where there is criticism that a CTG was not done but more common to find it was not done at the right time or it was misinterpreted. In particular, there is a frequent association of the poor interpretation of a CTG with the use of syntocinon. Doctors, by the very nature of how labour wards are organized, tend to come and go. The midwife stays with the woman. In coming and going, the doctor gets a fragmented view of the situation and may pay more attention to the machine than to the mother. A common error is to manage the CTG rather than the composite clinical situation. This is further exacerbated by frequent changes of shift by doctors – every four hours in some labour wards. It is important to evaluate changes over time in labour both in the clinical situation and with the CTG.

The features of a normal CTG are not disputed (see Figure 12.1). The normal fetal heart rate falls with gestation. Early this century, before the advent of EFM, it was thought that the normal fetal heart rate was 100–160 beats per minute (bpm). Greater experience with electronic monitoring has shown that it is actually 110–160 beats per minute (bpm). In 1987, the International Federation of Obstetrics and Gynaecology (FIGO) suggested a classification that included a normal baseline rate of 110–150 bpm at term.[12] Beard et al.[13] originally suggested that a baseline rate of 110–120 bpm was a reassuring feature. Not infrequently, this occurs with a steady baseline in a normal healthy fetus subsequently born in good condition. A rate of 150–160 bpm is less common at term. Such a fetus may be being exposed to a long labour, epidural anaesthesia, and syntocinon, with consequent stresses. In labour, a steadily rising rate warrants careful attention. It is important for the range of normality to be clarified because it is on this basis that a midwife would consider it necessary to inform a doctor of the situation.

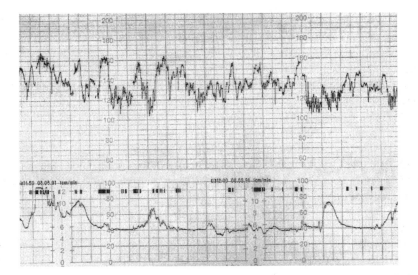

Fig. 12.1. Normal CTG.

Irrespective of the actual rate, the key to fetal health is accelerations and baseline variability: reactivity. Accelerations are associated clearly with fetal activity. Normal baseline variability indicates an intact central control through the autonomic nervous system. This appears to be very important as an indicator of fetal health. Changes in the baseline rate indicating changes in continuing fetal condition are important.

Decelerations are indicators of short-term events. Early decelerations suggest head compression that may occur with physiological events such as descent of the head in the late first stage and second stage of labour. Head compression also occurs with spontaneous or artificial membrane rupture and vaginal examination. An early deceleration is U shaped, inversely reflecting the contraction.

Late decelerations are a sign of hypoxia possibly due to myocardial ischaemia. They suggest a utero-placental problem and once established in labour it generally does not improve with time.

Variable decelerations suggest umbilical-cord compression. They vary in shape and timing because of anatomical plasticity of the umbilical cord. They are more frequent when the cushioning effect of the amniotic fluid is lost on account of membrane rupture or reduced amniotic fluid due to other reasons. The umbilical cord contains two arteries and a vein. The arteries carry blood away from the fetus to the placenta at higher pressure and are thick-walled. The veins return the blood to the fetus with lower pressure and the vessel is thin-walled. When the cord is compressed, the vein is compressed first, resulting in a reduction of circulating blood volume in the fetus. The autonomic nervous system responds to this by transiently increasing the pulse rate.

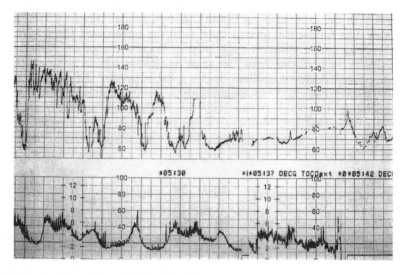

Fig. 12.2. Acute hypoxia: umbilical-cord prolapse.

This, however, is short lived as the artery then becomes compressed and there is a resulting fall in the heart rate. Release of compression results in an opposite effect. Well-grown, healthy fetuses can tolerate cord compression for many hours but changes in baseline rate and variability are signs of decompensation. The appearance of the deceleration is the still snap shot but the full CTG is the video evolution.

The concept of fetal distress as a description of a CTG is unhelpful. A CTG is better described in agreed terminology and the other clinical factors then taken into account. Some attempt should be made to attribute an underlying pathophysiology to the scenario. There are many false positives in CTG interpretation when the expression 'fetal distress' is abused. A CTG can be considered not normal for physiological, iatrogenic or pathological reasons. Physiological causes may be head compression, cord compression, maternal posture and rapid progress in labour. Iatrogenic reasons may be the use of Syntocinon, prostaglandins, other drugs or artificial rupture of the membranes. Pathological reasons for an abnormal CTG may be hypoxia, infection or intrinsic fetal disorders such as brain abnormality, cardiac abnormality and chromosomal abnormality. Effective CTG interpretation requires an understanding of these issues.

The following classification is a simplification and distillation of the FIGO recommendation.

Classification of fetal heart rate pattern intrapartum

Normal

Baseline heart rate between 110 and 150 bpm, baseline variability 10–25 bpm, two accelerations in 20 minutes and no decelerations.

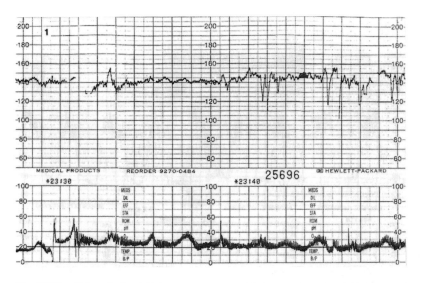

Fig. 12.3A Subacute hypoxia.

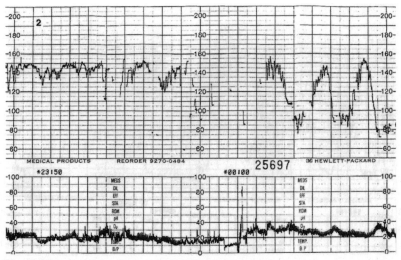

Fig. 12.3B

Suspicious

Absence of accelerations (first to become apparent, important) and any one of the following:

- Abnormal rate <110 or >150 bpm

- Reduced baseline variability <10 bpm and of greater significance if <5 bpm

- Variable decelerations without ominous features.

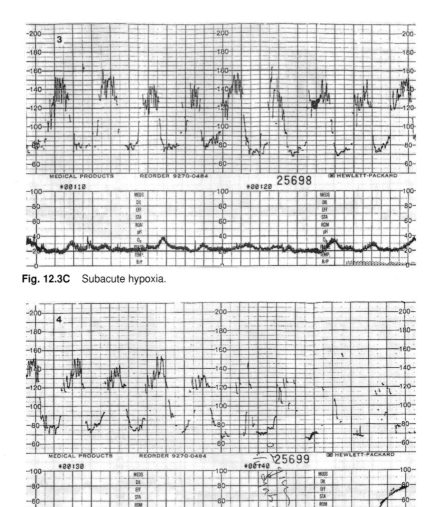

Fig. 12.3C Subacute hypoxia.

Fig. 12.3D

Abnormal

No accelerations and a combination of two abnormal features:

- Abnormal baseline rate and variability
- Repetitive late decelerations
- Variable decelerations with ominous features (duration >60 seconds, beat loss >60 beats, late recovery, late deceleration component, poor baseline variability in between and/or during decelerations).

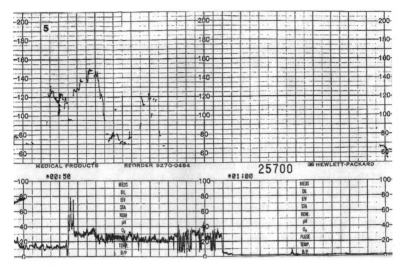

Fig. 12.3E

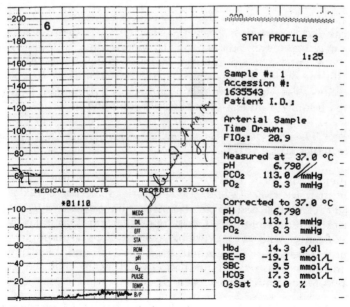

Fig. 12.3F

Fig. 12.3. Subacute hypoxia.

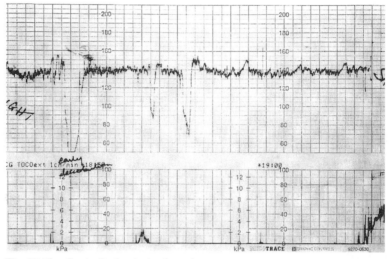

Fig. 12.4A Gradually developing hypoxia.

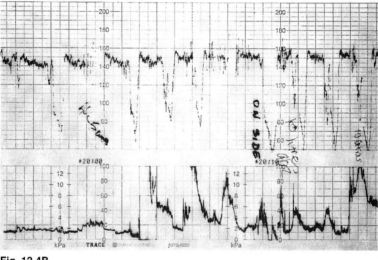

Fig. 12.4B

Other specific traces categorized as abnormal are sinusoidal pattern, prolonged bradycardia of <100 bpm and shallow decelerations in the presence of markedly reduced baseline variability (<5 bpm) in a non-reactive trace.

Adjunctive tests

As the CTG is an imperfect tool, there may be a need for an adjunctive test. The fetal scalp pH has been recommended. The Royal College of Obstetricians and

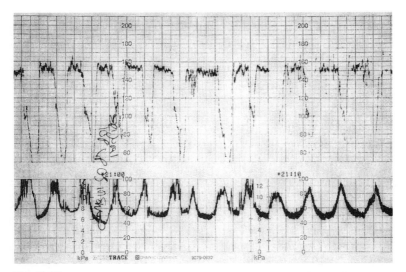

Fig. 12.4C

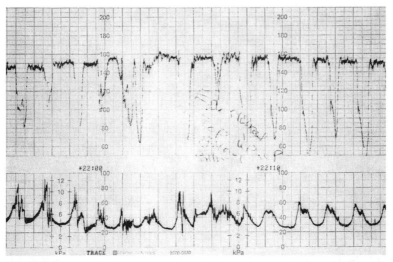

Fig. 12.4D

Gynaecologists working party on fetal monitoring has suggested that the fetal scalp pH should be used to clarify whether an abnormal CTG represents fetal acidaemia.[14] It is now over 30 years since this technique was introduced in the UK.[15] In 1985, a national survey showed that only 44% of obstetric units in the UK made use of the technique.[16] When the fetal heart rate is reactive and normal, the probability of fetal acidosis is extremely low. On the other hand, suspicious and abnormal fetal heart rate changes are not always associated with acidosis. When properly interpreted, assessment of CTG changes in most cases proves of equal value to pH in predicting outcome.[17] An

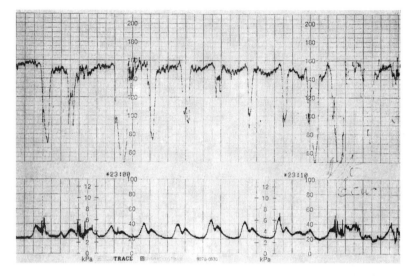

Fig. 12.4E Gradually developing hypoxia.

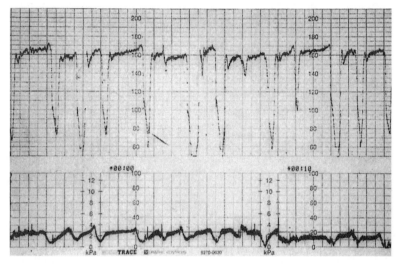

Fig. 12.4F

inexperienced person in a centre with fetal-scalp blood sampling (FBS) facilities might perform FBS frequently for their own reassurance. As they gain more experience they realize which trace is associated with a good pH and will perform it less. This learning experience is at the expense of the woman who finds the procedure uncomfortable and undignified. There are also rare but possible complications of scalp laceration, fetal bleeding and puncture of the fontanelle with loss of cerebrospinal fluid.

Fetal blood sampling may be a useful adjunct because even with the worst deceleration pattern of tachycardia with reduced variability and decelerations only

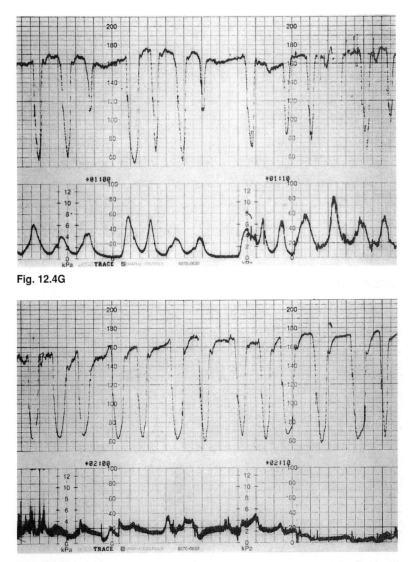

Fig. 12.4G

Fig. 12.4H

50–60% of the fetuses are acidotic.[13] A wall chart correlating different fetal heart rate patterns to the percentage of fetuses that are likely to become acidotic is available in most labour wards. It is clear from the chart and from other studies that when the fetal heart rate pattern exhibited accelerations, the chance of fetal acidosis was zero. When normal baseline variability is observed in the last 20 minutes before delivery, the babies were in good condition at birth irrespective of the other features of the trace.[18] Fetal acidosis is more common when there is a loss of baseline variability with tachycardia or late decelerations.[19,20] The fact that there are different fetuses showing

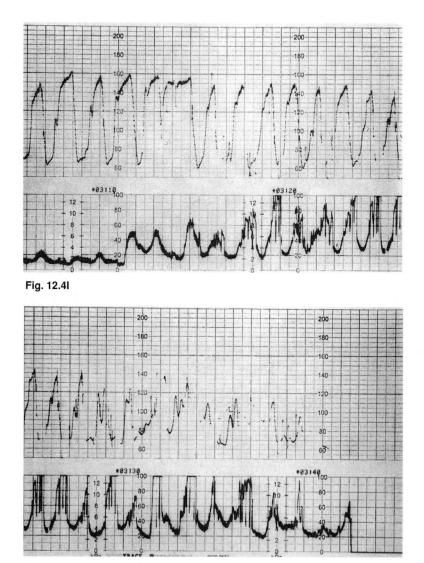

Fig. 12.4I

Fig. 12.4J

Fig. 12.4. Gradually developing hypoxia.

different levels of acidosis for a given fetal heart rate pattern is a reflection of the duration of the suspicious/abnormal fetal heart rate (FHR) pattern before the FBS. The time required for a fetus with a previously normal CTG to become acidotic has been related to the intervening FHR pattern.[21] The human fetus is very resilient – in many cases, it took over 100 minutes. It is recognized that in fetuses with less placental reserve such as those with IUGR, thick scanty meconium stained fluid[22] and post-term

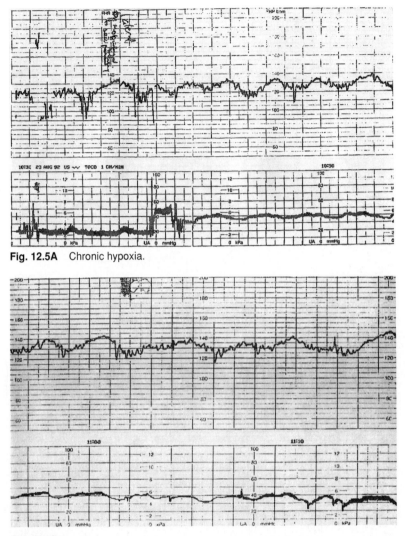

Fig. 12.5A Chronic hypoxia.

Fig. 12.5B

infants, the rate of decline of the pH is steep compared with term infants appropriately grown and with abundant, clear amniotic fluid.

Assessing pH alone in a fetal blood sample is not enough to identify the fetus at risk and more comprehensive blood gas analysis of base deficit or lactate is required. During the early stage of hypoxic threats to the fetus, the transfer of carbon dioxide from the fetal to the maternal circulation is reduced, leading to its accumulation. This results in a respiratory acidosis manifested by a low pH and a high pCO_2. Respiratory acidosis is usually transitory, particularly when corrective measures are taken, and can be managed conservatively providing the CTG

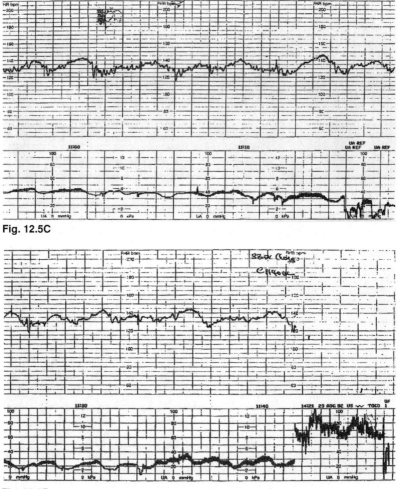

Fig. 12.5C

Fig. 12.5D

Fig. 12.5. Chronic hypoxia.

improves. The base deficit is unaffected. With a further reduction of perfusion from the fetal to the maternal circulation, the oxygen transfer becomes affected, leading to anaerobic metabolism and metabolic acidosis in the fetus. This is manifested by a low pH, pCO_2 and bicarbonate, and an increasing base deficit. It is metabolic acidosis that is damaging to the tissues. Transitory low pH values of respiratory type are not uncommon in low-risk labours, and acidotic pH values are seen in umbilical cord arterial blood in babies born with good Apgar scores because of this. It has been shown that 73% of babies with a cord pH of under 7.10 had a one-minute Apgar score of more than seven and 86% had a five-minute Apgar score greater than seven.[23] These findings are probably due to respiratory acidosis, which does not

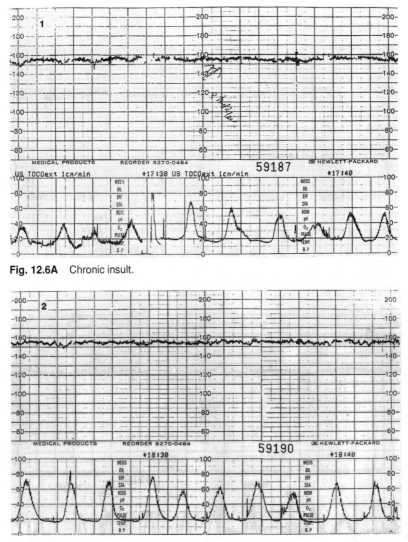

Fig. 12.6A Chronic insult.

Fig. 12.6B

correlate well with the fetal or neonatal condition. A comprehensive blood-gas analysis including pCO_2, base excess and preferably lactic acid is desirable and more predictive. Caution should be exercised in using equipment that measures only pH. It is possible to determine the lactic acid level by the bedside with 20 μl of blood using the lactic card.[24] Intrauterine infection with a high metabolic rate presents a greater oxygen demand to the fetus and metabolic acidosis can develop with minimal interruption of placental perfusion.

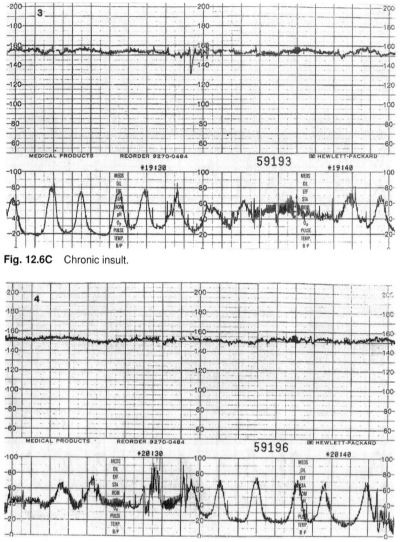

Fig. 12.6C Chronic insult.

Fig. 12.6D

Acute hypoxia

Abruption, umbilical-cord prolapse, scar dehiscence and uterine hyperstimulation may give rise to acute hypoxia (Figure 12.2). Severe interruption of placental transfer results in prolonged fetal bradycardia. At other times prolonged bradycardia occurs without obvious reason. In all circumstances, it is associated with rapidly progressive acidosis. In the case of uterine hyperstimulation, the situation is reversible. With a continuing bradycardia of less than 80 bpm, the pH is likely to decline at a rate of

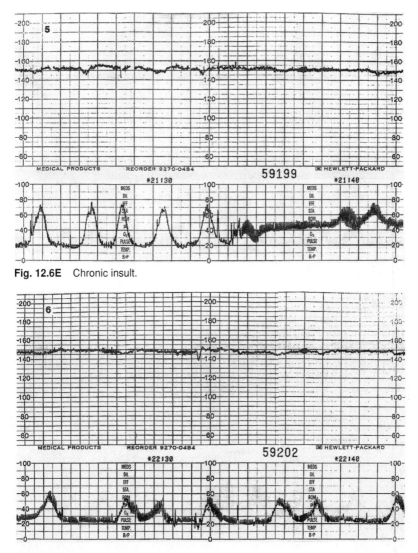

Fig. 12.6E Chronic insult.

Fig. 12.6F

approximately 0.01 per minute.[25] Urgent delivery is indicated. Twenty minutes of such hypoxia places the fetus at risk of lasting neurological damage, and attempting to perform a pH will result in critical delay. Such deliveries should be distinguished from other urgent deliveries by their immediacy. The use of the term 'immediate' has proved useful. The Standing Joint Committee of the Royal College of Obstetricians and Gynaecologists, with the Royal College of Anaesthetists, has recently agreed definitions in this respect, and classified a grade 1 – an emergency – as a Caesarean section performed because of an immediate threat to the life of the woman or her fetus. There has been general agreement that such deliveries should take, at most, 30 minutes

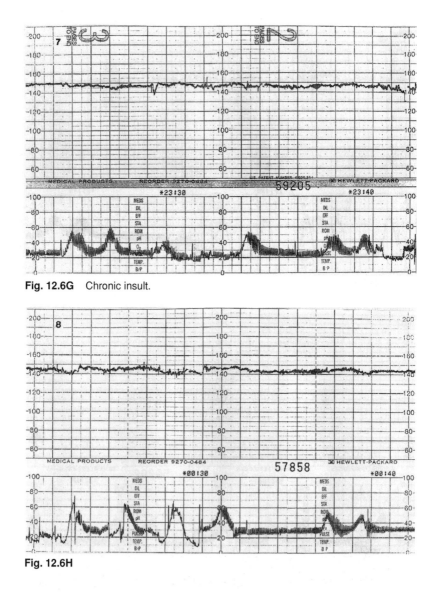

Fig. 12.6G Chronic insult.

Fig. 12.6H

from decision to delivery. The interval should be much shorter than this if some preparations have already been made; a high-risk woman in labour should already be in a state of preparedness for an emergency procedure, as should the staff.

Subacute hypoxia

The pH may deteriorate rapidly in a fetus who has previously had a reactive trace without an increase in the baseline FHR if the decelerations are pronounced, with large

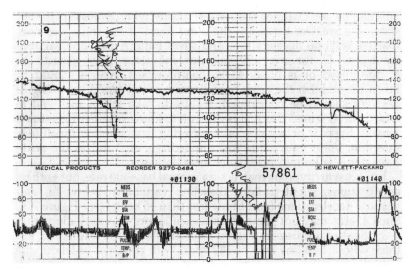

Fig. 12.6I

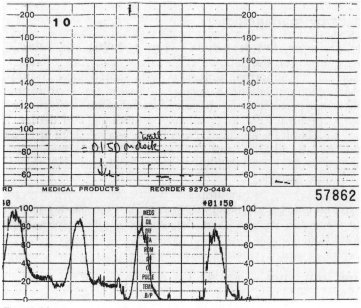

Fig. 12.6J

Fig. 12.6. Chronic insult.

dip areas (ie drops of more than 60 beats for over 90 seconds), with the FHR recovering to the baseline only for short periods of time (ie less than 60 seconds). Examples of such traces are shown in Figure 12.3. In these situations, a drop in pH can occur at 0.01 every three to four minutes. This decline in pH may be even steeper if the preceding trace was suspicious or abnormal or the clinical picture was one of high risk (IUGR, thick meconium with scanty fluid, or intrauterine infection). Further insults at this time – such as oxytocin infusion or a difficult instrumental delivery – may make the situation worse. Attempts at FBS in such a situation will delay a much-needed urgent delivery.

Gradually developing hypoxia

The fetus becomes hypoxic and acidotic in labour in association with compromise of perfusion to the fetal or maternal side of the placental circulation. With the exception of situations of acute hypoxia due to cord prolapse, scar dehiscence, abruption and prolonged bradycardia, it is unusual for a fetus that has shown accelerations and good baseline variability to become hypoxic without developing decelerations in labour. The decelerations indicate the presence of *stress* to the fetus, whether from the challenge of poor perfusion or mechanical pressure. Provided the baseline fetal heart rate has not started to rise and there is no reduction in the baseline variability to less than five beats, there is little to be gained by performing fetal blood sampling as the pH is likely to be normal. If the baseline FHR has risen by 20–30 beats and is not showing any further rise with a reduction in variability to less than five beats, *distress* is probable. Despite the fetus having increased its cardiac output to a possible maximum by increasing the FHR the functioning of the autonomic nervous system controlling the baseline variability is compromised by hypoxia. The time course of this process may be referred to as the *stress to distress period*. This period varies from fetus to fetus depending on the physiological reserve. This reserve is critically low in high-risk situations of postmaturity, IUGR, intrauterine infection and in those with thick meconium and scanty amniotic fluid.

When the FHR shows hypoxic features suggestive of distress, it is important to perform an FBS for pH and blood gases as the fetus may be or become acidotic. Initially, this will be a respiratory followed by metabolic acidosis. Once the FHR shows a distress pattern, the time taken for metabolic acidosis to develop is unpredictable. After a certain duration of the distress pattern – *the distress period* – the FHR starts to decline in a rapid stepwise pattern, culminating in terminal bradycardia and death (*the distress to death period*). The stress to distress interval (20.00 hours to 00.00 hours; ie 4 h), the distress period (00.00 hours to 03.00 hours; ie 3 h) and the distress to death period (03.00 hours to 03.40 hours; ie 40 minutes) are illustrated by Figure 12.4. Clinical interpretation of FHR patterns will identify the onset of stress, distress and the stress to distress period. It will also identify the fetus in the distress period. An accurate prediction of the distress period cannot be made based on the FHR pattern. During the final decline phase (distress to death period), when the fetal heart rate drops irretrievably within a short period, it is often too late to intervene.

The value of FBS may be at the onset of the distress period and again 30–40 minutes later or earlier depending on the baseline variability and the type of decelerations. The previous recommendation of immediate delivery when a pH is less than 7.20 (acidosis) and a repeat sample in 30 minutes or less when the pH is 7.20–7.25 (pre-acidosis) remains valid. Previous recommendations were that when the pH was greater than 7.25, repeat sampling was not required unless the FHR deteriorated. This approach may generate a false sense of security when the trace does not deteriorate although the pH is declining. The current FIGO recommendation is to repeat the pH in 30 minutes even when the first pH was in the normal range as this may indicate its rate of decline. A decision for delivery can be made considering the rate of decline of the pH, the clinical risk factors (IUGR, thick meconium), parity, current cervical dilatation and rate of progress of labour.

Chronic hypoxia

A non-reactive FHR pattern showing a baseline variability of less than five beats with shallow decelerations (less than 15 beats for 15 seconds) even with a normal baseline rate, indicates severe compromise and delivery should be expedited without delay to avoid fetal death (see Figure 12.5). A non-reactive trace with a baseline variability of less than five beats but without decelerations lasting more than 90 minutes indicates the possibility of already existing hypoxic compromise or damage due to other reasons (eg cerebral haemorrhage). This needs further evaluation if the pH is normal. In these circumstances fetal death may occur suddenly without further warning of a rise in baseline FHR or decelerations (see Figure 12.6). Hence, a non-reactive trace for greater than 90 minutes is abnormal and is an indication for further evaluation to rule out hypoxia.

When not to do fetal blood sampling

Frequently, the FHR changes observed might be due to factors other than hypoxia. Dehydration, ketosis, maternal pyrexia and anxiety can give rise to fetal tachycardia but do not usually present with decelerations. Occipito-posterior position is known to be associated with more variable decelerations without hypoxic features demonstrated by normal baseline rate and variability. Oxytocin can cause hyperstimulation resulting in FHR changes usually of a decelerative nature. Prolonged bradycardia can be due to postural hypotension following epidural analgesia. FHR changes should be correlated with the clinical picture before action is taken. In many instances, remedial action – such as hydration, repositioning of the mother or stopping the oxytocin infusion – will relieve the FHR changes and no further action is necessary. When the FHR changes persist despite such action, an FBS or one of the stimulation tests is warranted. At times, FBS may not be necessary because the trace is reassuring, or it may show a low result transiently and later show a good result; the pH may be low transiently due to respiratory acidosis. Above all, when the trace is ominous or the clinical picture is poor, it is better to deliver the baby rather than waste time with FBS. At times, a false reassurance leads to an unsatisfactory outcome. Fetal scalp blood sampling is often not appropriate under the following circumstances:

1. When the clinical picture demands early delivery (Figure 12.7): 42 weeks gestation, cervix 3 cm dilated, thick meconium with scanty fluid.
2. When an ominous trace prompts immediate delivery (Figure 12.8).
3. When the FHR trace is reassuring (Figure 12.9).
4. When the changes are due to oxytocic overstimulation.
5. When there is associated persistent failure to progress in labour.
6. During or soon after an episode of prolonged bradycardia.

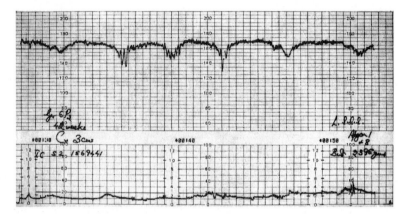

Fig. 12.7. Clinical picture demands early delivery.

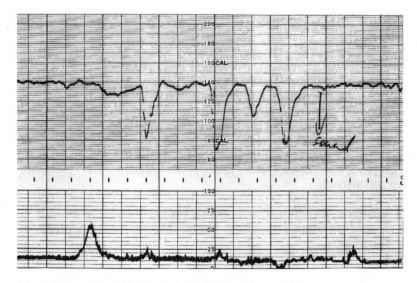

Fig. 12.8. Ominous trace prompts immediate delivery.

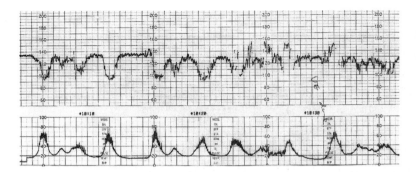

Fig. 12.9. A reassuring trace.

7. If spontaneous vaginal delivery is imminent or easy instrumental vaginal delivery is possible.

Following these principles will help to avoid unnecessary FBS, operative deliveries and fetal morbidity from undue delay in delivery.

Alternatives to fetal blood sampling

In practice, FBS might not be performed because the facilities or the expertise are not available. The woman also might resist what is an undignified and uncomfortable procedure. If this is so, alternative methods should be considered. A retrospective observation and correlation of the scalp-blood pH to the presence or absence of accelerations at the time of FBS led to the scalp stimulation test.[26,27] When the scalp was stimulated by pinching with a tissue forceps, if an acceleration was present it was unlikely that the pH was below 7.20.[28,29] On the other hand, if there were no accelerations to such a stimulus, only 50% had acidotic values (7.20–7.25) and others had normal values. Therefore, this test was useful in identifying those who were not at risk, although it was not good in predicting those who are likely to be acidotic. In centres where facilities do not exist for scalp FBS, such a test is useful in reducing the number of Caesarean sections for 'fetal distress', and in centres where it is performed it will reduce the number of samples performed. When there is difficulty in obtaining a sample during a procedure, observation of an acceleration is very reassuring and the procedure can be discontinued.

The Royal College of Obstetricians and Gynaecologists Study Group has recommended that fetal scalp blood sampling facilities should be available in any hospital where EFM is performed.[14] However, clinicians who understand the clinical situation and the fetal heart pattern may make a decision without resorting to FBS and without an increase in the Caesarean section rate for fetal distress.[30] In many situations it is wiser to proceed to delivery without wasting precious time. It has been shown that if the decision to delivery interval in situations of fetal distress is 35 minutes as opposed to 15 minutes then the admission rate to the special care baby unit is doubled.[31] FBS is not always possible because of lack of facilities or an undilated cervix with a high head. Decisions based on the clinical situation complemented by information from the CTG remain critical.

Induction and augmentation of labour

Induction of labour is performed to start labour when there is reason to believe that the pregnancy would be better to be concluded than to continue. This may be done for many reasons, but the key principle is that it is safer for the mother and/or the baby for delivery to take place. The induction procedure carries a risk, so a risk–benefit analysis should be considered. In the circumstances when the indication is pre-labour rupture of the membranes, the procedure is sometimes called 'stimulation'. When labour has already started but is slow on account of poor uterine contractions, the use of oxytocin in these circumstances is called 'augmentation'. Augmentation is a better word than acceleration. The augmentation process may be an integral part of an active management of labour strategy. In any of these scenarios, an oxytocic drug is used to increase the frequency, duration and amplitude of contractions. This inevitably reduces fetal oxygenation, and fetal surveillance must be careful.

The duration of induced labour can be predicted reasonably by the assessment of three inter-related factors: gestational age, parity and cervical score. The response to oxytocic stimuli depends on how favourable these factors are. Oxytocic stimuli are digital examination, membrane rupture (spontaneous or artificial), and administration of prostaglandin or oxytocin. Oxytocic treatment should be a complementation of the intrinsic situation with external stimuli. In a favourable condition, stretching of the cervix or artificial membrane rupture may suffice to trigger labour. In a less favourable situation, with more hours of labour in prospect, it is better to leave the membranes intact initially and use prostaglandin, which is supplied in the UK as Prostin gel (Upjohn) or as Propess pessaries (Ferring Pharmaceuticals). The advantage of Propess is that it can be withdrawn easily as it has a retrieval thread; however, it is slower to act and may be less effective in unfavourable cases. The manufacturers recommend that Prostin gel should only be given twice and should be given with a six-hour interval. This is a guideline and further treatment may be authorized by a consultant. In some hospitals, prostaglandin is given late in the evening and in others in the early morning. Whenever it is given, steps should be taken to ensure effective fetal surveillance and the availability of a labour ward bed when active labour supervenes. A CTG should be performed before the first treatment and when contractions begin. It is beneficial for the woman to mobilize in the interim.

The insertion of Prostin is repeated six hours later, with the same fetal surveillance. If labour then fails to begin, a consultant should undertake a review and consider whether to wait, administer more Prostin, rupture the membranes or perform a Caesarean section. This will depend largely on the fetal/maternal condition and the view of the woman. If effective contractions have begun then the later process may include membrane rupture and oxytocin infusion. In all circumstances, care must be taken not to hyperstimulate the uterus by cumulative treatment, which is too precipitate. At the end of labour, it should be remembered that the uterus may still be slow to contract and there is a risk of a postpartum haemorrhage. In these circumstances, an injection of Syntometrine at delivery and a continuing infusion of oxytocin should be considered.

There is no agreed standard method of giving oxytocin for induction or augmentation of labour. The Royal College of Obstetricians and Gynaecologists recommends a starting dose of one milliunit (mU) per minute to a maximum of 12 mU/min.[32] The increment should be in one to 2 mU at intervals of 30 min. Twelve milliunits may not be enough for a nulliparous woman with a fetus in an occipito-posterior position. Infusion pumps delivering fluid in millilitres (ml) per hour are used generally. Oxytocin is supplied as Syntocinon in vials containing international units, which are then diluted in a carrier infusion fluid. This is usually one litre of normal saline or dextrose saline. If 10 units are dissolved in one litre then there are 10 mU in 1 ml. Infusion pumps are set in ml/hour, which requires conversion into mU per minute. With 10 units of Syntocinon in one litre running at 12 ml per hour, 2 mU/min are delivered. The administration of Syntocinon should be separate but in parallel with the intravenous fluid regimen.

Augmentation of labour should be performed with the same precautions as induction. There should be an indication, and fetal surveillance should be meticulous. The true maximum dose of oxytocin is that which makes the uterus contract efficiently without causing hyperstimulation or fetal hypoxia. In the circumstances of augmentation of labour, vaginal examination should be carried out around every two hours to judge the response and make a plan for delivery. EFM is desirable when oxytocics are being given; if the trace becomes abnormal, the oxytocin should be stopped and treatment reviewed. In the interim, the woman is placed on her side to counteract any effect of reduced placental blood flow. Although given by many, it is doubtful whether inhaled oxygen has any beneficial effect. If it has been necessary to discontinue oxytocin twice in a nulliparous woman and the cervix is not dilating, Caesarean section is advisable. Again, it should be remembered that the poorly contracting uterus predisposes to a postpartum haemorrhage, and care should be taken after delivery to ensure efficient uterine contraction.

Twin labour and delivery

Twins face increased risks of many kinds. Monochorionic and monoamniotic (ie in a single sac) twins are at much increased risk. The risk of cord entanglement and mechanical problems at delivery is so great with monoamniotic twins that Caesarean section is the preferable option. The hazards faced by monochorionic, diamniotic twins are less clear but there is a risk of intrapartum twin-to-twin transfusion syndrome and some fetal medicine specialists recommend elective Caesarean section. Today, more twins are being delivered by caesarean section than previously; however, skills must be retained for vaginal breech delivery – this may include the second twin presenting as a breech. In litigation cases, the second twin is injured more often than the first. This is most often because of problems at delivery. The second twin may be smaller than the first. If the discordancy is thought, before labour, to be 25% or more, the risk of asphyxia to the second twin is high and Caesarean section should be considered. Strenuous efforts should be made to monitor the second twin in labour. This may be difficult because it lies behind the leading twin. There is also no information available about the amniotic fluid of the second twin. Delivery of the first twin is usually uncomplicated, particularly if it is in a cephalic presentation. This delivery should be by the midwife. The risk to the second twin increases after delivery of the first. Great efforts must be made to locate and follow the fetal heart of the second twin: the maternal pulse should be distinguished from it. Patience should be exercised in awaiting further contractions. A normal CTG and the absence of bleeding are reassuring, and the skill and experience of the doctor is essential at this stage. The risk of postpartum haemorrhage is much increased because of the overstretched uterus in multiple pregnancy and effective steps must be taken with oxytocin injection and infusion.

Breech labour

Labour in breech presentation carries many additional hazards that are particularly prominent in footling or complete breech. Umbilical-cord compression is the most prominent of these, resulting in variable decelerations. Meconium passage has less significance in breech presentation, being related to compression of the fetal abdomen, particularly in the late first stage and the second stage of labour. Should a CTG be abnormal due to hypoxia in a breech then delivery is a more reasonable option rather than FBS. Breech extraction involves more manipulation than (minimally) assisted breech delivery and should only be done by an experienced operator.

There has been a recent report of a large randomized study suggesting that elective Caesarean section is safer than planned vaginal delivery for the fetus in a breech presentation at term.[32] Skills in vaginal delivery of the breech-presenting baby are being lost – with more Caesareans being done, younger staff have less opportunity to gain experience. They are less confident and consequently so is the pregnant woman. Individualization of care remains important.

Previous Caesarean section

The late pregnancy assessment in this situation has been covered in another chapter. Trial of labour with a scar should be planned, spontaneous and carefully supervised. Uterine scar dehiscence is unusual if oxytocic drugs are not misused and labour is not allowed to continue for too long. EFM is important – FHR abnormalities can be a sign of impending scar dehiscence.

Third stage of labour

This is the time from birth of the baby until the placenta and membranes have been delivered. It is the time when there is greatest risk of haemorrhage because of the nature of haemochorial implantation. Postpartum haemorrhage (PPH) is a potentially serious complication. The placental bed is like a raw wound and the main mechanism of haemostasis is the lattice-like framework of the myometrium constricting the placental bed. The discovery of the oxytocic quality of extract of rye in 1955 opened up a therapeutic possibility. This was later synthesized and manufactured as ergometrine. It was suggested that the routine use of an injection of ergometrine after delivery of the placenta would reduce haemorrhage and this is indeed the case. In many hospitals, there is an active management of the third stage, including such an injection when the baby is being born followed by controlled cord traction when the uterus responds. Some women are at more risk than others – those with long labour, induced labour, previous PPH, twins and polyhydramnios. They should be strongly advised to have such treatment. There is evidence that in the low-risk group, treatment is also beneficial; however, such women are accepted for an opt-out if they are aware of the risk. They then have what is termed a 'natural' third stage of labour. An unfortunate result of the use of oxytocic drugs during the third stage is an increased incidence of retained placenta.

There are two main categories of PPH: atonic and traumatic. Atonic (90% of cases) is due to failure of the uterus to contract; traumatic (10% of cases) is due to damage to the genital tract. The comparison of clinical background is important. The uterus that is slow to contract before delivery will be so after. Atonic haemorrhage is more common in the uterus overstretched by multiple fetuses, polyhydramnios and a big baby. Induced labour or augmented labour, particularly when it has become very prolonged, is a clear association. Traumatic haemorrhage is associated with traumatic delivery – whether assisted or not – and previous uterine surgery. There may well be a combination of atonic and traumatic haemorrhage. Both must be considered carefully in the acute situation.

Immediate management is lifesaving. A call for help to mobilize senior staff from Obstetrics, Midwifery, Anaesthetics and Haematology is important. Because poor uterine contraction is likely to be contributing, a hand should placed on the lower abdomen and the fundus of the uterus rubbed to stimulate a contraction. Irrespective of whether nothing, oxytocin or ergometrine have already been given as part of routine management, ergometrine (0.5 mg) should be given intramuscularly.

Intravenous access must be secured. A large bore cannula of at least 16 gauge should be inserted into a forearm vein. Blood is withdrawn for haemoglobin estimation and crossmatch of blood. Immediate infusion of one litre of Hartmann's solution should be given. An infusion of normal saline with 100 units of Syntocinon added to one litre should be commenced at 20 drops per minute. In the proportion of cases that are due to poor contraction, this first series of manoeuvres will stop the bleeding. If significant further bleeding occurs, more detailed examination of the genital tract is necessary. Traumatic damage is likely and the source must be found. Problems arise because of delays in treatment moving to the next step.

A further 0.5 mg of ergometrine should be given intravenously. Fundal massage should be continued. Good light with lithotomy position and analgesia should be obtained for detailed vaginal and cervical inspection. Perineal, vaginal and cervical trauma should be repaired as indicated. Prostaglandin $F_2\alpha$ (Haemabate) is used as a second-line oxytocic. It can be injected systemically or into the myometrium through the anterior abdominal wall. It is also used intramuscularly and can be given in repeated doses.

If haemorrhage is severe or persistent, a central venous pressure line should be placed. This is particularly useful when oliguria persists in spite of adequate volume replacement or in severe pre-eclampsia. A positive venous pressure of 10 cm of water should be maintained. Initial infusion may be of Hartmann's solution or normal saline, but a colloid becomes necessary in order to maintain volume within the intravascular space. Haemaccel (Hoechst) or Gelofusine (Consolidated Chemicals), which are both chemically modified solutions of degraded gelatin, is the best choice initially, but should be followed by whole blood and fresh frozen plasma. The only difference between them is that Haemaccel contains over 10 times more calcium than Gelofusine. The calcium can lead to clotting in warming coils when Haemaccel is mixed with citrated blood or fresh frozen plasma. In cases of massive, rapid haemorrhage, uncrossmatched group 0-negative blood should be given. In the face of massive haemorrhage with a developing coagulation defect, fresh, whole blood is ideal but is no longer available because of the difficulties of screening for infection (such as AIDS) in donated blood while it remains fresh. A substitute of its component parts should be given as packed red cells, fresh frozen plasma and platelets (after five or six units of blood)

The collaboration of the duty haematologist is important. Accurate fluid management with central venous pressure measurement, urinary catheterization and careful fluid balance recording is critical. Serious sequelae develop because of too slow a response to the danger signals. Continuing haemorrhage necessitates an examination under anaesthesia, initially vaginally and followed by laparotomy, if indicated. At laparotomy, a senior doctor will have to decide whether uterine artery ligation is possible. The ultimate solution is hysterectomy. In an emergency situation, this may have to be subtotal, leaving the uterine cervix in place. The family should be kept fully informed of the decision making.

Conclusion

The public have high expectations for the birth of the next generation. Technology and modern medicine have provided the tools necessary to achieve these expectations. Knowledge and the application of skills needs to be updated constantly through continuing education. Guidelines and evidence-based medicine provide an infrastructure for care but this must be tailored by experience and wisdom. Good communications are indispensable and an essential part of the strategy in reducing complaint and litigation.

References

1   *Guidelines for Monitoring the Availability and Use of Obstetric Services*. United Nations Children's Fund, World Health Organization, United Nations Population Fund, 1997.
2   Department of Health. *Why Mothers Die*. Report on the Confidential Enquiries into Maternal Deaths in the UK 1884–1996. London: HMSO, 1998.

3   *Confidential Enquiry into Stillbirth and Deaths in Infancy.* Fourth Annual Report: Concentrating on Intra-partum Deaths 1994–1995. London: Maternal and Child Health Research Consortium, 1997.
4   Royal College of Obstetricians and Gynaecologists, Royal College of Midwives. *Towards Safer Childbirth,* 1999.
5   Expert Maternity Group. *Changing Childbirth.* London: HMSO, 1993.
6   Enkin M, Kierse MJNC, Neilson J *et al. A Guide to Effective Care in Pregnancy and Childbirth,* 3rd Edition. Location of Publisher: Publisher, 2000.
7   Department of Health. *An Organisation with a Memory.* Report of an Expert Advisory Group on Learning From Adverse Events in the NHS, Chaired by the Chief Medical Officer. London: The Stationery Office, 2000.
8   Gibb D, Arulkumaran S. *Fetal Monitoring in Practice.* Oxford: Butterworth–Heinemann, 1993.
9   Ennis M, Vincent CA. Obstetric accidents: a review of 64 cases. *British Medical Journal* 1990, 300: 1365–1367.
10 Gaffney G, Sellers S, Flavell V, Squier M, Johnson A. Case control study of intrapartum care, cerebral palsy, and perinatal death. *British Medical Journal* 1994; 308: 743–750.
11 MacDonald D, Grant A, Sheridan-Pereira M, Boylan P, Chalmers I. The Dublin randomised controlled trial of intrapartum fetal monitoring. *American Journal of Obstetrics and Gynecology* 1985; 152: 524–539.
12 FIGO. Guidelines for the use of fetal monitoring. *International Journal of Gynaecology and Obstetrics* 1987; 25: 159–167.
13 Beard RW, Filshie GM, Knight CA, Roberts GM. The significance of the change in the continuous fetal heart rate in the first stage of labour. *Journal of Obstetrics and Gynaecology of the British Commonwealth* 1971; 78: 865–881.
14 Spencer JAD, ed. Recommendations Arising from the 26th Study Group in Intrapartum Fetal Surveillance. London: RCOG Press, 1993: 387–393.
15 Beard RW, Morris ED, Clayton SG. pH of foetal scalp capillary blood as an indicator of the condition of the fetus. *Journal of Obstetrics and Gynaecology of the British Commonwealth* 1967; 74: 812–822.
16 Wheble AM, Gillmer MDG, Spencer JAD, Sykes GS. Changes in fetal monitoring practice in the UK 1977–1984. British Journal of Obstetric and Gynaecology 1989; 96: 1140–1147.
17 Parer JT. In defense of FHR monitoring's specificity. *Obstetrics Gynaecology* 1982; 19: 228–234.
18 Paul RH, Suidan AK, Yeh SY *et al.* Clinical fetal monitoring. VII. The evaluation and significance of intrapartum baseline variability. *American Journal of Obstetrics & Gynaecology* 1975; 123: 206–210.
19 Bread RW, Filshie GM, Kinght CA. Roberts GM. The significance of the changes in the continuous fetal heart rate in the first stage of labour. *Journal of Obstetrics and Gynaecology of the British Commonwealth* 1971; 78: 865–881.
20 Schifrin BS, Dame L. Fetal heart rate patterns: prediction of Apgar score. *JAMA* 1972; 219: 1322–1325.
21 Fleischer A, Schulman H, Jagani N *et al.* The development of fetal acidosis in the presence of an abnormal fetal heart rate tracing. 1. The average for gestation age fetus. *American Journal of Obstetrics & Gynecology* 1982; 144: 55–60.
22 Starks GC. Correlation of meconium stained amniotic fluid, early intrapartum fetal pH and Apgar scores as predictors of perinatal outcome. *Obstetrics & Gynaecology* 1980; 55: 604–609.
23 Sykes, GS, Molloy, PM, Johnson P *et al.* Do Apgar scores indicate asphyxia? *Lancet* 1982; i: 494–495.
24 Nordstrom L, Arulkumaran S, Chua S *et al.* Continuous maternal glucose infusion during labor: effects on maternal and fetal glucose and lactate lends. *American Journal of Perinatology* 1995; 12: 357–362.
25 Ingemarsson I, Arulkumaran S, Ratnam SS. Single injection of terbutaline in term labor. 1. Effect on fetal pH in cases with prolonged bradycardia. *American Journal of Obstetrics & Gynecology* 1985; 153: 859–865.
26 Clarke SL, Gimovsky ML, Miller FC. Fetal heart rate response to scalp blood sampling. *American Journal of Obstetrics & Gynecology* 1983; 144: 706–708.
27 Clarke SL. Gimovsky ML, Miller FC. The scalp stimulation test: a clinical alternative to fetal scalp blood sampling. *American Journal of Obstetrics & Gynecology* 1984; 148: 274–277.
28 Arulkumaran S, Ingemarsson I, Ratnam SS. Fetal heart rate response to scalp stimulation as a test for fetal wellbeing in labour. *Asia Oceania Journal of Obstetrics & Gynaecology* 1987; 13: 131–135.
29 Clarke SL, Paul RH. Intrapartum fetal surveillance: the role of fetal scalp blood sampling. *American Journal of Obstetrics & Gynecology* 1985; 153: 717–720.
30 Dunphy BC, Robinson JN, Sheil OM *et al.* Caesarean section for fetal distress, the interval from decision to delivery, and the relative risk of poor neonatal condition. *British Journal of Obstetrics & Gynaecology* 1991; 11: 241–244.
31 Induction of Labour. Guideline No 16. London: Royal College of Obstetricians and Gynaecologists, 1998.
32 Hannah ME, Hannah WJ, Hewson SA, Hodnett ED, Saigal S, Willan AR, for the Term Breech Trial Collaborative Group. Planned Caesarean section versus planned vaginal birth for breech presentation at term: a randomised multicentre trial. *Lancet* 2000; 356: 1375–1383.

▶13

Operative Obstetrics

Roger V Clements

Introduction

The title of this chapter might reasonably include a number of diagnostic antenatal procedures as well as cervical cerclage. Apart from brief mention of ovarian tumours in pregnancy, the chapter will concentrate, for reasons of space, on operative intervention in labour. In the past 30 years, there has been marked reduction in operative vaginal delivery, with an increasing reluctance to perform the more difficult manoeuvres. There are three principle reasons for the change. Firstly, obstetricians in training now spend less time in the labour ward and have less opportunity to learn the more difficult vaginal manoeuvres, and in most hospitals Kjelland's forceps delivery is no longer taught. Secondly, operative vaginal delivery involving rotation, by whatever method, is perceived as a high-risk undertaking for both baby and mother. Thirdly, Caesarean section has become a much safer alternative.

There will soon be few obstetricians left who can claim to be trained in the art of rotational forceps delivery and few who are competent at vaginal breech delivery. Whilst there may be a genuine alternative to operative vaginal delivery in Caesarean section, the same cannot be said for breech delivery. Although some obstetric units would claim to have a policy of no vaginal breech delivery, the reality is that no unit can in fact avoid it; there will always be mothers who refuse Caesarean section for a breech; there will be second twins presenting as breeches and there will be those who at home or in the labour ward progress so rapidly that the breech is on the perineum before the obstetric attendant appears. There will therefore be breech deliveries – but decreasing numbers of doctors and midwives with any adequate skills to perform them.

Ovarian tumours in pregnancy

The great majority of ovarian swellings in the first trimester of pregnancy are functional, follicular or corpus luteum cysts. They seldom grow beyond 6 cm, and 90% of them resolve spontaneously and are undetectable by the 14th week. Ovarian tumours requiring surgery are uncommon; most are asymptomatic and discovered on routine ultrasonography. Malignancy is exceptionally rare and estimates vary from 1:10 000 to 1:25 000 pregnancies.

Torsion is more common than in the non-pregnant but is still rare; haemorrhage and rupture are rarer still. Symptomatic tumours, suggestive of torsion, haemorrhage or rupture demand intervention as for the non-pregnant. In the absence of either symptoms or the suspicion of malignancy, operative intervention is best postponed until about 18 weeks. Not only does this reduce the risk of miscarriage but it also avoids unnecessary surgery for functional tumours that resolve. There is nothing to be gained by waiting longer, and surgery *after 20 weeks* carries with it a risk of inducing a premature delivery. When an ovarian tumour is discovered in the last trimester, the operation may sometimes be better postponed, so as to achieve greater fetal maturity.

Operative technique is similar to that employed in the non-pregnant save only that a longitudinal incision is essential.

Episiotomy

The perceived benefits of episiotomy over perineal tears have not been substantiated by evidence.[1] Neither is there yet any evidence that episiotomy reduces the incidence of damage to the anal canal and rectum. Unfortunately, most of the literature that attempts to address that issue does not distinguish between midline and medio-lateral episiotomy.

Few indications remain, therefore, for episiotomy. These would include:

 patient request

shoulder dystocia

fetal distress

forceps (and sometimes vacuum-assisted) delivery

vaginal breech delivery.

The most frequent cause of complaint and litigation in relation to episiotomy is the retained swab. All labour ward records should require a declaration from the doctor or midwife repairing the perineum that a swab count has been completed and is correct. In no other branch of surgery would it be possible to undertake such a procedure without a full two-person swab and instrument count before and after the procedure.

The second area of complaint is the poor functional outcome that sometimes follows the repair of episiotomy or tear. The dyspareunia which results is often caused by poor healing and the persistence of granulation tissue in the wound; sometimes it is because the repair is too tight and the introitus too narrow. Much depends on the skill and experience of the operator but there is now good evidence that the choice of suture material influences the outcome. There is some advantage in using a subcuticular suture in the reduction of immediate postpartum pain.[2] Catgut and soft gut are no longer acceptable as suture materials. In 1986, soft gut was shown to increase by 26% the incidence of dyspareunia persisting beyond three months, compared with 19.5% when untreated catgut was used.[3] The use of polyglycolic acid (Dexon and Vicryl) produces a 40% reduction in short-term pain when compared with catgut, but there is no difference in the prevalence of longer-term dypareunia.[4]

Damage to the rectum and anus

The nomenclature used in the discussion of damage to the rectum and anus is complex and unsatisfactory. Different systems of classification have been used in the American and the British literature. A one-day meeting entitled 'Obstetric anal sphincter injury: is it time to rethink practice as we enter the Millennium?' was held in Birmingham, UK, on 14 January 2000; it produced a consensus statement on prevention and management of post-obstetric bowel incontinence and third degree tear,[5] and a new classification was suggested (see Box 13.1).

Box 13.1   The new classification for damage to the rectum and anus

First degree	Vaginal epithelium only
Second degree	Injury to perineal muscles as well
Third degree	Injury to include the anal sphincters:
	a) less than 50% of the external anal sphincter
	b) more than 50% of the external anal sphincter
	c) to include internal anal sphincter injury as well
Fourth degree	Injury to anal sphincters and ano-rectal epithelium

---

The reported incidence of third degree tears ranges from 0.6% to 2.3%,[6] and it seems likely that the condition is under-reported. Occult or unrecognized mechanical disruption of the anal sphincter is a major contributor to the subsequent development of anal incontinence.[7] Between 26% and 35% of women undergoing their first vaginal delivery develop occult sphincter injury.[8] It is essential that any woman with a perineal injury should be examined carefully in the immediate post-delivery period, to ascertain the extent of the injury. If there is any question of damage to the rectum or anus, the diagnosis should be made by a fully-trained obstetrician, by careful digital examination.[5] The consensus statement further recommends that all women having an instrumental delivery or who sustain a perineal tear should undergo digital rectal examination by an individual fully trained in the recognition of third degree tears to detect a sphincter injury. Failure to recognize a significant sphincter injury is the principle cause of successful litigation.

If subsequent ano-rectal incontinence is to be reduced to a minimum, the repair which follows must be executed with proper skill and care. In the resting state the tone of the internal sphincter keeps the anal canal closed. When the sphincter is interrupted as it is by a third degree tear, its two ends become separated widely into a sickle shape (Figure 13.1). The principle of repair of a third degree tear therefore is to paralyse the sphincter first, allowing it to relax. This is achieved by general or regional anæsthesia; it cannot be achieved by local infiltration. Once the sphincter is relaxed, its two ends can be grasped and sutured (Figures 13.2 and 13.3). Provided the steps in repairing a third degree tear are achieved and provided the suture material remains in place long enough to facilitate complete healing, the restoration of continence is usually

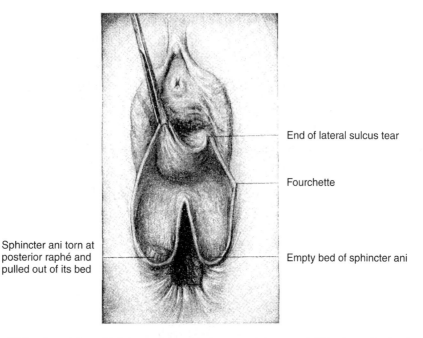

End of lateral sulcus tear

Fourchette

Sphincter ani torn at
posterior raphé and
pulled out of its bed

Empty bed of sphincter ani

Fig. 13.1. Complete or third degree tear: critical survey of the wound. This shows the depth of the wound and how the flap of the vagina may be raised. The split in the rectum and the sphincter, torn out of its bed and ruptured at the side (not always in the midline) are plainly visible. Reproduced, with permission, from Greenhill JP. *Obstetrics*, 13th edition. WB Saunders Co., 1965.

complete. The immediate repair of a third degree tear more often than not results in a patient with normal continence.[9] In a review of the literature, Schofield and Grace[9] demonstrated that primary repair results in the restoration of full continence in 66% of recognized anal sphincter injuries. Conversely, only 49% of women recovered full continence after a secondary repair. Most of the complaints arising from this injury relate to:

▶ failure of recognition that the sphincter is damaged

▶ failure to repair the damage adequately.

The consensus statement[5] advises that the repair should be by a 'trained professional' in a well-equipped operating theatre under appropriate anæsthesia. There should be antibiotic cover using metronidazole and a broad-spectrum agent against aerobic bacteria. The repair should be performed using PDS or Vicryl – *not* with catgut. Prolene should be avoided because of the risks of migration.

As with all other perineal repairs, a swab count followed by a vaginal and rectal examination should be conducted at the end of the procedure. It is important to ensure that there is no significant bleeding before the legs are lowered and the procedure considered complete. Ice packs may help to reduce the bruising and stools should be softened by generous fluid intake and bulk laxatives.

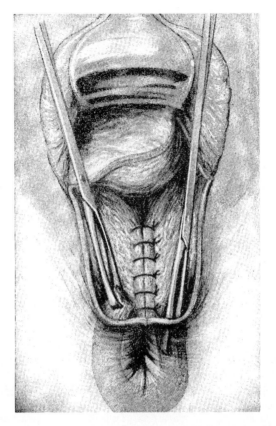

Fig. 13.2. Reaching down into the bottom of the sphincter pit. The bottom of the sphincter pit is touched with the fingers and with an Allis or tissue forceps the retracted end of the sphincter ani is drawn up. It is usually a part of the retracted torn levator. Reproduced, with permission, from Greenhill JP. *Obstetrics*, 13th edition. WB Saunders Co., 1965.

Should the repair break down, no attempt should be made to repair it whilst there is any sign of wound sepsis.

Fear of perineal injury and the loss of continence is now an increasing factor in maternal request for abdominal delivery:

> Until anal sphincter injury is more fully understood and researched it is likely that the increase in rate of Caesarean sections will continue and that as recently suggested, it may be difficult to decline a patient's request for Caesarean section to avoid pelvic floor damage during childbirth on the basis of the current evidence.[10]

The mechanics of labour

No attempt at operative vaginal delivery can be undertaken safely without a thorough understanding of the mechanics of labour and the relationship between the fetal head

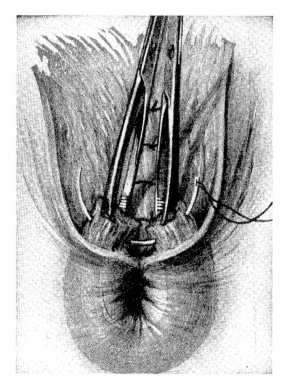

Fig. 13.3. Uniting the sphincter ani. To ensure broad apposition of torn muscle, the needle should pass well to the side, and two, even three, figure-eight sutures may be placed; one of these should unite the fascia surrounding the muscle. This is the most important part of the operation. Reproduced, with permission, from Greenhill JP. *Obstetrics*, 13th edition. WB Saunders Co., 1965.

and the maternal bony pelvis. Although much information can now be obtained on the size of the fetus (by ultrasonography) and the size of the pelvis (by modern X-ray and other methods), this information is of little help in forecasting the outcome of labour. In the developed world, the difference between success and failure in achieving safe vaginal delivery is not usually determined by the absolute size of the baby or mother but rather by the degree of extension or flexion of the fetal head. The *attitude* of the baby in turn determines rotation within the pelvis and most occasions of cephalo-pelvic disproportion are the result of malrotation and deflexion. These are important considerations when contemplating operative vaginal delivery.

The examination of many sets of hospital records suggests that both midwives and junior doctors lack competence in determining both the *position* and *descent* of the fetal head.

Position is determined by reference to the sutures and fontanelles and is best recorded by a diagram. In recent years, it is increasingly common to find – whilst reviewing cases in which things have gone wrong – no sensible account of fetal

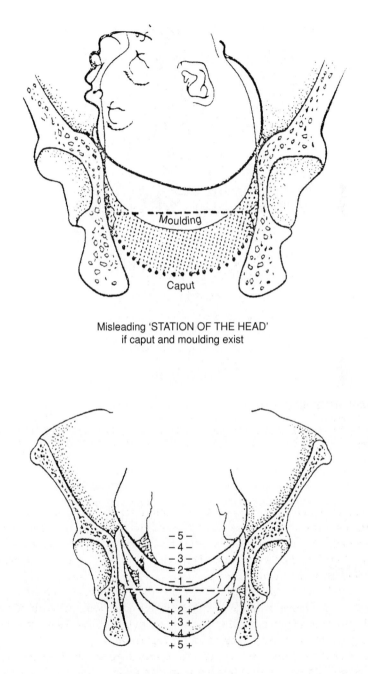

Misleading 'STATION OF THE HEAD'
if caput and moulding exist

STATION OF THE HEAD

Fig 13.4   Caput and moulding. Reproduced, with permission, from Crichton D. A reliable method of establishing the level of the fetal head in obstetrics. *South African Medical Journal* 1974, 17 April, p. 787.

position at any time during labour, even though four, five or six vaginal examinations may have been performed.

Descent of the fetal head should be described by both abdominal palpation (head level) and by vaginal examination (station). The design of the partogram should require that head level is recorded in fifths palpable and at each vaginal examination the *station* of the head is separately recorded. Because caput and moulding may distort findings on vaginal examination (Figure 13.4), it is essential that both methods of recording are used. In the presence of moulding and caput, the abdominal examination to determine fifths palpable is the more reliable observation. Maternal obesity and distress may make the observation difficult but an epidural block in preparation for an operative delivery will usually facilitate the observation. In general, station and head level have a constant relationship. In the absence of caput and moulding, with an average-sized baby in an average-sized pelvis, the plane of the brim (judged abdominally) corresponds to the plane of the ischial spines (judged vaginally):

> If the lowest point of the head is at the ischial spinal level, the largest diameter is probably just through the pelvic brim, provided there is no marked moulding or caput formation.[11]

Moulding and caput will suggest a lower station than is appropriate for the level of the head as felt abdominally. In neglected obstructed labour, the head may be visible at the vulva whilst remaining unengaged, with more than three-fifths palpable abdominally.

Forceps delivery

Proper documentation and comparison of data has been hindered by inconsistent definitions. These have been clarified by the American College of Obstetricians and Gynaecologists.[12] The American classification is reproduced in Box 13.2.

The high forceps operation is not included in the definition and is no longer an acceptable procedure. It refers to the application of the forceps to the unengaged head when the lowest part of the fetal skull has not reached the ischial spines.

Indications

Forceps delivery should not be conducted without proper indication. The indications are:

 maternal distress

fetal distress

inadequate maternal effort.

All are somewhat subjective and defy proper definition. Maternal distress includes maternal exhaustion, patient request and those conditions that are thought to

Box 13.2 Classification of forceps delivery according to station and rotation	
Type of procedure	Classification
Outlet forceps	Scalp is visible at the introitus without separating the labia
	Fetal skull has reached the pelvic floor
	The sagittal suture is in the Antero-posterior diameter or right or left occiput anterior or posterior position.
	Fetal head is at or on the perineum.
	Rotation does not exceed 45°.
Low forceps	Leading point of fetal skull is at station ≥+ 2 cm, and not on the pelvic floor.
	Rotation ≤45° (left or right occiput anterior to occiput anterior, or left or right occiput posterior to occiput posterior).
	Rotation >45°
Mid forceps	Station above 2 cm but head engaged.

contraindicate prolonged expulsive effort such as heart disease, epilepsy, retinopathy and intracranial pathology.

Fetal distress means no more than that the fetal condition, as judged by the cardiotocograph (CTG), is causing anxiety.

Inadequate maternal effort is reflected in a prolonged second stage but the older concepts of second-stage limits have been confused by the introduction of epidural blocks. The risk factor in the second stage of labour is maternal pushing which, if prolonged, will cause deterioration in the fetal condition and induce fetal acidaemia. With an effective epidural block, the mother no longer has a desire to push and at this stage although the cervix is fully dilated, the fetus is no more at risk than at the end of the first stage of labour. Provided only that the CTG remains normal, it is probably no longer appropriate to set strict time limits even to the pushing phase of the second stage of labour, but after 45 minutes the fetal pH will begin to fall.[13]

Common errors in forceps delivery

The most frequent causes of both fetal and maternal injury during forceps delivery are:

▶ operator inexperience

▶ repeated attempts by junior doctors, often with different instruments

▶ delay in the decision – delivery interval

mistaking head level

 mistaking head position.

Very occasionally, forceps delivery is attempted before full dilatation of the cervix, resulting in maternal injury.

Unless the operator is certain of the position of the fetal head, the level of the fetal head, and has sufficient experience and competence, operative delivery should not be undertaken.

Outlet forceps

In outlet forceps delivery, the head is visible without parting the labia, the sagittal suture is in the antero-posterior diameter of the pelvis and the head is on the perineum with the only remaining barrier the maternal soft tissues. In principle, the mother should be in the lithotomy position but experienced operators may feel comfortable and confident with the mother in a dorsal position if the forceps delivery is sufficiently low. The operator should maintain continuous verbal and eye contact with the mother, explaining every step to her. The forceps are assembled in front of the perineum and if there is no pre-existing analgesia the perineum and vulva should be infiltrated with a local anæsthetic agent.

The left blade of the forceps is first selected. The position and level of the fetus are checked again and the left blade is applied, followed by the right. Traction is applied with a uterine contraction. With the head so low in the pelvis the direction of traction is usually close to the horizontal. Traction should never be greater than that exerted by the operator flexing the forearm. Placing the index finger between the blade also protects from the use of excessive force. Descent should occur with the first traction; if it does not a careful reassessment should be undertaken. Outlet forceps delivery requires little traction force.

If the indication for forceps delivery is the maternal condition, it may not be necessary to perform an episiotomy. However, in a primigravid patient with a prolonged second stage an episiotomy is usually an integral part of the procedure. A medio-lateral incision is appropriate. After the head has emerged, the blades of the forceps are removed and the body delivered normally. The vagina and perineum should be examined for injury and if necessary vaginal repair conducted immediately by the operator.

Low forceps

In low forceps delivery, the head is at or near the pelvic floor but may not be visible without parting the labia and the perineum does not distend with contractions. The lowest bony part is at least 2 cm below the ischial spines. The sagittal suture may not be in the antero-posterior diameter but will not be more than 45° from it. The head may well be occiput posterior.

The mother should be in the lithotomy position and the operator should be seated facing the perineum. The position and station of the fetal head should be checked and the operator should not attempt to apply the obstetric forceps until the position is certain. If deviation from the antero-posterior diameter is minimal, it may be possible to ease the head round by digital rotation. Alternatively, less than 45° rotation can be undertaken with conventional forceps (such as Neville Barnes or Simpson). The advantage of these forceps is that traction subsequently can be exerted in the correct direction because of the pelvic curve. Again, the left blade is applied before the right. If there is any difficulty applying the forceps, the situation must be reassessed fully. In the absence of a contraction, any minor malrotation of the head is corrected. Again, if the head does not turn easily the situation is reassessed.

With a contraction, traction is exerted downwards towards the floor. When the head has reached the perineum the appropriate upward movement is applied to achieve delivery in a horizontal plane, with extension of the head. An episiotomy is performed when the head distends the perineum. If during traction the forceps blades adopt a rather more horizontal position, this suggests that the head is in the occipito-posterior position. A generous episiotomy is then essential because the widest diameter is more posterior and the occiput will exert pressure posteriorly, increasing the possibility of damage to the anus and rectum.

If an occiput posterior position is recognized at the outset, the operator will need to decide whether to embark on full rotation or deliver the baby face to pubis. If the head is low, it may be less traumatic to both mother and baby to complete delivery in the occiput posterior position. In these circumstances, the forceps are applied exactly as if the head were occiput anterior.

Difficulty in achieving the correct position of the forceps, failure to turn the head with minimal force, failure of descent with the first pull are all danger signals that demand full reassessment. Particularly in the presence of major degrees of caput and moulding, the operator must check that assumptions about head level and position are correct. After each contraction, the fetal heart must be checked. If after three contractions, with traction and bearing-down effort, the head is not delivered, Caesarean section should be performed.

Mid-cavity forceps

In these circumstances, the leading bony part of the head is above the pelvic floor. The head is engaged abdominally with no more than one fifth palpable. Forceps delivery should not be undertaken if two fifths or more of the head are palpable.[14] Station of the head is below the ischial spines but less than 2 cm below. The occiput is unlikely to be anterior and is most likely transverse – deep transverse arrest. There is also likely to be some asynclitism with one parietal bone leading the other. It is this type of delivery requiring rotation from the mid-pelvis, which demands the greatest skill.

The instrument most frequently used for the purpose is Kjelland's forceps. The procedure requires training, skill and frequent practice. Epidural analgesic block is preferred but the delivery can be effected with pudendal block. Before embarking on the procedure, the operator must satisfy himself that the fetus is in good condition and must have no doubt about the precise position and station of the fetal head. If there is doubt about position, it is usually possible to feel an ear by passing the index finger anteriorly between the fetal head and the symphysis pubis. In the transverse position of the fetal head the anterior ear is usually readily palpable and assists the operator in determining the position of the occiput.

The procedure is then explained to the mother and the forceps are assembled with the buttons towards the occiput. The anterior blade is then selected and applied to the fetal head. Whether the operator applies the blade directly or by wandering is a matter of personal choice. The posterior blade then follows, applied directly and with great care, it is eased into position in front of the sacrum. The forceps blades will then lie at different levels because of the asynclitism. This is corrected by adjusting the blades within the sliding lock so that they lie at the same level. Between contractions, the head is rotated gently using only the force of the wrist. If there is any difficulty or obstruction, the operator must carefully reassess the position. On occasion, it may not be possible to rotate the head at the level of arrest and it may have to be displaced upwards or downwards in order to achieve sufficient room to rotate.

Once rotation is completed successfully, the position of the sutures and fontanelles is again checked without removing the forceps. Since Kjelland's forceps do not have a pelvic curve the direction of traction is posterior and towards the floor. In order to apply traction appropriately, it is usually necessary for the operator to kneel or to sit on a very low stool, close to the ground. Some operators remove the Kjelland's forceps at this point and apply conventional curved forceps. In my view, this is poor practice, for it adds to maternal discomfort and trauma; occasionally the head will revert to its previous malrotated position once the Kjelland's forceps are removed. The fetal heart is assessed following rotation and before traction is applied. The rest of the delivery is then conducted as for a low forceps procedure. Episiotomy should only be performed when the head distends the perineum. Episiotomy performed before rotation frequently leads to a spiral tear of the vagina which may prove difficult to repair. If delivery is not achieved in five contractions with bearing-down effort, the procedure should be abandoned and Caesarean section performed.

Trial of forceps

The only circumstances in which it is permissible to attempt forceps delivery, remove the blades and proceed to Caesarean section is in the context of a trial of forceps. If the operator has any doubt about the outcome, he should not embark upon a forceps delivery without full preparation for Caesarean section. That means that the operation should begin in a fully-equipped operating theatre with sufficient anæsthesia to proceed directly to Caesarean section with the theatre staff and the anæsthetist prepared to proceed immediately to Caesarean section. The mother must also be informed that, in the event of failure, Caesarean section will immediately be performed. There will be no time for explanations or consent when the attempt at operative vaginal delivery fails.

The operator who embarks upon a forceps delivery without these precautions may be tempted, in the event of difficulty to have 'one last pull' rather than admit defeat. Mature judgement is required; the inexperienced operator must err on the side of caution. In the words of Ian Donald:

> Trial of forceps is like lion taming; it is not the sort of exercise one would willingly undertake in expectation of failure.

Failed forceps

The application of forceps and failure to deliver, without full preparations for a trial, is an obstetric disaster. Most failed forceps arise as the result of 'disobeying the ground rules, inexperience and lack of discipline'.[15] Contributory factors include failure to locate the occiput correctly, unrecognized brow presentation, incomplete dilatation of the cervix and cephalo-pelvic disproportion. O'Grady[16] distinguishes between two types of failure: failure in the initial application of the instrument and failure in extraction once the instrument has been applied correctly:

> Errors in clinical judgement, lack of sufficient skill, or unforeseen difficulties contribute to both categories of failure.[16] (Page 60.)

In the context of training, a junior doctor may fail to deliver the baby, having applied the forceps; it is, of course, permissible for the trainer to continue and complete the delivery. What is not acceptable is for a series of junior doctors, often with different instruments to attempt vaginal delivery repeatedly without preparation for Caesarean section.

Ventouse delivery

With the decreasing skills and increasing reluctance to use the obstetric forceps ventouse delivery is increasing in popularity. Whilst the instrument requires much less training to achieve basic proficiency and whilst it is, by design, less likely to damage mother and baby, it should not be assumed that it is totally safe. Beyond basic instruction, formal training in the use of the instrument is rare and most junior doctors acquire their experience by self-instruction. Litigation arising out of the ventouse occurs principally because of:

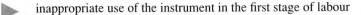 inappropriate use of the instrument in the first stage of labour

prolonged and repeated traction

injury to the baby

soft-tissue injury to the mother.

It is difficult to conceive of a proper indication for the ventouse in the first stage of labour in modern obstetrics. Lack of progress with no sign of fetal compromise is properly managed by oxytocic stimulation of the uterus. If the indication for delivery is fetal distress, the ventouse is not an appropriate instrument. With cervix still remaining, the likely time scale for ventouse delivery is not appreciably faster than a Caesarean section and the stress on the baby incomparably greater. Fetal distress in the first stage of labour is managed by Caesarean section, not by operative vaginal delivery.

Indications for the ventouse in the second stage of labour include delay, fetal distress, and elective shortening of the second stage for fetal or maternal benefit. Most would regard the ventouse as too slow for use in severe fetal distress but some claim that with modern instruments and an experienced operator, the application-delivery interval may by no longer than for forceps.[17]

Special indications for the more skilled operator include delay in the second stage with malposition of the fetal head, and delivery of the second twin with the head not yet engaged.

Success with the ventouse is closely related to patient selection, which should take into account the following:

- The history of the pregnancy and labour
- The degree of moulding
- The station of the head
- The position of the head.

With the head visible or on the perineum, success is likely even with severe moulding and some malposition. With the head at the level of the ischial spines and in the absence of fetal distress or malposition, safe delivery is usually readily accomplished. However, with head only at station zero, the additional risk factors of fetal distress, malposition or severe moulding call for increased caution, and the delivery should either be by Caesarean section or, in the hands of a suitably experienced operator, a trial of ventouse delivery, conducted exactly as a trial of forceps. If the leading part of the fetal head is above the ischial spines, Caesarean section is the preferred option, save only in the case of the second twin. The practice of applying the ventouse to a high head so as to bring it down to a level where forceps can safely be applied is not acceptable

If the labour has been slow and the second stage complicated by delay with a suspected large baby, a difficult extraction is likely. It is in these circumstances that shoulder dystocia is most commonly encountered.

Whilst the literature is clear that ventouse deliveries are less likely than forceps deliveries to result in fetal injury, it should not be supposed that the instrument is free of danger. Subgaleal bleeding is strongly related to ventouse delivery; cephalo-haematoma, primary subarachnoid haemorrhage, epidural, intradural, central tentorial and basal subdural haemorrhages are all reported.[18] Most fetal injuries resulting in litigation result from prolonged traction, repeated traction or repeated re-application of the cup. O'Grady[19] warns (p. 184):

> In vacuum extraction operations, safety is best ensured by careful cup placement and by strictly limiting the surgeon's efforts in terms of number of traction efforts, cup displacements, and the total period of cup application... For forceps, meticulous adherence to traction technique and limiting the total number of efforts are similarly appropriate. It is well to understand that more than **85% of ultimately successful deliveries with either instrument occur with four or fewer traction efforts**.

Vacca[20] reviewed the literature concerning the measurements of traction and the safe limits and concluded that objective measurement was not possible. He concludes (on page 68):

> Ultimately it is the operator who decides how much extra force, in addition to the normal compression forces of labour, will be exerted on the fetal head as a result of vacuum extraction. The difference between excessive, average or minimum force in delivery may depend primarily on the attending obstetrician's knowledge of how to correct abnormalities and to deliver along the path of least resistance. The least additional force to effect delivery with vacuum extraction will result from flexing median applications of the cup, followed by traction in the line of the axis of the birth canal. Total force will be reduced if a limit is placed on the duration of the procedure and on the number of pulls.

Finally, much emphasis is laid upon the reduction in maternal soft-tissue injury with the ventouse, as compared with forceps. Because the instrument does not distend the perineum, there is less tendency for ano-rectal injury and soft-tissue damage at the vulva. However, some of the most extensive soft-tissue injuries I have encountered in litigation practice have been as the result of maternal soft tissue (vagina or cervix) becoming trapped and avulsed by the ventouse cup. It is essential that before any traction is applied, the operator ascertains that nothing other than fetal scalp is included within the vacuum cup.

Breech delivery

There are two essential components to good risk management in breech presentation:

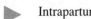 Antenatal selection for vaginal breech delivery

Intrapartum care by a competent practitioner.

Reference has already been made to the impossibility of pursuing a policy of 'no vaginal breech delivery'. It simply cannot be done, and any obstetric department which claims to do it is failing to face the reality that breech deliveries will occur; the skills base required for their proper selection and conduct will be lost if such mistaken policies are pursued.

Prenatal selection for mothers for vaginal breech delivery has been discussed elsewhere but may be summarized here:

 Size of the baby

Size of the maternal pelvis

Fetal attitude

 Counselling and consent.

Babies presenting as a breech whose birth weights are estimated above 3.5 kilos should not be delivered vaginally. Maternal size was traditionally estimated by erect lateral pelvimetry but that is no longer fashionable. Some modern textbook authorities regard X-ray measurements are unnecessary but a view still prevails[21] that pelvimetry may have a role as part of the selection process for the mode of delivery for women with breech presentation.

The attitude of the baby is every bit as important as its weight, and extension of the head, demonstrated on ultrasound, is a clear contraindication to vaginal breech delivery. The footling breech is also unsuitable for vaginal breech delivery because of the very high risk of prolapse of the umbilical cord.

There is clear evidence that external cephalic version at term substantially reduces the incidence of breech birth and Caesarean section.[22] In UK reported series, the success rate for version is about 40%.

For those in whom external version fails, full counselling of the mother to include all of the risks and benefits of vaginal versus abdominal delivery is essential. The task is not easy, for a careful review of the literature has until recently produced no convincing statistics and:

> Although fetuses presenting by the breech have an increased perinatal mortality, because of the paucity of randomized controlled trial data it has proved impossible to separate out the independent risks of the breech position itself, and the problems of the delivery, from the problems which stem from the fetus being abnormal. The perinatal mortality remains increased even when delivery is by caesarean section, and this is true even after correction for gestational age, congenital defects and birth weight.[23] (Page 1026.)

Nevertheless, certain hazards are inherent in vaginal breech delivery:

 Prolapse of the cord

 Arrest of the head

 Precipitate head delivery

 An obligatory period of anoxia.

Although prolapse of the cord is not peculiar to breech delivery, it is very much more common than in cephalic presentation. Prolapse of the cord becomes increasingly common in those varieties of breech presentation that fit the pelvic brim poorly, with the highest incidence in the double footling presentation.

Recently, a multicentre study of 2083 women at term with breech presentation[24] has demonstrated that in the group assigned to elective Caesarean section, perinatal mortality, neonatal mortality and serious neonatal morbidity were significantly lower than for the planned vaginal birth group. The authors conclude that:

Planned caesarean section is better than planned vaginal birth for the term fetus in the breech presentation; serious maternal complications are similar between the two groups.[24]

It remains to be seen whether other trials confirm this observation.

Once the decision has been made to permit vaginal breech delivery, the less operator interference with the process, the safer it becomes.

In the first stage of labour, the mother should be asked to report early, in case of cord accidents when the membranes rupture. A vaginal examination to exclude cord prolapse at the time of membrane rupture is essential. Induction of labour has a poor reputation in breech presentation and spontaneous onset of labour carries a much better prognosis for success. An intravenous line should be introduced early and blood taken for cross-matching because of the high risk of Caesarean section. Electronic fetal heart monitoring is essential throughout breech labour and an epidural block a distinct advantage. There is no place for fetal blood sampling in breech labour. Since there is an obligatory period of near-total asphyxia towards the end of labour when the fetal head engages, significant fetal distress in the first stage of breech labour demands Caesarean section, not procrastination with blood sampling. The blood is more difficult to obtain and it may be different from that obtained from scalp skin:

If, having understood the normal mechanisms of CTG changes in a breech, there is good indication for pH measurement then there is good indication for caesarean section.[25] (Page 124.)

The use of oxytocin in the first stage of breech labour is both controversial and problematic. Whilst oxytocin may be appropriate in primary dysfunctional labour it is generally unwise to employ the drug in secondary arrest or with any slowing down of the labour process after 4 cm dilatation. Delay at that stage should be seen as a clear indication that the breech may, after all, be too big. Failure to make expected progress in dilatation of the cervix or in descent of the breech should prompt a careful reassessment of whether vaginal breech delivery is safe.

In the second stage of vaginal breech delivery, there should be present an experienced obstetrician and an anæsthetist. It is a common error to encourage maternal effort before full dilatation of the cervix. The desire to push may be triggered by the appearance of the breech in the vagina before the cervix is fully dilated. The consequences may by disastrous if the body of the baby is delivered through an incompletely dilated cervix for the head will surely be trapped by it.

Under no circumstances should there be any traction upon the body of the breech. Not until the umbilicus is born should the operator touch the baby and then only to assist the descent of the legs by flexion of the knee joint. The fetal condition may at this time be conveniently checked by palpation of the cord. It is essential that, in the succeeding phases of the delivery of the baby's body, the fetal back should be uppermost. If it is not, the operator should gently hold the body of the baby in a towel and turn the baby, but without exerting traction. When the tip of the scapula is delivered, it is permissible to search for the arms, which will usually be found flexed in front of the baby's body. The arms are then readily disengaged with a finger. Only in the rare circumstances of nuchal displacement of the fetal arms (ie arms above the head) is it necessary to perform the Løvset manoeuvre. Nuchal displacement is almost always a consequence of traction on the body of the breech and in spontaneous breech delivery will rarely be encountered.

Once the arms are delivered, the baby should be allowed to hang by its own weight until the hairs on the nape of the neck are visible. At that point the operator is called upon to intervene. The safest method of delivery of the head is a combination of the Burns Marshall manoeuvre[26] and the application of obstetric forceps. The Mauriceau–Smellie–Veit manoeuvre is inferior and unsafe. In this manoeuvre, the operator passes his right hand along the ventral surface of the baby and places his middle finger in the baby's mouth. His index and ring finger grasp the baby's shoulders. The left hand is passed along the dorsal surface of the baby and the middle finger presses upon the occiput, so as to flex it, the index and ring fingers grasping the shoulders. In this way, the head may be brought down and flexed but the procedure is inferior to the obstetric forceps because:

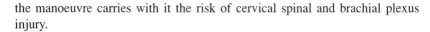 the operator has less control

the manoeuvre carries with it the risk of cervical spinal and brachial plexus injury.

The interval from the moment the umbilicus is born (and the cord therefore obstructed) until delivery of the mouth and nose should not exceed 10 minutes. During this time, the fetus will be severely short of oxygen but provided there has been no previous compromise, the baby should be capable of resuscitation to normality.

If the fetal head does not descend and the obstetric forceps cannot be applied easily, disaster is imminent. The fetal head will usually be arrested at or above the pelvic brim and probably still in the transverse position. The obstetric forceps are at this point of no use and should be abandoned. Unless the fetal head can be brought down quickly into the pelvis and the mouth and nose made available for resuscitation, the baby will die of asphyxia. Whilst this situation should never be encountered with proper antenatal screening it is the one circumstance in which the Mauriceau–Smellie–Veit manoeuvre, combined with suprapubic pressure and the McRoberts position (see below) may be of assistance. With a generous episiotomy it may be possible for the operator to draw the baby's head into the pelvis whilst still in the transverse position and to rotate it, with traction, and achieve safe delivery.

Breech extraction

Breech extraction differs from the description given above for it implies active traction upon the breech from the beginning. The traction inevitably results in extension of both the arms and the head and increases significantly the mechanical difficulties for the baby. Breech extraction therefore should never be practised upon a term baby. The only place for breech extraction is in the context of twin delivery (see below) where the second small twin may, on occasion, be safely delivered by this method.

Twin delivery

A single amniotic sac and discordant growth with a 25% difference in ultrasound estimated weight might be indications for abdominal delivery. In other circumstances, provided the first twin presents longitudinally, vaginal delivery may be permitted. If the first twin presents by the breech the conditions necessary to satisfy a singleton breech delivery should be fulfilled.

During the first stage of labour, it is essential that both twins are monitored electronically. In practice, this is best achieved, once the membranes of the first twin are ruptured, by the application of a scalp electrode to the first twin, so as adequately to differentiate the two fetal hearts. The threshold for intervention, particularly if there is abnormality in the CTG of the second twin, should be much lower than in singleton pregnancy. The second twin is at much higher risk and if already showing signs of stress in early labour, must be rescued by Caesarean section.

Otherwise the first stage of labour for the first twin is managed much as any other labour. It is because the position of the second twin, following delivery of the first, is unpredictable that special precautions are necessary. The position of the second twin, whilst the first is still *in utero* is irrelevant for, with delivery, the second twin, previously longitudinal and cephalic, may suddenly become transverse and undeliverable. In the second stage of twin delivery, therefore, there must be present in the labour ward:

▶ an obstetrician capable of all forms of operative intervention

▶ an anaesthetist

▶ at least one paediatrician, preferably two.

Even if an epidural block is not in place, there should be an intravenous infusion already running before the start of the second stage, so that oxytocin can be introduced, if necessary, without delay; and so that, in the event of a Caesarean section, the anæsthetist will have immediate intravenous access.

Once the first twin is delivered (usually by a midwife) and ergometrine withheld, the doctor must immediately palpate the mother's abdomen so as to determine the lie of the second twin. An ultrasound machine should be available in the room and, if there is any difficulty in identifying the lie and presentation of the baby, ultrasound should be employed. If the lie of the second twin is not longitudinal, the doctor should gently perform external version; it matters little whether the baby is turned to a cephalic or breech presentation. Once longitudinal, uterine activity is awaited. During this time it is essential that the fetal heart is monitored. Provided the fetal heart is satisfactory, there is no immediate hurry. If contractions do not begin again within about 10 minutes, an oxytocin infusion should be started so as to encourage uterine contractions. Once the uterus is contracting, the presenting part will usually descend and delivery will occur spontaneously. Provided that the fetal heart remains normal, the membranes of the second twin should be preserved as long as possible. There is no particular advantage in rupturing the membranes in such circumstances.

If the membranes rupture spontaneously, a vaginal examination should immediately be performed to exclude cord prolapse. If monitoring of the fetal heart indicates the need to intervene, it will be necessary to rupture the membranes and expedite delivery. Under these circumstances breech extraction may be permissible; if the head presents and is too high for the obstetric forceps, the ventouse may be applied in the reasonable certainty that there is no mechanical obstruction to the delivery. It may be necessary to correct the lie by internal version but this manoeuvre requires general anæsthesia. The alternative is Caesarean section. It is for this reason that an anæsthetist must be present for every twin delivery and facilities must be appropriate for the rapid induction of general anæsthesia. There is little point in having an obstetrician capable of intervention and an anæsthetist ready to administer a general anaesthetic if the delivery is conducted in a place where such manoeuvres are inappropriate. Twin delivery must be performed in a delivery room capable of accommodating general anæsthesia, or at the very least, within a few yards of such a venue.

Common causes of litigation in relation to twin delivery are:

▶ failure to intervene in the first stage of labour because of CTG abnormalities, particularly in the second twin

▶ delay in delivery of the second twin.

This delay is most frequently due to:

▶ the absence of key experienced personnel at delivery

▶ artificial rupture of the second amniotic sac before the presentation is appropriate

▶ lack of preparedness for Caesarean section.

Whilst the delay in delivery of the second twin is most often due to the absence of a key member of the team, it sometimes occurs because, although all the members of the team are present, the circumstances for the induction of general anæsthesia are thought to be inadequate and the patient has to be moved, often over a long distance and on to a different floor, to achieve abdominal delivery. It is absolutely essential that at the beginning of the second stage of twin labour all of the preparations are in place for immediate induction of anæsthesia and abdominal delivery, should that become necessary.

Shoulder dystocia

Difficulty in delivering the shoulders vaginally after the delivery of the head is referred to as shoulder dystocia.

> Shoulder dystocia, although it represents only 0.15%–0.38% of all vaginal deliveries, is a bona fide obstetric emergency for it holds an inordinate perinatal and maternal morbidity in both motor and behavioural function.[27]

Of all the labour ward emergencies in the developed world, obstetricians generally fear true and severe shoulder dystocia more than any other. The time scale for successful management is so short.

The circumstances required to produce shoulder dystocia are a baby whose shoulder girdle exceeds its head diameter. This is not common, even in large babies. Provided the shoulder girdle is no larger than the head, simple rotation in the birth canal will deliver it.

The principles of physics as applicable to shoulder delivery were described by Woods in 1942.[28]

The classic description of shoulder dystocia was made by Morris[29] in 1955. Since that time a number of manoeuvres have been described to overcome this potentially disastrous difficulty and a number of risk factors have been established to warn of the probability of shoulder dystocia

Definition

There is no agreed definition of 'shoulder dystocia'. The term simply means difficulty in delivering the shoulders. O'Leary,[30] in a textbook devoted entirely to the subject, reviews definitions and concludes:

> ... most investigators agree that it has occurred when the standard delivery procedures of gentle downward traction of the fetal head and moderate fundal pressure fail to accomplish delivery. The problem with this definition is that the qualifiers 'gentle' and 'moderate' lack precise definition. (Page 2.)

Classification according to the severity of shoulder dystocia was not attempted until the 1990s. There are two approaches. O'Leary[30] grades the condition according to its response to treatment, a necessarily retrospective analysis (Table 13.1). Gibb[31] takes a simple approach to classification (Table 13.2) depending upon the anatomy.

Table 13.1.   O'Leary:[30] Severity of shoulder dystocia and suggested treatment

Stage	Treatment

I. Mild	Suprapubic pressure with or without rotation
	    Directed posterior (Mazzanti)
	    Directed to one side (Rubin)
	    Woods' manoeuvre
	    Rubin's manoeuvre (reverse Woods')

II. Moderate	Posterior shoulder delivery Hibbard manoeuvre
III. Severe	McRoberts' manoeuvre McRoberts' manoeuvre combinedwith rotations and suprapubic pressure
IV. Undeliverable	Cephalic replacement (Gunn–Zavanelli–O'Leary manoeuvre)

Table 13.2. Gibb:[31] Classification of shoulder dystocia

There are three types of shoulder dystocia:

- A tight squeeze of a chunky baby with a degree of uterine inertia, in which case the rotation mechanism is present although relatively ineffective: this may be perceived by the midwife as 'some difficulty with the shoulders', and is relatively easily resolved
- Unilateral dystocia
- Bilateral dystocia (the most serious)

The anatomy of shoulder dystocia

Assuming a normal female pelvis, the fetal head usually engages in the pelvis in the transverse position so that the baby is facing either to the left or to the right of the mother; thus it descends in the birth canal until undergoing rotation so as to be born facing backwards. The shoulders do not follow this rotation of the baby so that after the fetal head is freed the head tends to be turned by the muscles of the neck so as to face sideways again. The shoulders are generally considered to engage and descend in either the antero-posterior or an oblique diameter of the maternal pelvis.

When the anterior shoulder fails to descend below the symphysis pubis the shoulder becomes obstructed. Occasionally, both shoulders lie above the pelvic inlet, the posterior shoulder being held up by the sacral promontory. These two conditions are illustrated in O'Leary's diagram (Figure 13.5). Bilateral shoulder dystocia is exceptionally rare and when it occurs the baby cannot usually be delivered vaginally without harm. In both the classifications of O'Leary[30] and Gibb,[31] bilateral shoulder dystocia is managed by cephalic replacement rather than by any vaginal manoeuvre. When vaginal manoeuvres are discussed in relation to shoulder dystocia, they should be understood to be concerned with *unilateral* shoulder dystocia.

Incidence and risk factors

The incidence of shoulder dystocia is difficult to determine from the literature and widely varying rates are quoted: between 0.15% and 1.7% of all vaginal deliveries. Gibb suggests an incidence of 0.2–1.2%[31] and Roberts, in a recent review article,[32] quotes figures varying between 0.23% and 1.1% (page 201).

Gibb[33] lists the following antecedents of shoulder dystocia, which should put the obstetric attendants on notice of its likely occurrence:

➤ Maternal obesity

➤ Diabetes mellitus

➤ Gestational age of greater than 41 weeks

➤ Previous shoulder dystocia

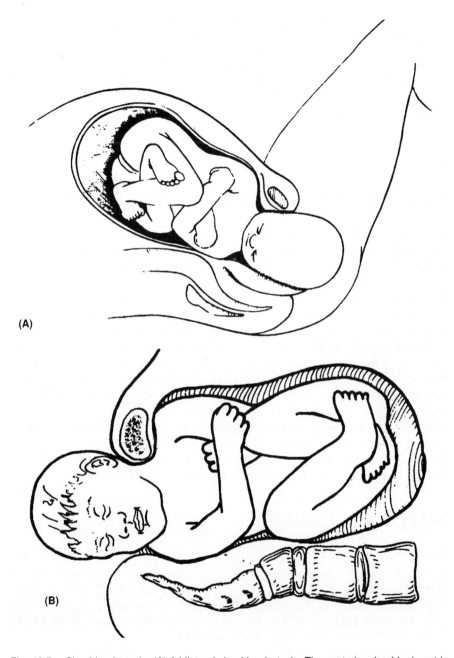

Fig. 13.5. Shoulder dystocia. (A) A bilateral shoulder dystocia. The posterior shoulder is not in the hollow of the pelvis. This presentation often requires a cephalic replacement. (C Pauerstein [ed.] *Clinical Obstetrics*. New York: Churchill–Livingstone, 1987.) (B) Unilateral shoulder dystocia is usually easily dealt with by standard techniques. (Harris B. Shoulder dystocia. Clinical Obstetrics and Gynaecology 1984; 27: 106.) Reproduced, with permission, from O'Leary JA. *Shoulder Dystocia and Birth Injury: Prevention and Treatment.* McGraw–Hill, 1992: 108.

▶ Previous big baby

▶ Recognized macrosomia of the present pregnancy

▶ Prolongation of the late first stage of labour

▶ Prolongation of the second stage of labour

▶ Operative delivery (see page 233[33]).

O'Leary divides the risk factors into three:

▶ Preconceptual (Table 13.3)

▶ Antepartum (Table 13.4)

▶ Intrapartum (Table 13.5)

Table 13.3. Key preconceptual historical risk factors

1. Maternal birthweight
2. Prior shoulder dystocia
3. Prior macrosomia
4. Diabetes – pre-existing
5. Obesity
6. Multiparity
7. Prior gestational diabetes
8. Advanced maternal age

Table 13.4. Antepartum risk factors

1. Glucose intolerance or excess
2. Excessive weight gain
3. Macrosomia
4. Short stature
5. Abnormal pelvic shape
6. Abnormal pelvic size
7. Post-datism

Table 13.5. Intrapartum risk factors

1. Prolonged second stage
2. Protracted descent
3. Arrest of descent
4. Failure of descent
5. Macrosomia
6. Moulding
7. Need for mid-pelvic delivery

The older textbooks suggest that shoulder dystocia cannot be predicted but the impressive list of risk factors above demonstrates that shoulder dystocia can reasonably be expected when these risk factors occur in combination. It is not necessary for diabetes to be fully developed – gestational diabetes also carries a significant risk.

Prevention

The prediction of birth weight is at present imprecise and the margin of error seems to increase in proportion to fetal size. Even if birth weight could be accurately predicted Caesarean section for all babies weighing more than 4 kilos would not solve the problem because almost half of all shoulder dystocias occur during the delivery of babies weighing less than 4 kilos and most babies weighing more than 4 kilos are delivered without injury. But when does fetal size become critical? Roberts,[32] reviewing the literature, demonstrated the influence of fetal size on the incidence of shoulder dystocia and the additional effect of diabetes. The baby of the diabetic mother is of a different shape from that of the non-diabetic, such that for babies above 4 kilos the incidence of shoulder dystocia in the non-diabetic is 10% and for diabetics is 23.1%. Above 4.5 kilos the incidence in the non-diabetic rises to 22.6% and in the diabetic to 50%. Whilst there is no consensus in the literature that Caesarean section should be performed at any particular birth weight, it would seem reasonable to warn mothers whose babies are estimated to weigh more than 4.5 kilos, particularly if they are diabetic, that there is a high risk of shoulder dystocia. In those circumstances, most would probably prefer abdominal delivery.

The other major factor influencing risk is a history of shoulder dystocia in a previous pregnancy. In a small retrospective study of 51 cases,[34] Smith and Pearson found a recurrence rate of 9.8% – 17 times the background rate amongst all deliveries. They recommended only that the woman 'should have her ante-natal notes flagged to alert the obstetric and midwifery staff to the increased possibility of recurrence'.

In such circumstances, every effort should be made to estimate the birth weight of the baby in the index pregnancy; the mother should be warned of the significantly increased risk of shoulder dystocia in her circumstances.

For most cases, Roberts summarizes the position:[32]

> It is a truism to state that if a vaginal delivery does not occur, neither will a shoulder dystocia, but our predictive capabilities are not yet sufficiently developed to justify a policy of abdominal delivery to prevent this complication of a vaginal birth. Every birth assistant should be prepared for the moment when an infant's shoulders impact by developing a sequence of manoeuvres that he or she intends to use in this situation. (Page 213.)

Management

For the majority of shoulder dystocias, therefore, the key to prevention is not abdominal delivery but preparedness for shoulder dystocia. In most shoulder dystocias, correct procedure will prevent injury; and only in the most extreme cases of bilateral shoulder dystocia is injury truly inevitable.

A number of manoeuvres are now well-established and clearly recommended in midwifery and obstetric textbooks. Perhaps more important is the recognition of those manoeuvres which are *harmful* and which should be avoided.

Firm downward traction on the fetal head whilst the anterior shoulder is firmly impacted upon the symphysis pubis is likely to damage the child's brachial plexus. O'Leary[30] advises:

> Initially most obstetricians apply downward pressure to the head in an effort to dislodge the impacted anterior shoulder from under the pubic symphysis. This gentle downward tug is a standard manoeuvre for effecting delivery of the anterior shoulder in the otherwise normal vaginal delivery, so it is understandable why it is done so often for shoulder dystocia. However, its common use does not make it right. We teach our residents that when shoulder dystocia is diagnosed, they must not touch the baby's head again until after the shoulder impaction is corrected. Pulling on the head, even gently, risks brachial plexus injury. (Page 107.)

Excessive downward traction on the fetal head causes Erb's palsy. Alternative methods of delivery must therefore be learned in advance and practised whenever shoulder dystocia occurs. The key is for the midwife or doctor to be prepared and to have a strategy for dealing with the crisis.

In addition to stressing the importance of avoiding excessive traction, the midwifery texts recommend a change of maternal posture. For example:

> A position should be chosen which allows space for manoeuvring the baby towards the mother's sacrum. If she is on a bed turn the mother into the left lateral position with her buttocks at the end of the bed. If the lithotomy position is used, the buttocks should be slightly beyond the edge of the bed. In many cases a change of position is the only treatment required.[35] (Page 440.)

The author goes on to recommend:

- a generous episiotomy
- rotation of the shoulders into the antero-posterior diameter of the outlet
- suprapubic pressure
- elevation of the head to deliver the posterior shoulder
- rotation of the shoulders to take advantage of the fact that the posterior shoulder is already in the pelvis.

This last manoeuvre was first recommended by Woods in 1942[28] and refined by Rubin[36] in 1964.

Most texts emphasize the importance of maternal posture and supra-pubic pressure in releasing the anterior shoulder from beneath the pubic symphysis before applying traction. The optimal maternal posture was devised by William A. McRoberts of Houston, Texas,[37] and first described by Gonik et al.[38] in 1983. The mother is asked to adopt a position in which her knees and hips are maximally flexed with hips externally rotated, so that her knees are pushed up towards her shoulders (Figure 13.6).

The McRoberts position does not increase the dimensions of the pelvic brim but does aid delivery because:

- the anterior shoulder is elevated
- the fetal spine is flexed
- the posterior shoulder is pushed over the sacrum
- maternal lordosis is straightened

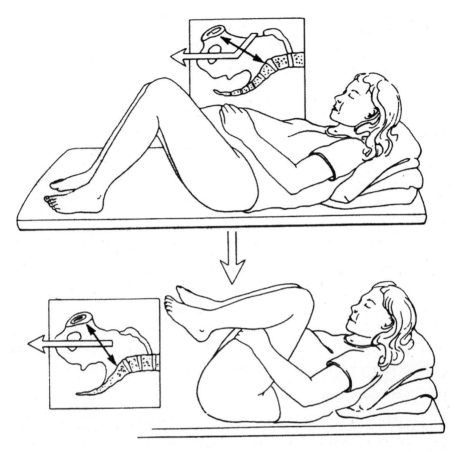

Fig 13.6. McRoberts manoeuvre. Hyperflexion of the patient's thighs changes the relationship of the pelvis to the lumbar spine, facilitating delivery of the fetal shoulders. From Beckmann CR, Ling FW, Barzensky BM *et al.* (eds.): *Obstetrics and Gynecology for Medical Students*. Baltimore: Williams and Wilkins, 1992, and reproduced with permission.

▶ the sacral promontory is removed as a point of obstruction

▶ the weight bearing force is removed from the sacrum

▶ the inlet is opened to its maximum

▶ the inlet is brought perpendicular to the maximum expulsive force.

Midwife authors tend to favour 'all fours' as an alternative to McRoberts.[39] Once the mother is in the optimum position the first manoeuvre to be attempted is suprapubic pressure.[40] At this point, the operator is acting within a time constraint for the baby, with its head delivered and its trunk firmly fixed in the birth canal cannot breathe and cannot obtain oxygen through the cord. O'Leary advises:[30]

In most cases, delivery can be accomplished without injury to the fetus if the physician is familiar with certain manipulative and operative techniques. Once the head has been delivered, the respiratory tract cleared of mucus and fluid, and the baby permitted a free airway, time becomes less important as long as the fetal heart is normal and shows no distress. Delivery of the impacted shoulders may then be performed unhurriedly and without panic. A scalp electrode from the electronic fetal monitor will determine the urgency of delivery due to cord compression and manipulation.

When there is difficulty, the simplest and least traumatic measures should be attempted; for instance manipulative methods of extracting from below and strong pressure applied to the suprapubic area from above. We condemn the practice of effecting shoulder delivery by strong traction on the baby's head once it is delivered, for by such unwise pulling, injury to the brachial plexus or even to the cervical spine may result.

The frequent question is, how much time do I have before brain damage will occur? Over 10 years ago Wood et al described serial pH determinations between delivery of the head and trunk. The pH declined at a ratio of 0.04 U per minute. Thus, there is adequate time to proceed in a well-organized manner, knowing that cephalic replacement is ultimately available. Delays greater than 7 to 10 minutes may be associated with low Apgar scores and perinatal asphyxia. (Pages 109, 110).

Thus, there is time for more than one attempt at an operative manoeuvre. If maternal repositioning and suprapubic pressure do not succeed, most authors suggest rotation of the fetal shoulders within the birth canal so as to rotate the baby's trunk, taking advantage of the fact that the posterior shoulder is already in the pelvis. If whilst maintaining gentle traction (without lateral flexion) the baby's trunk is rotated, the erstwhile posterior shoulder becomes anterior, remaining in the pelvis and the previously obstructed anterior shoulder is delivered into the hollow of the sacrum. The obstruction is thus overcome.

An alternative manoeuvre is to deliver the posterior arm but this requires a generous episiotomy and anæsthesia so as to allow the operator to place a hand within the already crowded space of the posterior vagina. In delivering the arm, the operator may fracture the baby's humerus but this is a small price to pay for it normally heals without long-term consequence.

Gibb summarizes the steps to be taken if shoulder dystocia is to be overcome safely:[29]

During antenatal assessment late in pregnancy in women at risk, the case sheet should be clearly marked: '**Big baby: Beware shoulder dystocia**'. The primary warning should appear in the part of the notes used for admission in labour.

With or without antepartum warning signals, intrapartum signals may appear . . . a doctor with appropriate experience in this management should be alerted and be in or just outside the room during delivery of the head. In most cases such assistance will not be necessary. It is much better to mobilize assistance that is not required than lack the essential life-saving assistance in the emergency. If it is, then a clear plan of action a 'Shoulder Dystocia Drill' can be implemented. All units should have this written down in the labour ward protocol and all staff must be familiar with it. From a review of the literature and logical analysis, there is a general agreement on the following procedures and their sequence as a shoulder dystocia drill:

1 **help should be summoned in the form of the most experienced obstetric doctor and an anaesthetist . . .**

2 the woman should be placed in the McRoberts position on in the all-fours position ...

3 an episiotomy must be done and liberally extended if it has been done already ...

4 pressure is exerted suprapubically to try to dislodge the anterior shoulder ...

5 when anaesthesia is adequate, then manipulation should be undertaken to rotate the shoulders ...

6 if rotation fails, then attempts should be made to deliver the posterior shoulder. (Pages 51, 52.)

In severe cases, and particularly where the shoulder dystocia is bilateral, all of these manoeuvres may fail, and the only alternative available then is cephalic replacement (the Zavanelli manoeuvre) first described in the middle 1980s in the United States but seldom employed. There are few successful references to it in the literature.

For the vast majority of shoulder dystocia, a solution can be found by employing the vaginal manoeuvres outlined above.

The fifth annual report of the Confidential Enquiry into Stillbirths and Deaths in Infancy focused upon the problems of shoulder dystocia. That report,[41] published in May 1998, recommended (page 78):

> Anticipate the possibility of shoulder dystocia if there is evidence of a big baby, especially in association with maternal obesity or glucose intolerance.
>
> If, following delivery of the head, there is immediate head retraction (the 'turtle sign') or restitution does not occur with the next expulsive contraction then immediate action is necessary. Call for assistance. The most senior available obstetrician should be alerted and a paediatrician must be in attendance. Additional midwifery staff may be needed to assist with the delivery. The mother should be given a brief, clear explanation of the problem and the proposed course of action.
>
> McRoberts' manoeuvre should be carried out by flexing the woman's legs right back so that her thighs are on her anterior abdominal wall. Suprapubic pressure should be applied to disimpact the anterior shoulder.
>
> If obstetric assistance is not available and these manoeuvres fail, then it is reasonable to try delivery in a squatting position, or on all fours, using downward traction to release the posterior shoulder.
>
> If a generous episiotomy, McRoberts' manoeuvre and suprapubic pressure have not achieved delivery of the body, an obstetrician or midwife should attempt to get access to the posterior shoulder.
>
> **(FUNDAL PRESSURE OR INCREASINGLY FORCEFUL TRACTION ON THE HEAD SHOULD BE AVOIDED.)**
>
> By this stage, the first attending paediatrician should have called for assistance of his or her most senior available colleague and, whenever possible, a neonatal nurse experienced in resuscitation.
>
> Complete and accurate clinical notes are essential, especially of the time when help is called for.
>
> Reiteration of delivery ward protocols for shoulder dystocia to labour ward and paediatric staff at regular intervals may be helpful.
>
> Symphysiotomy, deliberate clavicular fracture or the Zavenelli procedure have not been included in this sequence because they are not widely used in the UK. However, shoulder dystocia is a desperate situation for the fetus, so obstetricians and midwives should be aware of all the possible techniques for effecting delivery.

Brachial plexus injury without dystocia

Since the early 1990s, reports have begun to appear in the American literature of brachial plexus injury in the absence of *recorded* shoulder dystocia. In 1993, Jennett *et al.*,[42] from Phoenix Arizona, USA, reported a series of 39 infants diagnosed as having incurred brachial plexus impairment. Seventeen were associated with recorded diagnosis of shoulder dystocia, whereas 22 had no such recorded association. The authors commented:

> It has been postulated that intrauterine pressures associated with uterine anomalies could be a factor. Although the presence of such anomalies could not be determined from the available data, uterine maladaptation associated with young maternal age and nulliparity might well be associated with a higher incidence of intrauterine pressures resulting in nerve impairment. Spontaneous vaginal delivery was more than twice as common in the non-shoulder-dystocia group, suggesting less probability of difficulty in delivery. Certainly, the brachial plexus impairment in a 2572 gm infant delivered by cesarean section from a transverse lie would have a high probability of intrauterine maladaptation as a cause.

The theory in Phoenix, therefore, was that some form of uterine 'maladaptation' was responsible for those cases of brachial plexus injury that could not be explained by shoulder dystocia. Hankins and Clark,[43] from Salt Lake City, Utah, USA, suggested an alternative when they reported a single case in which brachial plexus injury had occurred in the posterior shoulder without recording of shoulder dystocia. They speculate on the mechanism – that the posterior shoulder may become temporarily lodged behind the sacral promontory, yet delivery of the head results from maternal expulsive efforts or use of instruments.

Other authors reported brachial plexus injury without shoulder dystocia but without suggesting a mechanism. Sandmire and DeMott[44] reported a retrospective study from 1985 to 1994 and analysed them according to the Caesarean section rates of the obstetricians in their study. They reported 19 brachial plexus injuries associated with shoulder dystocia and a further 17 in cephalic deliveries in the absence of recorded dystocia; newborns with shoulder dystocia-associated brachial plexus injury were larger than those having the same injury without shoulder dystocia.[44]

Jennett and Tarby[45] returned to the question of uterine 'maladaptation' in a further paper in 1997. Other authors[46] also reported brachial-plexus injury without recorded shoulder dystocia but again did not suggest a mechanism. A group from Los Angeles[47] published in 1998 a paper whose purpose was to determine whether Erb's palsies occurring in the absence of shoulder dystocia differ from those occurring after shoulder dystocia. They found that the characteristics of the children concerned did differ in certain respects: smaller birth weight, an increased incidence of both precipitate labour and clavicular fracture; speculating that:[47]

> Pressure of the fetal shoulder against the symphysis pubis during the ante-partum period may also lead to clavicular fracture.

But in a term fetus the only opportunity for the anterior shoulder to impact upon the symphysis pubis is when the fetal head is already partially delivered.

Many of these reports have as their logical basis the failure of *reported* shoulder dystocia in the births of babies found later to be suffering from Erb's palsy. The danger of drawing conclusions from matters *not* recorded is self-evident. A further difficulty was pointed out by a correspondent in the *American Journal of Obstetrics and Gynecology* following the papers by Gherman and Ouzounian:[48]

> In their recent article Gherman *et al* found that 17 of 40 (42.5%) cases of Erb's palsy occurred 'without shoulder dystocia' and that these infants had more fractured clavicles and were more likely to be permanently injured. The authors concluded that this group of injuries occurred from 'an in utero insult' and not neck traction. The authors define the 'shoulder dystocia' group on the basis of 'the need for ancillary obstetric maneuvers other than gentle downward traction after delivery of the fetal head'.
>
> Another explanation for their results is very possible. What if the operator experienced shoulder dystocia and managed it by pulling hard on the infant's neck to achieve delivery? In a retrospective review of hospital charts that type of case would not be classified as 'shoulder dystocia' in this study because no other maneuvers were performed. The excessive neck traction could result in more fractures and permanent Erb's palsy than occurs in infants who were managed by applying classic shoulder dystocia maneuvers.
>
> Although the authors have attempted to further understand the etiology of Erb's palsy, these retrospective data do not do that. Only a prospective, well-documented study will provide the indisputable data to identify the etiologies of Erb's palsy.

The authors in reply conceded, 'We agree that there is inherent ascertainment bias in our retrospective study.'

This body of literature makes it possible for the defendants to seek to defeat a claimant's case where there is:

▶ no recorded shoulder dystocia

▶ injury to the posterior shoulder.

In the presence of macrosomia, anterior shoulder injury and recorded shoulder dystocia, it remains more likely than not that the injury was caused by traction. The issue before the court then will be whether the traction applied was reasonable, necessary and appropriate or whether in applying such traction the defendant doctors and midwives were failing to meet a reasonable standard of care.

Caesarean section

The rate of Caesarean section has risen from about 3% in the 1950s to 15% in 1994–1995.[49] The Confidential Enquiry for the triennium 1994–1996[50] reported 93 deaths from Caesarean section of which 17 were elective, compared with some 63 emergency Caesarean sections. When counselling women of the risks of Caesarean section, compared with the more dangerous types of vaginal delivery such as breech, multiple pregnancy and labour with a Caesarean section scar, it is important to discuss with the mother the difference between a Caesarean section carried out electively and one carried out as an emergency in labour when things go wrong. The problem for the obstetrician in these circumstances is that the true risk of elective Caesarean section is difficult to ascertain from the literature. In the previous triennial report, the maternal mortality for elective Caesarean section was of the order of 1 in 10,000. Chamberlain[51] commenting on the trends in mortality at Caesarean section over the past 20 years commented:

> Further analysis of the 1982–84 figures showed that the incidence of direct deaths from elective Caesarean section was only 0.09 per 1000 operations compared with 0.37 per 1000 emergency operations. (Pages 873, 874.)

The author goes on:

> A similar difference was found in the previous triennium, but the 1982–84 report does not show the reason for the high mortality amongst the emergency group. Undoubtedly the conditions for which the operation is performed carry greater risks among women undergoing emergency procedures. (Page 874.)

The authors for the Confidential Enquiry for the Triennium 1991–1993[52] note:

> There was a dramatic fall, of nearly 44% in the number of deaths following elective sections but a doubling of the number after unplanned emergency procedures. In the latter case a common finding was that the junior staff took too much responsibility, or had it devolved to them. (Page 140.)

The authors go on:

> In previous reports the estimated fatality rate per thousand Caesarean sections has been quoted. However, because of known inaccuracies in the available denominator data it is not possible on this occasion to derive valid estimates. (Page 141.)

Nevertheless, the mortality would appear to be about 1 in 10,000.

Technique

There is no space here for a full discussion of the technique of Caesarean section, just to point out some of the pitfalls for the unwary. The choice of incision may be critical. The classical operation is now mostly of historical interest but at least one indication persists. In the term fetus with a transverse lie and a prolapsed arm, it is not possible to extract the baby through any other type of incision.

In all other circumstances, the incision should be in the lower segment and in the great majority a transverse incision heals best. The skin incision must be adequate and should be symmetrical; it is of much greater importance that the uterine incision should also be symmetrical for an asymmetric incision in the uterus may result in damage to a major uterine vessel. Any dextrorotation of the uterus should be corrected or allowed for. When the lower segment is thin, the incision should be made with great care so as not inadvertently to cut the baby. The aim is to observe the membranes bulging through the incision before their careful perforation and then opening of the incision with the fingers. At the lateral extremities the direction of pull should be upwards. Only rarely should it be necessary to use scissors to extend the wound and then great care must be taken not to injure the lateral structures and to extend the wound in a 'U' shape.

If the lie of the baby is not longitudinal at the beginning of the operation, every effort should be made to correct the lie before the uterus is opened. The alternative is internal podalic version through the lower segment incision but this may be difficult if the baby is lying with its back towards the pelvis. In those circumstances, the operator cannot tell at the beginning how large an incision may be required and a longitudinal midline incision, beginning in the lower segment is preferred.

The traditional transverse lower segment incision may not be suitable for extraction of the premature breech or transverse lie. In such circumstances, the lower segment may be poorly formed, and an incision made across its entire width may prove inadequate to extract the fetal head although the body of the baby will escape without difficulty. The operator, having made an inadequate incision, is then left to struggle with the head of the premature breech, causing extensive bruising and perhaps intracranial injury; the alternative of an inverted T is better but the wound heals poorly. In circumstances such as this, the correct incision is a vertical lower uterine segment incision, which can, if necessary, be extended upwards without unnecessary injury to baby or mother.

The operation, particularly when performed under spinal or epidural block, should be conducted with a lateral tilt or a wedge under the side of the patient, so as to avoid supine caval occlusion.

At Caesarean section late in labour, the fetal head or the breech may be deeply engaged in the pelvis and prove difficult to extract. Forceful entry of the surgeon's hand into the lower segment under these circumstances may cause catastrophic extension of the wound upwards into the uterine vessels and downwards into the vagina. Such injuries can and should be prevented by the simple expedient of asking an assistant to elevate the presenting part from below with a hand in the vagina. The omission of this simple step results in much (usually successful) litigation for maternal injury, for the resulting haemorrhage may be very severe and difficult to control.

Time

The other frequent cause of complaint, in relation to Caesarean section, is the time taken to organize the operation. Several attempts have been made to categorize requests for Caesarean section in labour with such terms as crash, immediate, urgent, soon etc. Such classification is not particularly helpful. What is important is that when Caesarean section is ordered in emergency circumstances (for fetal distress, prolapsed cord, maternal haemorrhage etc.) the person making the decision must indicate clearly the urgency with which the operation needs to be carried out. The time taken to perform Caesarean section in urgent circumstances must be monitored in every department and a 'emergency Caesarean section drill' carried out, from time to time, to improve performance. It is also helpful to audit the weakest link, the last member of staff to arrive on each occasion. If the same member of the team is always the last on the scene, the problem can be addressed and performance improved.

Urinary tract trauma

Urinary tract trauma is an occasional subject of litigation. Injuries to the bladder, particularly in repeat Caesarean section, are common because of the difficulty in separating the bladder from the scarred lower segment. Provided that the damage is noticed at the time and the bladder repaired, there are seldom long-term consequences. Injury to the ureter is a different matter. It is difficult to conceive of circumstances (save only in the presence of the most abnormal pelvic anatomy) in which ureteric injury at Caesarean section could be excusable. The left ureter is most at risk because of the dextrorotation of the uterus. However, if the operator is careful to note the anatomy before the incision is made, to reflect the bladder fully and to follow the instructions given above for the performance of the incision, the ureter should be nowhere near the incision. Most ureteric injuries occur because there is a catastrophic extension of the left side of the wound. This occurs either because the operator has chosen the wrong incision or because, having failed to elevate the presenting part from below, the hand inserted deep into the pelvis to elevate the baby tears the uterus both upwards and downwards.

Rupture of the uterus

There are only three circumstances in which rupture of the uterus commonly occurs:

▶   rupture of a previous scar

▶   rupture of the multiparous uterus, usually as the result of the abuse of oxytocin

▶   direct trauma with obstetric forceps.

With the demise of Kjelland's forceps rotation, the last group is now vanishingly small.

Rupture of the multigravid uterus may occur spontaneously if there is unsuspected cephalo-pelvic disproportion. More often, it occurs because Syntocinon has been administered unwisely and in too high a dose, often following a previous administration of prostaglandin. At the National Maternity Hospital in Dublin oxytocin is used aggressively for the treatment of slow labour in the primigravida but the proponents warn: [53]

> Rupture of uterus is such an exceptional event in primigravidae that for practice purposes it can be assumed not to occur ... whereas primigravidae are rupture proof, multigravidae are rupture prone. The inherent tendency of the multigravid uterus to rupture is a factor which must be taken into account whenever the potential risks of epidural anaesthesia are under consideration. (Pages 24, 25.)

Oxytocin should be used with the greatest care to augment slow labour in the multigravid woman.

By far the most common circumstances in which rupture of the uterus leads to litigation is the rupture of the previous Caesarean section scar. There are no reliable figures for scar rupture because of the inevitable favourable bias of published series. Hospitals with poor results do not publish them. The perception is generally that the risk is of the order of 1%.[54] But the American College of Obstetrics and Gynaecology estimated the risk as 2%.[55] It is said often that provided the baby could be born within 30 minutes the consequences of scar rupture may not be severe; the baby may be rescued intact. Indeed, it may, but it is not always so. In a personal series, investigated for litigation, I have reviewed 18 ruptured scars, 17 following lower segment Caesarean section and one following myomectomy. In each case, Syntocinon was used to augment the contractions of labour. In this series, five mothers were injured and 14 babies were either injured or died. In two cases, both mother and baby were injured. The maternal injuries included two hysterectomies (one with brain damage following prolonged shock) and three bladder injuries, including one vesico-vaginal fistula. The 14 fetal injuries included four stillbirths, four neonatal deaths and six survivors with cerebral palsy.

Before setting out on an enterprise as dangerous as vaginal birth after Caesarean section (VBAC), it is not unreasonable to expect that the mother should be informed of the risks:

> I am not aware of any credible VBAC study that did not report adverse outcome. Nor am I aware of any VBAC proponent who would not advise patients of the risk of uterine rupture during labour.[56]

Reviewing labour after Caesarean section at the Coombe Hospital in Dublin, Turner[57] advised:

> Ideally, the obstetrician and the mother should base their decisions about the management of pregnancy and delivery on the recent results from their own hospital.

The mother in such circumstances must be told of the risk; there is only one risk. The only risk peculiar to labour after Caesarean section is that of scar rupture. In every other respect, labour is the same as for any other woman. The mother must be told of that risk, the obstetrician's understanding of the incidence of that risk and the possible consequences. The mother should also be told the only other alternative to labour, that of elective Caesarean section. It is not unreasonable also to inform her of the relatively increased risk of emergency, as compared with elective, Caesarean section. Provided that this information is given honestly, many women will still decide in favour of vaginal delivery for many women have a strong drive towards vaginal delivery and will accept certain risks. It should, however, be for the woman to decide; complacency on the part of the obstetrician is misplaced. It is the mother and her baby who are at risk.

Once in labour, the main controversy concerns the advisability of oxytocin augmentation. It is true to say that:

> The published series indicate high vaginal delivery rates and low scar dehiscence rates in association with oxytocin usage.[55] (Page 1213.)

But of course published series do not necessarily reflect practice in the average obstetric unit. It is probably true that oxytocin, used responsibly, is no more dangerous than spontaneous labour but it is abundantly clear to anyone with extensive experience of litigation that oxytocin is not necessarily used responsibly and the penalties for its misuse in these circumstances are so much heavier than with an intact uterus. Oxytocin, if it is to be used at all, must be used with the utmost care and in association with continuous fetal heart monitoring. Equal attention should be paid to the tocograph as to the cardiograph and great care taken to make sure that the uterus is not overstimulated. Contrary to popular mythology, there are no other reliable signs of scar rupture. Pain in the scar even without epidural block is not often reported before the scar actually ruptures. Fetal distress is usually seen as a consequence of scar rupture, not as the herald of it.

Conclusion

The most common causes for complaint and litigation arising in labour ward practice are:

▶ Fetal death or injury as a consequence of:

  ▶ the mismanagement of labour, often with Syntocinon

  ▶ failure to recognize CTG abnormalities and to act on them

  ▶ mismanagement of operative vaginal delivery or shoulder dystocia.

▶ Maternal injury as a consequence of:

  ▶ failure to recognize injury to the anal sphincter and to repair it

  ▶ rupture of the uterus.

References

1   Sleep J, Roberts J, Chalmers I. Care in the second of labour. In: I Chalmers, M Enkin and MJNC Kierse (eds.) *Effective Care in Pregnancy and Childbirth*. Oxford: Oxford University Press, 1989: 1129–1144.
2   Grant A. Repair of episiotomies and perineal tears. *British Journal of Obstetrics and Gynaecology* 1986; 93: 417–419
3   Spencer JAD, Grant A, Elbourne D. A randomised comparison of glycerol-impregnated chromic catgut with untreated chromic catgut for repair of perineal trauma. *British Journal of Obstetrics and Gynaecology* 1986; 93: 426–430.
4   Jarvis GJ. Perineal damage following childbirth. *Clinical Risk* 1999; 5(5): 181–184.
5   Keighley MRB, Radley S, Johanson R. Consensus on prevention and management of post-obstetric bowel continence and third degree tear. *Clinical Risk* 2000; 6(6): 231–237.
6   Walsh CJ, Mooney EF, Upton GJ, Motson RW. Incidence of third degree perineal tears in labour and outcome after primary repair. *British Journal of Surgery* 1996; 83: 218–221.
7   Sultan AH, Kamm MA, Hudson CN, Thomas JM, Bartram CI. Anal sphincter disruption during vaginal delivery. *New England Journal of Medicine* 1993; 329: 1905–1911.

8   Sultan AH. Obstetrical perineal injury and anal incontinence. *Clinical Risk* 1999; 5(6): 193–196.

9   Schofield PF, Grace R. Faecal incontinence after childbirth. *Clinical Risk* 1999; 5(6): 201–204.

10   Kelleher C, Braude P. Recent advances: Gynaecology. *BMJ* 1999; 319: 689–692.

11   Ritchie JWK. Obstetric operations and procedures. In: CR Whitfield (ed.) *Dewhurst's Textbook of Obstetrics and Gynaecology for Postgraduates*, 5th edn. Oxford: Blackwell Science, 1995: 390.

12   American College of Obstetricians and Gynaecologists. *Operative Vaginal Delivery*. Technical bulletin no. 196. Washington DC, 1994.

13   Pearson JF, Davies P. The effect of continuous lumbar epidural analgesia upon fetal acid–base status during the second stage of labour. *Journal of Obstetrics and Gynaecology of the British Commonwealth* 1974; 81: 975–979.

14   Cardozo LD, Gibb DMF, Studd JWW, Cooper DJ. Should we abandon Kjelland's forceps? *BMJ* 1983; 287: 315–317.

15   Chamberlain GVP. Operative vaginal delivery. In: G Chamberlain (ed.) *Turnbull's Obstetrics*, 2nd edn. London: Churchill Livingstone, 1995: Chapter 27.

16   O'Grady JP. Instruments and indications. In: *Modern Instrumental Delivery*. Baltimore: Williams & Wilkins 1988: Chapter 2.

17   Vacca, A, Grant A, Wyatt G, Chalmers I. Portsmouth operative delivery trial. *British Journal of Obstetrics & Gynaecology* 1984; 90: 1107–1112.

18   Govaert P. *Cranial Haemorrhage in the Term Newborn Infant*. Cambridge: Mac Keith Press, 1993.

19   O'Grady JP. Instrumental delivery. In: JP O'Grady, ML Gimovsky (eds.) *Operative Obstetrics*. Baltimore: Williams & Wilkins, 1995: Chapter 9.

20   Vacca A. *Handbook of Vacuum Extraction in Obstetric Practice*. London: Edward Arnold, 1992.

21   Ikhena SE, Halligan A, Naftalin NJ. Has pelvimetry a role in current obstetric practice? *Journal of Obstetrics and Gynaecology* 1999; 19(5): 463–466.

22   Hofmeyr GJ. Breech presentation and abnormal lie in late pregnancy. In: I Chalmers, M Enkin, MJNC Keirse (eds.) *Effective Care in Pregnancy and Childbirth*. Oxford: Oxford University Press, 1989: Chapter 42.

23   Penn ZJ. Breech presentation. In: JK James, PJ Steer, CP Weiner, B Gonik (eds.) *High Risk Pregnancy: Management Options*, 2nd edn. London: WB Saunders Co., 1999: Chapter 58.

24   Hannah H, Hannah WJ, Hewson SA, Hodnett ED, Saigal S, Willan AR, the Term Breech Trial Collaborative Group. Planned Caesarean section versus planned vaginal birth for breech presentation at term: a randomised multicentre trial. Lancet 2000; 356: 1375–1383.

25   Gibb D, Arulkumaran S. *Cardiotocographic Interpretation: Clinical Scenarios. Fetal Monitoring in Practice*, 2nd edition. Oxford: Butterworth–Heinemann, 1997: Chapter 8.

26   Donald I. Breech presentation. In: *Practical Obstetric Problems*, 5th edn. London: Lloyd–Luke, 1979: Chapter 13.

27   Hopwood HG. Shoulder dystocia: 15 year's experience in a community hospital. *American Journal of Obstetrics and Gynaecology* 1982; 144: 162–166.

28   Woods CE. A principle of physics as applicable to shoulder dystocia. *American Journal of Obstetrics and Gynaecology* 1943; 45: 796–804.

29   Morris WIC. Reports of Societies. *Journal of Obstetrics and Gynaecology of the British Empire* 1955; 62: 302.

30   O'Leary JA. Delivery technique. In: *Shoulder Dystocia and Birth Injury: Prevention and Treatment*. New York: McGraw–Hill, 1992: Chapter 8.

31   Gibb DMF. Shoulder dystocia: the obstetrics. *Clinical Risk* 1995; 1: 49–54.

32   Roberts L. Shoulder dystocia. In: J Studd (ed.) *Progress in Obstetrics and Gynaecology*, vol. 11. London: Churchill Livingstone, 1994: 201–216.

33   Gibb DMF. Operative delivery. In: RV Clements (ed.) *Safe Practice in Obstetrics and Gynaecology: A Medico-Legal Handbook*. London: Churchill Livingstone, 1994: Chapter 18.

34   Smith RB, Pearson JF. Shoulder dystocia: what happens at the next delivery? *British Journal of Obstetrics and Gynaecology* 1994; 101: 713–715.

35   Williams J. Obstetric emergencies. In: VR Bennett, LK Brown (eds.) *Myles Textbook for Midwives*, 12th edn. London: Churchill–Livingstone, 1993: Chapter 27.

36   Rubin A. Management of shoulder dystocia. *Journal of the American Medical Association* 1964; 189(11): 835–837.

37   McRoberts WA. Manoeuvres for shoulder dystocia. *Contemporary Obstetrics and Gynaecology* 1984; 24: 17.

38   Gonik B, Stringer CA, Held B. An alternative maneuvre for the management of shoulder dystocia. *American Journal of Gynaecology* 1983; 145: 882–888.

39   McDonald SE, Stirk FD. Shoulder dystocia: the midwife's role. *Clinical Risk* 1995; 1: 61–65.

40   Johnstone FD, Myerscough PR. Shoulder dystocia. *British Journal of Obstetrics and Gynaecology* 1998; 105: 811–815.

41   Shaw RW. *Focus Group — Shoulder Dystocia. Confidential Enquiry into Stillbirths and Deaths in Infancy.* Maternal and Child Health Research Consortium, 1998: Chapter 8.

42   Jennett RJ, Tarby TJ, Kreinick CJ. Brachial plexus palsy: an old problem revisited. *American Journal of Obstetrics and Gynecology* 1992; 166: 1673–1677.

43   Hankins GDV, Clark SL. Brachial plexus palsy involving the posterior shoulder at spontaneous vaginal delivery. *American Journal of Perinatology* 1995; 12(1): 44–45.

44   Sandmire HF, DeMott RK. The physician factor as a determinant of Cesarean birth rates for the large fetus. *American Journal of Obstetrics and Gynaecology* 1996; 174: 1557–1564.

45   Jennett RJ, Tarby TJ. Brachial plexus palsy: an old problem revisited again. *American Journal of Obstetrics and Gynecology* 1997; 176: 1354–1357.

46   Peleg D, Hasnin J, Shalev E. Fractured clavicle and Erb's palsy unrelated to birth trauma. *American Journal of Obstetrics and Gynecology* 1997; 177: 1038–1040.

47   Gherman RB, Ouzounian JG, Miller DA, Kwok L, Murphy Goodwin T. Spontaneous vaginal delivery: a risk factor for Erb's palsy? *American Journal of Obstetrics and Gynecology* 1998; 178: 423–427.

48   Spellacy WN. Erb's palsy without shoulder dystocia [Letter]. *American Journal of Obstetrics and Gynecology* 1998; 179(2): 561.

49   Department of Health. NHS *Maternity Statistics, England: 1989–1990 to 1994–1995.* Department of Health Statistical Bulletin, December 1997.

50   Department of Health. *Why Mothers Die. Report on Confidential Inquiries into Maternal Deaths in the United Kingdom 1994–1996.* London: HMSO, 1998.

51   Chamberlain GVP. Maternal mortality. In: G Chamberlain (ed.) *Turnbull's Obstetrics*, 2nd edn. London: Churchill Livingstone 1994: Chapter 50.

52   Department of Health. *Report on Confidential Inquiries into Maternal Deaths in the United Kingdom 1991–1993.* London: HMSO, 1996.

53   O'Driscoll K, Meagher D, Boyland P. Primigravidae v. multigravidae. In: *Active Management of Labour: The Dublin Experience*, 3rd edn. London: Mosby, 1995: Chapter 1.

54   Dickinson JE. Previous Caesarean section. In: DK James, PJ Steer, CP Weiner, B Gonik (eds.) *High Risk Pregnancy Management Options*, 2nd edn. London: WB Saunders, 1999: Chapter 67.

55   ACOG Committee Opinion. Vaginal delivery after a previous Caesarean birth. No. 143, October 1994. *International Journal of Obstetrics and Gynaecology* 1995; 48: 127–129.

56   Gleicher N. Mandatory trial of labour after Caesarean delivery: an alternative viewpoint [Letter]. *Obstetrics and Gynaecology* 1991; 78(4): 727.

57   Turner MJ. Delivery after one previous Cesarean section. *American Journal of Obstetrics and Gynecology* 1996; 176(4): 741–744.

▶14

Cerebral Palsy and Intrapartum Events

Peter R F Dear and Simon J Newell

> It is incident to physicians, I am afraid, beyond all other men, to mistake subsequence for consequence.
>
> **Samuel Johnson, 25 November 1734**

Introduction

There is universal agreement that some permanent neurodisability is the result of hypoxic–ischaemic injury to the previously normal fetal brain occurring during the course of labour and delivery; but there is very little agreement beyond that. In population terms, there is no widespread agreement about the contribution of birth asphyxia to neurodisability or about the spectrum of neurodisability that might be attributable to perinatal hypoxic–ischaemic events. In individual cases, attributing disabilities to intrapartum events is often problematic, and in the field of litigation, sincerely held but opposing views are common.

The problem of assigning a cause to disabilities is too important – both for the individual and society – to allow these difficulties to frustrate continuing attempts to improve our understanding of the mechanisms and epidemiology of perinatal hypoxic–ischaemic brain injury. The tools available to help unravel these mysteries are developing apace, particularly brain imaging techniques and those for studying brain metabolism and biochemistry, and it is likely that we are on the threshold of a much greater understanding. In the meantime, it is important to apply the best available knowledge to the consideration of causation of disabilities, whether in the clinic or in the court. The purpose of this chapter is to explore what is known about the relationship between intrapartum events and subsequent disability, especially – but not exclusively – cerebral palsy.

What is cerebral palsy?

Cerebral palsy (CP) is essentially a disorder of motor function, manifesting as abnormal muscle tone, contraction and strength, brought about by an acquired defect of the developing brain. The different patterns of motor dysfunction will be discussed in detail later. The developing brain may be injured by various insults at various times and so CP is best regarded as a final, common expression of diverse pathological processes. Injury acquired around the time of birth as a result of a lack of oxygen or blood flow, or both, is the main focus of this article. Observable signs of CP usually become apparent between birth and two years of age. CP is a non-progressive disorder in the sense that the brain injury responsible for it is a discrete event. The physical signs change over time, however, as a result of the maturation of the nervous system. The motor abnormalities of CP are associated commonly with impaired mental function, epilepsy and sensory abnormalities. A compact definition might run as follows: 'Cerebral palsy is [an] umbrella term covering a group of non-progressive but often changing, motor impairment syndromes secondary to lesions or anomalies of the brain arising in the early stages of its development'.[1]

Magnitude of the problem

CP is the most common motor disability in childhood.[2,3] It has been estimated that more than 100,000 Americans under the age of 18 have a degree of neurological morbidity attributable to CP.[4] The prevalence of CP in the UK has been reported recently as 2.45[5] and as 2.1[6] per 1000 neonatal survivors. In the latter survey, 33.4% of patients could not walk independently, 23.1% had severe learning difficulty and 8.9% severe visual disability. Similar prevalence figures have been reported from different countries at various times during the past 40 or so years.[7-13] Allowing for a 15% mortality in infancy and childhood, the estimated cumulative incidence at seven years of age is 4.6 per 1000.[14] There is evidence of a rising incidence of CP, mainly accounted for by an increase in survival rates among low birthweight infants.[5,9,11,15]

Low birthweight infants now account for around half of all CP cases,[5,11,16] but this article will mainly address the relationship between intrapartum events and CP in term infants.

Historical perspectives

Opinions on the relationship of CP to intrapartum events go back a long way. The most frequently referenced supporter of the proposition that birth events are the major cause of CP was William Little, a London orthopaedic surgeon. In 1862, Little reported on 47 cases of spastic CP and concluded that obstetric factors were paramount in all.[17] Sigmund Freud, writing some 35 years after Little's article was published, offered the alternative view that the cause of much CP lay in the prenatal period and that problems at birth were a consequence of that pre-existing abnormality.[18]

Since Little's time, professional views on the link between intrapartum asphyxia and CP have evolved gradually. Around 50 years ago, some 30% of CP cases were thought to be of pre-partum origin and around 60% of intrapartum origin.[19] Twenty or so years ago, the figure for pre-partum origin was reported to be about 38%, and for intrapartum origin about 46%.[20] However, a contemporary survey of the views of healthcare professionals discovered that the risk of CP was overestimated by a factor of ten compared with published figures.[21] The current view is that less than 17% of all types of CP originates during birth.[22-25] Some of the difficulties involved with drawing inferences about causation from epidemiological research will be discussed later in the article.

The public perspective has not been elicited formally as far as we can ascertain; however, if medical undergraduates are any guide, most people are probably closer to William Little than to present-day epidemiologists. In any event, the parents of children with CP often feel the need to pursue the possibility of a negligent perinatal causation, for a number of reasons. These include the high cost of providing adequately for a disabled person compared with what is available from the state, and the failure of some members of the medical profession to take time to listen to and answer parents' concerns about the cause of their child's disabilities.

Medical litigation is a very costly business and a very anxiety-provoking and time-consuming one for the clinical staff concerned. The overall expenditure on clinical negligence by the NHS in England in 1998 was around £84 million (one quarter of 1% of NHS annual expenditure) and the rate of closed claims increased during the 1990s at a rate of about 7% per annum.[26,27] The steepest rate increase has been in claims arising from obstetrics and gynaecology; and awards made to children believed to have been damaged by intrapartum events as a result of obstetric negligence are among the highest made by the courts in relation to clinical negligence. During 1995, the National Health Service Litigation Authority (NHSLA) was created to deal with substantial claims against the Health Authorities in the UK. Their data do not include cases settled before 1995 or those born in the incident year who have not yet lodged a claim. The figures demonstrate a considerable increase in claims for CP (Figure 14.1), and increasing numbers of claims alleging deafness, intellectual deficit, and behavioural problems related to birth asphyxia (NHSLA, personal communication, 2000).

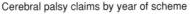

Cerebral palsy claims by year of scheme

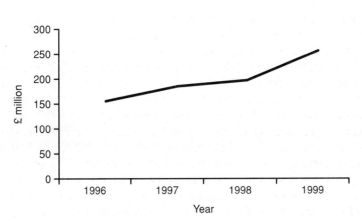

Fig. 14.1. Current settlements and outstanding settlements held in reserve, 1995–1999. The rate of increase is underestimated, as data do not include cases in recent years where no claim has yet been made (NHSLA, June 2000).

In terms of justice to both providers and consumers of obstetric and neonatal services, it is imperative that court judgments are informed by the best available data and interpretation.

Establishing a causal link between disability and intrapartum events

Proving that observed associations are causally related is an infamously difficult problem in philosophy and science. Showing that a case of CP has been caused by intrapartum asphyxia is no exception. To be sure of causality, it would be necessary to know that without the intercession of intrapartum asphyxia, the CP would not have occurred. The main impediments to attaining this knowledge are as follows:

- CP can occur without the intercession of intrapartum asphyxia. So, the concurrence of intrapartum asphyxia and CP is not of itself proof of causation.

- Generally, it is impossible to be certain that the brain was normal before the onset of labour, using the investigational tools in common use.

- Fetuses with abnormal brains may withstand the stresses of birth poorly and give the outward show of having suffered intrapartum asphyxia when in fact they have not. To quote Freud: 'Difficult birth in itself in certain cases is merely a symptom of deeper effects that influenced the development of the fetus.'[18]

- It is difficult to define and quantify intrapartum asphyxia using the investigational tools in common use. Concluding when asphyxia has been severe enough to cause brain injury, therefore, is a challenging task.

- Intrapartum asphyxia does not necessarily lead to permanent brain injury and fetuses almost certainly vary in their susceptibility to incur brain injury, as a result of their genetic endowment and prior environmental influences.

So, at the present time establishing causality with certainty is rarely possible, although it may become so in due course as a consequence of developing investigational techniques. Certainty, though, is an elusive state of mind in the practice of Medicine, and rather more so in the practice of Law. In both disciplines, probabilistic reasoning is the prevailing methodology and in many questions of causality relating to intrapartum asphyxia and CP, there is enough evidence to support the formation of a probabilistic view. Much of what is known in general about the role of intrapartum asphyxia in causing CP is the result of epidemiological study.

Epidemiological methods

Broadly speaking, there are two epidemiological approaches. One is to take a cohort of individuals with CP and a comparison group of unaffected individuals, and look back at their birth histories for evidence of intrapartum asphyxia – a *retrospective* approach. The other is to take a group of individuals with evidence of birth asphyxia and a comparison group without such evidence and to follow them to look for evidence of disability – a *prospective* approach. Both approaches are problematic.

Retrospective methods suffer from the following problems:

> Defining the disabled cohort prejudges the question of the spectrum of CP and other disability that might arise from intrapartum asphyxia, so that some causally related adverse outcomes might be excluded from the outset. Even definitions of CP vary significantly between studies.[28]

> Defining a potentially damaging severity of intrapartum asphyxia is difficult and the attribution of cause will vary considerably according to how this is defined.

> Retrospective data gathering is often unreliable as the required data are not always collected systematically and often are in the wrong form.

> Even when reliable data are obtained, they are often outmoded by the passage of time (for example, data relating to the diagnosis of intrapartum asphyxia collected before the widespread introduction of fetal heart rate monitoring).

Prospective methods suffer from the following problems:

> Defining a potentially damaging severity of intrapartum asphyxia is difficult and the attribution of cause will vary considerably according to how this is defined.

> A very large cohort must be followed in order to guarantee a sufficient number of affected individuals. This is expensive.

> Very long-term follow-up is necessary if the full spectrum of adverse outcome is to be realized. This is expensive.

Both prospective and retrospective methodologies have been employed in the search for causal links between intrapartum asphyxia and CP,[22,29-31] but because of the problems outlined above, interpretation of the findings is often difficult. For example, one of the most influential and quoted studies is that undertaken by Blair and Stanley in Western Australia.[22] In that retrospective study, the cohort of children chosen was limited to those with *spastic* CP, thus removing the possibility of finding other forms of disability linked to intrapartum asphyxia. Another example is to be found in the much-analysed and much-quoted findings of the Collaborative Project concerning a cohort of babies born in 12 teaching hospitals in the United States between 1959 and 1966.[32-35] Although this study has provided valuable insights into the relationship between adverse intrapartum events and subsequent CP, it antedates electronic fetal monitoring and magnetic resonance brain imaging, which now would be considered almost indispensable adjuncts to clinical observation in the diagnosis of intrapartum hypoxia and its consequences. Research into the aetiology of CP that has not employed magnetic resonance brain imaging should not be regarded as definitive.

The burden of proof

The degree of certainty sought by scientists is very different from that required by the civil courts. In medical research, statistical tests are used in order to evaluate associations, and it is generally necessary to achieve 95% confidence that there is a seminal link between two events before causality is accepted. It is now customary to present the strength of an association as an odds ratio with a related 95% confidence interval.[36] For example, it might be said that the odds ratio for CP when there is clear evidence of significant intrapartum hypoxia is 20, with a 95% confidence interval of 2 to 180. In lay terms, this means that babies who show clear evidence of significant intrapartum hypoxia are 20 times more likely to suffer from CP than those who do not. The 95% confidence interval indicates that although the best estimate is '20 times more likely' we can only be 95% confident that the real effect lies between '2 and 180 times more likely'. The requirement for proof of this degree is onerous but deemed imperative to the rigours of good science. Even in medical science, however, this level of proof may be excessive – who would not want to try a treatment for a life-threatening disease which was only 90% likely to be effective?

In comparison, the level of certainty required by the civil court seems lenient. No doubt there are many good reasons for this in terms of justice. From the point of view of expert medical evidence, one good reason to lower the burden of proof is that the confidence intervals around a single case are very much wider than they are around a sample large enough for scientific study. Medical experts often have difficulty in coming to terms with giving a medico-legal opinion which is based on the 'balance of probability' rather than the more robust scientific assurance which they suppose underpins most of their medical opinions. A moment's reflection, however, will expose the fact that although the science may be good, its application to an individual patient is usually no more robust a process than can be represented by the phrase 'on the balance of probability'. Therefore, in both clinical and medico-legal practice the challenge is to apply good population science to an individual case, which may or may not be epitomized by the samples studied and reported in the literature.

The notion of a spectrum of disability arising from intrapartum events

CP is regarded rightly as the archetypal adverse outcome of damaging intrapartum hypoxia, but by many it is apparently held to be the only adverse outcome.[37] By analogy with other corporal responses to injury, it seems more likely that there would be a spectrum of adverse outcomes, particularly in view of the diverse functions of the central nervous system. After all, no one expects every person who receives a damaging blow to the head to suffer identical disability. Biological systems are inherently complex and are likely to respond to injury in a way that is non-linear and difficult to predict. Large differences in the physiological state of fetuses at the time of asphyxial insults and in the nature and duration of the insults are also bound to exist.

It would be very surprising indeed if, despite these complexities, the only adverse outcome of intrapartum asphyxia was CP.

The task of ascertaining the complete spectrum of adverse outcome of intrapartum hypoxic brain injury is a vexed one that can only be accomplished by very large, long-term, longitudinal follow-up studies, interpreted with an open mind. To illustrate the magnitude of the problem, we will take a fabricated example. Imagine that there is a twofold increased risk of schizophrenia among individuals who have been damaged by intrapartum hypoxia compared with the general population. The prevalence of schizophrenia in the population is around 2%; therefore, in the sample damaged by intrapartum hypoxia it would be around 4%. In order to have a 90% chance of showing this with a statistical significance of 5%, it would be necessary to recruit a sample of over 1200 subjects who had suffered from potentially damaging intrapartum hypoxia and to follow them into adulthood. It is easy to see how the scale of this problem is likely to have prevented the full spectrum of adverse outcome of intrapartum hypoxia from emerging in the literature to date. As an interesting footnote to this discussion, a recently published paper has drawn attention to a probable link between schizophrenia and perinatal hypoxia.[38]

Diagnosing intrapartum hypoxia

Some degree of fetal hypoxia during the process of birth is common. Uterine contractions raise the pressure within the uterus to the extent that the flow of maternal blood through the placenta is diminished or ceases,[39-41] and as a result feto-maternal gas exchange is reduced.[42] In the course of normal labour, the reduction is not critical and the normal fetus copes easily. When some complication of labour occurs or when there is some pre-existing abnormality of the placenta or the fetus, a potentially damaging severity and duration of fetal hypoxia may develop. This concept of 'potentially damaging' hypoxia is a useful one. The human fetus possesses a remarkable ability to withstand hypoxia without sustaining permanent injury, and it is really only possible to say that hypoxia has resulted in permanent injury through follow-up – or to a less accurate extent, by employing advanced forms of brain imaging. So, when there is evidence of intrapartum hypoxia in a child who develops signs of CP, or other possibly related disability, the first of several causation questions to be asked is, was the intrapartum hypoxia of sufficient severity to have caused brain injury? That is, was it of potentially damaging severity?

This question is best addressed using a combination of two approaches. One is to assess the *circumstantial* evidence for intrapartum hypoxia, and the other is to look for more or less direct evidence of acute injury to the brain that might have a permanent effect.

Circumstantial evidence of intrapartum hypoxia of potentially damaging severity

This will always be a controversial area because in respect of almost everything that can be measured to provide evidence of intrapartum hypoxia, there is considerable overlap between babies who have encountered potentially damaging asphyxia and those who have not. This applies to complications of pregnancy, labour and delivery, fetal heart-rate abnormalities detected on the cardiotocograph (CTG), fetal and cord blood pH values, Apgar scores and resuscitation measures. In every case, it is very difficult to develop useful, non-controversial definitions of abnormality that can be used to define potentially damaging intrapartum hypoxia. In both clinical and medico-legal practice, however, what is needed are criteria which define a population sufficiently at risk of having encountered potentially damaging hypoxia to warrant further investigation, and the Holy Grail of a perfect test is probably not worth pursuing. As this article is written from a paediatric perspective, we will concentrate on cord blood pH values and the condition of the baby at birth and during the early neonatal period.

Cord blood pH

When a fetus experiences asphyxia of potentially damaging severity during the hours immediately preceding birth, it is virtually certain that umbilical arterial blood will show an abnormal degree of metabolic acidaemia. This is the result of excess lactic acid production by tissues forced to try to meet their energy needs by anaerobic (without oxygen) metabolism. Lactic acid accumulates in fetal tissues and blood because it diffuses relatively slowly across the placenta.[43-46] Lactic acid can be measured in the blood, but its presence is usually inferred from the combination of a lowered pH and a raised base deficit, indicating a metabolic acidosis. Umbilical-cord blood or very early neonatal samples may be used.[47] This is the basis for the assertion that evidence of metabolic acidosis is an essential criterion for establishing that an asphyxial event of potentially damaging severity has occurred during the few hours preceding birth, and in this sense the pH can be used as a test for *when* damaging asphyxia may have occurred.

The problem is that there is no pH value that separates cleanly those babies who have experienced potentially damaging intrapartum asphyxia from those who have not. As with virtually every test based on a continuous variable, deciding on a cut-off value involves a trade-off between the proportion of unaffected cases who have a positive test (known as 'false positives') and the proportion of affected cases who have a negative test (known as 'false negatives'). Inevitably, as one improves the other gets worse, and where the balance is set depends on the purpose for which the test is being used. A recently published consensus statement[48] set the cut-off value at a pH of 7.0 (along with a base deficit of 12 mmol/L). This value was clearly biased towards reducing the number of false-positive results. In clinical and medico-legal practice, no diagnosis can be made or refuted on the basis of a single laboratory measurement and the idea of a set cut-off is naïve.

In support of the recommended cut-off value, two original articles are quoted.[49,50] In the first of these studies, the entry criterion was a pH value of less than 7.0 and so it was of no use in determining a cut-off value. In the second study, where several cut-off values were explored, 67% of babies who suffered unexplained seizures (which was the main proxy used to indicate significant asphyxia) had a cord arterial blood pH of less than 7.0 but the remaining 33% had a pH between 7.0 and 7.2. This shows that the recommended cut-off value of 7.0 is too low and will exclude a significant number of babies who have encountered potentially damaging intrapartum asphyxia.

If our understanding of brain injury from intrapartum hypoxia is to improve, it is important to avoid setting diagnostic criteria that exclude a substantial proportion of genuine cases. There are good population data on the frequency distribution of cord artery pH values,[51–55] and a more reasonable approach, which is applied to most tests in medicine, would be to set a cut-off value that identifies a population sufficiently likely to have the condition in question to warrant further investigation. The 10th centile for umbilical artery pH in the general population is reported as around 7.15[52] and the 2.5th centile in a population of normal newborns is reported as around 7.1.[51]

As useful as cord pH information is, it is not always available.

Cord pH is not measured universally, even in high-risk cases in university departments of obstetrics in Canada and the USA, for example,[56] and not universally valued.[57,58] There is no published survey of the practice in the UK, but informal enquiries indicate that cord-blood sampling is undertaken reliably and systematically in very few centres. It is even less likely to have been undertaken in the past.

Finally, it is necessary to consider the validity of the method used to assess metabolic acidosis. If cord blood is used, a good arterial specimen is needed. The arterial blood coming from the fetus indicates the level of fetal metabolic acidosis. If there is free flow through the umbilical cord, the difference between the blood gases in the arterial blood and the umbilical venous blood returning from the placenta is small. If cord blood flow is obstructed, however, the fetus may suffer marked hypoxia, while placental gas exchange continues. As a result, if venous blood is used when intrapartum asphyxia arises from cord compression[59–62] or is associated with cardiac failure in the fetus,[63] the cord pH may be near normal even in the face of marked acidaemia in cord arterial blood. Obtaining a good sample from the umbilical arteries is a task requiring quite a lot of skill and practice[59] and in many instances the blood obtained is either from the vein or else a mixed venous/arterial sample. In order to ensure that arterial blood has been obtained, it may be necessary to take a venous sample as well so that the results can be compared.[64] It may be useful to compare arterial and venous pH and pCO_2 values.[65] If a cord blood-gas result is to be used to inform about the likelihood of intrapartum hypoxia, a reasonable degree of certainty is required that it was a clean arterial sample; that it was taken from the cord no more than 60 minutes after birth[66,67] – preferably within 30 minutes;[68] that the correct amount of anticoagulant was used;[69] and that the analyser was working accurately.[58]

Condition at birth

Babies who have met with a potentially damaging severity of hypoxia during birth will almost invariably be in poor condition and have difficulty in making the transition to extra-uterine life. The only exception is the occasional instance of intra-uterine recovery from hypoxia following cessation of the cause – for example, ceasing syntocinon-induced hyperstimulation of the uterus.

Conventionally, the condition of babies at birth is measured by the Apgar score,[70] based on respiration, heart rate, skin colour, muscle tone and response to stimulation.

The response to resuscitation is measured by serial scoring as well as by noting the time to the first gasp and the establishment of regular breathing.

It is important to recognize that much of the formal research which informs our beliefs about the effect of intrapartum asphyxia on the condition of babies at birth comes from animal experiments involving acute total asphyxia.[71–73] This is where terms such as 'primary' and 'secondary apnoea' and the relationship between the duration of asphyxia and the interval to the first breath come from. It is easy to understand why acute and more or less complete hypoxia interferes with adaptation at birth, for we know that the brainstem structures responsible for driving respiration and other vital functions are among the best perfused and most metabolically active and therefore among the most susceptible structures to acute hypoxia and ischaemia,[74–78] albeit less susceptible than the adult brainstem.[79] Far less is known about how adaptation at birth is influenced by the effect of prolonged partial asphyxia, during which the brainstem is preferentially perfused relative to the cerebral hemispheres.[80–84] It would be perfectly reasonable to theorize that in those circumstances, recovery with resuscitation might be more rapid than is seen following acute anoxia, at least in terms of breathing and heart rate, and consequently skin colour. So, it may be that the clinical criteria that are appropriate for diagnosing intrapartum acute, total asphyxia may not be appropriate for diagnosing intrapartum prolonged partial asphyxia. If it is the case that babies damaged by *prolonged partial* asphyxia make a better recovery at birth than those damaged by *acute total* asphyxia, many contemporary assumptions about the causal relationship between intrapartum events and CP would be brought into question.

Encephalopathy

It is widely held to be true that in the aftermath of an intrapartum asphyxial event of potentially damaging severity there will inevitably be an acute disturbance of neurological function. When this neurological illness is genuinely the result of asphyxia, it is known as a post-asphyxial or hypoxic–ischaemic encephalopathy (HIE). This illness, which features abnormal movements, tone, posture and conscious level, is the outward sign of acute brain dysfunction brought about by hypoxia and ischaemia. During the encephalopathic illness, the energy state of the brain is disturbed, with loss of high-energy phosphates. Magnetic resonance spectroscopy can now demonstrate loss of cellular ATP and a fall in the ratio of high-energy phosphocreatine to low-energy inorganic phosphate. Intracellular concentrations of N-acetylaspartate, lactate, calcium and sodium are also elevated after asphyxia.[85–91] The severity and duration of these changes as measured by magnetic resonance spectroscopy correlate well with adverse long-term outcome.[85,88,92,93]

The timing of onset of signs of HIE following a potentially damaging episode of asphyxia differs between infants. Some are overtly encephalopathic from the moment of birth, whereas others appear to be almost normal for many hours before obvious signs of encephalopathy become apparent. These differences are not explained currently. It is tempting to suggest that they are accounted for by the timing of the determining insult in relation to birth, but a study of the timing of post-asphyxial encephalopathy following near-miss sudden infant death syndrome shows that there is genuine variability in the interval between asphyxial events and the ensuing encephalopathy.[94] In this study, some infants showed a delay of 36–96 h before neurological deterioration set in. Another study concentrated specifically on the timing of onset of seizures following perinatal asphyxia, finding that although the mean age at onset was about 10 hours, the range was 1–90 h.[95] The authors attempted to relate the onset of seizures to the estimated timing of the asphyxial insults but concluded that there was no reliable relationship.

The mechanisms of brain-cell death during asphyxia and subsequent HIE are the focus of intense interest because of the possibility of therapeutic intervention. It has been shown that some cells become necrotic during or soon after the asphyxial insult, as the result of energy failure. Other neurons die after a delay, with secondary energy failure as a result of apoptosis (programmed cell death; see Figure 14.2).[89,96–98] Apoptosis is possibly transduced by a cell-surface receptor known as Fas/CD95/ Apo-1.[99] Whether necrosis or apoptosis makes the greater contribution to neuronal loss seems to vary from one part of the brain to another. In experimentally asphyxiated piglets, for example, immature neurons seem prone to apoptotic death while terminally differentiated neurons die by necrosis.[98]

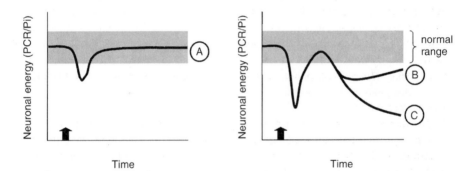

Fig. 14.2. Changes in cerebral energy levels. Time of asphyxial insult is marked by an arrow. Three patterns are shown: (A) Short-term energy loss with good recovery; (B) Severe initial energy loss with recovery, followed by secondary energy failure with some recovery; (C) Severe secondary energy loss that is likely to be fatal.

The contribution to neuronal loss by necrosis probably cannot be prevented (other than by preventing the damaging insult). The apoptotic element of neuronal loss, however, occurs beyond birth and its extent may be attenuated by therapy. For example, brain cooling after intrapartum asphyxia has been shown to reduce the delayed rise in cerebral lactate in asphyxiated newborn piglets.[90]

Although the occurrence of HIE is considered a necessary prerequisite for deducing that intrapartum asphyxia of potentially damaging severity has occurred, it is by no means inevitable that babies who suffer HIE will be permanently disabled. Hypoxic–ischaemic encephalopathy is graded conventionally into three bands of severity, according to the clinical features.[100] Grade I is a transient illness characterized by poor feeding and alternating periods of lethargy and irritability. Jitteriness is a feature but seizures are not. The prognosis for babies exhibiting signs limited to this grade of

HIE is good[100,101] and if disability follows, causes other than intrapartum asphyxia should be sought. Grade II HIE is a more prolonged illness that is characterized by a depressed level of consciousness, loss of muscle tone and spontaneous movement and seizures. Long-term adverse effects are seen in some 20–40% of babies who have suffered from this level of HIE.[102–104] Babies suffering from the most severe grade of HIE (grade III) are comatose, flaccid, unresponsive to pain and often exhibit decerebrate posturing. They frequently require circulatory and ventilatory support. There is a high mortality rate and a virtual certainty of severe disability among survivors.

Since the original descriptions of HIE and its outlook were published, a subgroup of babies who have suffered hypoxic/ischaemic injury confined to the basal ganglia of their brains have been described in whom the severity and duration of HIE was less than expected in relation to the severity of their disabilities.[105,106] Such infants may show prominent brainstem and extra-pyramidal signs in the newborn period.

Brain imaging during HIE may provide supportive evidence of an asphyxial aetiology and help determine the severity of injury. Ultrasound is least informative, often showing no abnormality despite permanent injury. In other cases, it may show evidence of brain swelling, increased echogenicity in the hemispheric white matter or basal ganglia or, occasionally, associated haemorrhage. Serial ultrasound, which shows the appearance and subsequent disappearance of brain swelling, is of some value in timing the asphyxia insult. Brain swelling is a variable phenomenon following asphyxial injury to the brain but when it occurs it is usually at its most obvious between 36 and 72 hours following the insult. It must be said, though, that systematic study of this phenomenon has not been undertaken.

Hypoxic–ischaemic injury to organs other than the brain

Although the brain is relatively susceptible to hypoxic–ischaemic injury compared with other organs, it is sheltered from injury during asphyxia by the redistribution of the circulation in its favour and at the expense of other organs.[81,107] It is not surprising, therefore, that when the brain is injured by intrapartum asphyxia, other organs also may be. The organs most often showing signs of injury are the kidneys, liver, gut, heart and lungs (see Table 14.1). Asphyxial injury to organs other than the brain is commonly termed 'systemic injury' in the literature. Evidence of compromised systemic blood flow during hypoxia can be seen in the fetus (Figure 14.3).

Trying to establish the incidence of these complications from the literature is a frustrating task because no two studies appear to have used the same criteria for defining either asphyxia or organ dysfunction. Estimates of the overall frequency of

Table 14.1. Effects of asphyxial injury to organs other than the brain

Organ	Effects
Kidneys	Renal failure, oliguria, haematuria, proteinuria
Liver	Abnormal liver function tests, abnormal blood clotting, hypoglycaemia
Gut	Necrotizing enterocolitis, mucosal haemorrhage
Heart	Heart failure, poor cardiac output, hypotension, mitral regurgitation
Lungs	Respiratory distress, pulmonary haemorrhage

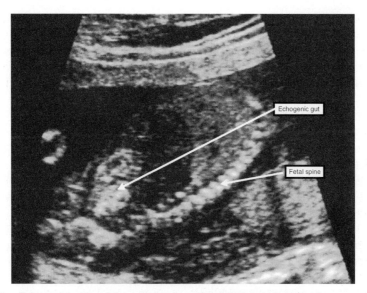

Fig. 14.3. Echogenic gut in a fetus suffering from chronic intra-uterine hypoxia.

systemic injury have been reported as 32% of all cases suffering from HIE[108] and 57% of cases with evidence of birth asphyxia as demonstrated by fetal distress, depression at birth and metabolic acidosis.[109] With regard to signs of renal injury, tubular proteinuria has been found in 72% of cases[110] and acute renal failure in 61%,[111] 43%,[112] 42%,[113] 30%[114] and 8%.[115] A general association exists between the degree of renal dysfunction and central nervous system injury, but this relationship does not reliably hold true in individuals.[116] Signs of liver injury, manifested by abnormal liver function tests, have been reported in 65% of cases of what was called 'severe asphyxia'.[117]

Since systemic injury is thought to be a consequence of redistribution of the circulation to the detriment of the supply of oxygen and blood to organs other than the brain, it seems likely that when asphyxia is so acute and severe as to overwhelm these protective mechanisms, the brain itself will be the first to suffer. There is some evidence for this in cases of asphyxia due to events such as uterine rupture. Phelan *et al.*[118] have reported 14 cases of severe brain injury without signs of systemic injury following such acute and catastrophic asphyxial insults.

Electroencephalography

The appearance of the neonatal electroencephalograph (EEG) varies greatly with gestational age and this must be taken into account when interpreting recordings.[119] In relation to HIE, the two main tasks for the EEG are to distinguish between seizures and other abnormal movements, and to assess prognosis.

It is sometimes difficult to decide whether abnormal movements observed in babies should be classified as seizures or whether they represent the release of brainstem motor centres from supratentorial control.[120] Clonic seizures with a normal background EEG for gestation are probably a benign phenomenon.[121]

In the context of overt HIE, the EEG has been shown to be a useful predictor of outcome when interpreted by those with experience.[121-126] Absent or very low voltage and the burst-suppression pattern correlate strongly with a poor outcome in term infants.[124-128]

Direct evidence of hypoxic–ischaemic brain injury

Discussed so far are observations that can be made at birth and during the early neonatal period which can be used to assess the likelihood that intrapartum asphyxia of potentially damaging severity has occurred. When taken in conjunction with the birth history and with observations made on the fetus during the course of labour and delivery, there is often enough evidence either to substantiate or contradict the notion that there has been a potentially damaging intrapartum event with reasonable certainty. None of this is direct evidence of brain injury, however, and we know that babies can show signs of distress *in utero*, can require a lot of resuscitation at birth, suffer from an encephalopathy and an episode of acute renal failure and still turn out to be normal. It is really only by looking at the brain with modern imaging techniques that direct evidence of brain injury can be obtained.

Magnetic resonance (MR) spectroscopy has already been referred to in relation to the mechanisms of brain injury during HIE. Proton MR spectroscopy is able to show abnormalities in the brains of babies who have suffered from intrapartum asphyxia when employed only a few hours after birth. In demonstrating which babies are likely to suffer a decline in cerebral high-energy phosphate concentrations, it may be able to provide an early direct indication of permanent brain injury.[129,130]

MR imaging (MRI) is also proving to be a useful tool for providing more or less direct evidence of brain injury in babies showing signs of HIE.[131,132] In one study of 73 term babies with HIE, all of whom showed abnormal signal intensity in the posterior limb of the internal capsule, were developmentally abnormal at one year of age, while a normal signal predicted a normal outcome in virtually every instance.[133] The technique of diffusion-weighted MRI[134] improves diagnostic accuracy and has been shown to improve the early detection of brain lesions in babies suffering from HIE[135] The correlation between the distribution and severity of brain injury shown using MRI and the clinical features in babies with HIE has been shown to be quite good.[136]

Interestingly, diffusion-weighted MRI applied to newborn babies who were born in good condition but then suffered from seizures has shown a high incidence of haemorrhagic or ischaemic lesions which were almost certainly acquired around the time of birth[137] – a reminder that there is still much to understand about the potentially adverse effects of the birth process.

Criteria which suggest that intrapartum asphyxia of potentially damaging severity has occurred

As is apparent from the foregoing discussion, devising a set of criteria that will distinguish clearly between babies who have experienced potentially damaging intrapartum asphyxia and those who have not is almost impossible. This is because of the overlap that exists between the two groups in many of the features used to indicate potentially damaging asphyxia. This has already been illustrated in respect of cord-blood pH. In many cases, the best that can be done is to balance the evidence in favour of potentially damaging asphyxia against the evidence opposing it. Table 14.2 summarizes the possible sources of evidence and indicates how each might be used to build up a case, either endorsing or contesting the diagnosis of significant intrapartum asphyxia.

Table 14.2. Summary of sources of information pertinent to the diagnosis of significant intrapartum asphyxia

Evidence suggesting that potentially damaging intrapartum asphyxia has occurred	Evidence suggesting that potentially damaging intrapartum asphyxia has *not* occurred
Complication of pregnancy known to predispose to intrapartum asphyxia	Normal pregnancy
Complication of labour or delivery known to predispose to intrapartum asphyxia	Normal labour and delivery
Evidence of fetal hypoxia or acidosis developing in labour; for example, on CTG or from fetal blood sampling	No significant CTG abnormality. Normal fetal scalp pH
Evidence of acidaemia on cord arterial blood	Cord pH in normal range
Poor condition at birth requiring advanced resuscitation	Good condition at birth
Encephalopathic illness in early neonatal period	No signs of encephalopathy
Ultrasound evidence of brain swelling	Normal ultrasound imaging
MR spectroscopic evidence of abnormal brain energy state and intracellular acidosis	Normal spectroscopy
MRI evidence of brain injury	Normal MRI
Electroencephalographic abnormality	Normal EEG
Signs of asphyxial injury to systemic organs	No signs of systemic injury

Clearly, every aspect of evidence is not available in every case and some points are weightier than others. In fact, the weightiest evidence from magnetic resonance spectroscopy and imaging is available least often (because the technology for spectroscopy is not widely available and imaging is not practical if the baby is ill in intensive care). There is also the difficulty of defining the *level* of abnormality that justifies inclusion in the left-hand column of the table. It is these issues that usually account for differences in opinion between experts – almost everyone would agree with the *principles* expressed in Table 14.2.

Patterns of hypoxic–ischaemic brain injury

No insult to a complex multicellular organism leads to a stereotypic response. Many factors relating to the anatomy, physiology and biochemistry of the individual and to the nature, duration and timing of the insult modulate the effects of hypoxia and ischaemia on the brain of the fetus and newborn infant. Although there is a growing body of descriptive data linking brain biochemistry and brain imaging to clinical outcome, it remains difficult to make inferences about the relationship between intrapartum asphyxia and cerebral damage because it is usually not possible to define the nature or severity of the hypoxic–ischaemic insult.

Much of our understanding of these matters comes from animal work in which more or less precise control of the hypoxic–ischaemic insult can be achieved – albeit that many models do not mimic precisely the patterns of intrapartum asphyxia seen in clinical practice. The animal model has the advantage of consistency and reproducibility of the consequences of an insult.[138] The main disadvantage of animal models is that there are marked interspecies differences in brain ontogeny at the time of delivery. For example, brain weight in the human infant is 27% of the adult value, whereas in the newborn rat the brain is 11% of adult weight; and, perhaps surprisingly, in the primate the brain is 75% of adult weight.[139] These and other limitations must be borne in mind when considering the data from animal work.[138,140]

In the next section, we will briefly consider the pathophysiology of cerebral damage and the factors that influence fetal susceptibility. Consideration will then be given to the current understanding of the different kinds of neurodevelopmental problem that may follow hypoxic–ischaemic cerebral damage in the term infant.

Factors influencing fetal vulnerability

The large variation in outcome following hypoxic–ischaemic brain injury is ill explained. Some factors are well recognized, however.

Brain maturity

It is well established that the newborn is better able to withstand hypoxia than the adult. In 1670, Robert Boyle observed that, placed in a jar with a burning candle, baby rats outlived adult rats.[141] Since then, the greater resistance of the immature brain to hypoxia has been demonstrated *ad nauseam* in a multitude of small furry animals.[142–145] A number of factors favour the immature organism:

▶ Lower cerebral metabolic rate

▶ Cerebral oxidative metabolism which can utilize a number of energy sources

▶ Ability to redistribute blood supply in favour of the brain, heart and adrenals

▶ Increased myocardial resistance to hypoxia

▶ Fetal haemoglobin.

In the first half of pregnancy, insults lead to lesions characterized by abnormal brain development. In the extreme, early embryogenesis may be disrupted leading to anencephaly. In the following months, the fetus may suffer defects of neuronal migration, leading to polymicrogyria or more subtle abnormalities such as band heterotopia, where a group of neurons arrested during their migration may be seen on an MR scan.[146]

Gestation has a profound effect upon susceptibility to hypoxic–ischaemic injury and the anatomical distribution of that injury. The immature brain is considerably less susceptible to damage. The immature brain which has not yet commenced rapid growth and is unmyelinated can withstand hypoxia for two or three times as long as the brain in the animal born at term.[138] This may at first seem to conflict with the epidemiological evidence of the high prevalence of CP in surviving pre-term infants.[147,148] Unfortunately, in the extremely pre-term infant, resistance to asphyxial damage cannot compensate for exposure to the fetal effects of maternal illness and the neonatal consequences of immaturity.[149]

The distribution of brain pathology brought about by hypoxia and ischaemia is determined principally by local cerebral blood flow and by the basal metabolic requirement of the tissue. It is not the purpose of this chapter to consider the pre-term infant. In this group, however, it is immediately apparent that the distribution of cerebral lesions responsible for CP and poor outcome differs markedly from that of the term infant. In the pre-term, the area of brain most likely to be damaged when the brain is subjected to ischaemia is the periventricular white matter, leading to periventricular leukomalacia (PVL; literally, softening of the white matter beside the ventricles).[149,150] The distribution of corticospinal fibres means that lower-limb function is more likely to be affected, resulting in CP predominantly of the diplegic form – in which the legs are exclusively, or more markedly, affected.

The importance of this observation to discussion of CP in term infants is that upon finding a diplegia or PVL in an infant born at term, it is important to give careful consideration to the possibility of antenatally acquired damage. In a study using MR brain imaging in 56 children with bilateral CP, injury to the subcortical white matter (parasagittal injury, see below) was more likely to be associated with neonatal encephalopathy, implying acute causation. On the other hand, when PVL with mild or moderate diplegia was seen in infants born at term, none had a history of neonatal encephalopathy, consistent with antenatally acquired damage.[146]

Maternal factors

Severe maternal illness, collapse or poisoning may directly lead to damage of the fetus. Other factors include pregnancy-related diseases such as hypertension and chorioamnionitis.[151,152] In developing countries, maternal anaemia, iodine-deficient hypothyroidism and other indicators of poor maternal nutrition represent important antenatal risk factors for encephalopathy.[153] The avoidance of these risk factors clearly is an important aim for health promotion in women of child-bearing age. These epidemiological data do not overcome the difficulty of determining when such factors are sufficient in themselves to have led to damage and when they act by predisposing the fetus to more severe damage secondary to hypoxic–ischaemic insult.

Fetal health

If fetal growth is restricted (ie if there is intra-uterine growth retardation/restriction [IUGR]), the fetus may less easily withstand the normal levels of hypoxia that occur during uterine contractions. This lack of reserve predisposes to hypoxic–ischaemic injury, especially during delivery[154] and partly explains the poorer outcome in the infant with IUGR.[155] These factors may be compounded by altered patterns of neurotransmitter activity in the central nervous system.[156]

Multiple pregnancy increases the risk of CP considerably – in twins, by a factor of 4.6–7.1. This effect remains marked in twins delivering with birthweights >2500 g, where the risk of CP is increased by factor of 3–4.5 compared with the singleton fetus.[157–159] A still greater risk is seen in pregnancy complicated by the death of one twin, and in triplets. Increased risk of low birthweight and prematurity are important contributors to this risk, but this does not explain the differences in outcome between twins and singletons delivered at term with normal birthweight.

Brain injury in the term infant

The insult

The severity of an asphyxial insult is a product of the degree and duration of hypoxia and ischaemia. Important differences occur with different patterns of asphyxia and these will be discussed below. It is important to recognize at the outset, however, that all levels of asphyxia sufficient to lead to cerebral damage are close to those that are lethal. In the absence of an ability to monitor fetal oxygen partial pressure (pO_2) in humans, the degree of hypoxia necessary to lead to damage is not known. In the monkey at term, reduction of blood oxygen to 30% of normal values results in no discernible change in cardiovascular or neurological status, even if this is maintained for some time.[160] In Myers' classic experiments, damage occurred when blood oxygen levels reduced to 5–15% of normal values were maintained for periods in excess of 30 minutes. Fetal oxygen levels below 5% of normal rapidly led to fetal death.

It is now appreciated that not only does the fetal response to differing severities and durations of asphyxia vary, but that this has important implications for the consequent pathology. This translates to different patterns of insult resulting in different neurodevelopmental outcomes. It would be naive to suggest there is a simple, reliable relationship between any form of asphyxia and specific long-term neurological problems in an older child. In broad terms, however, the following patterns of CP may be related to typical forms of hypoxic–ischaemic insult and brain pathology. Recognition of this has led to the use of two terms – 'prolonged partial asphyxia' and 'brief total asphyxia'.

Prolonged partial asphyxia

This term refers to a persisting low level of oxygenation of sufficient severity to lead to damage after a period of at least one hour.

In the animal model, this can be simulated through maternal hypotension or hypoxia or partial clamping of the iliac arteries or the umbilical cord. In clinical practice, intermittent cord compression or uterine hyperactivity may produce this picture. Again turning to Myers' laboratory, in the rhesus monkey prolonged partial asphyxia led to the familiar picture of HIE in the newborn. At birth, the onset of spontaneous respiration was delayed, seizures began on the first day of life that were associated with cerebral oedema, and subsequently there was recovery from the acute encephalopathy.[161]

After prolonged partial asphyxia, the degree of permanent cerebral damage varied but typically affected the parasagittal areas of the brain. Similar observations have been made in sheep exposed to one to two hours of prolonged partial asphyxia.[162,163] These parasagittal regions include subcortical white matter in the cerebral cortex running from front to back (see Figure 14.4). The affected area lies in a watershed or boundary zone in the brain. A watershed is the ridge of a hill that lies between the drainage areas of two rivers. The term is at first misleading. If however, one imagines that the natural process was reversed and that water flowed up the rivers, like blood up an arterial tree, feeding water to the hillsides, it would be apparent immediately that the watersheds would be the driest parts of the landscape. In the brain, the parasagittal subcortical white matter is on the boundary zone of perfusion of the anterior, posterior and middle cerebral arteries, lying at the watershed of the three arterial circulations.

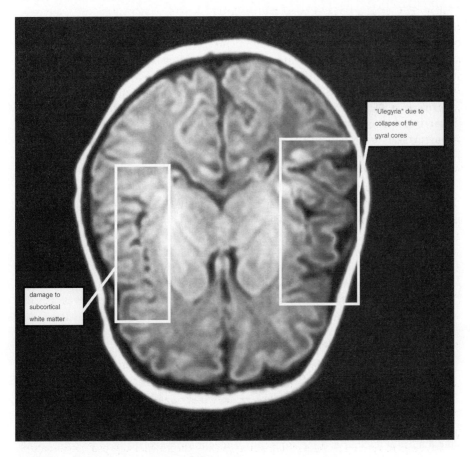

"Ulegyria" due to collapse of the gyral cores

damage to subcortical white matter

Fig. 14.4. Bilateral watershed injury (MR image).

Circulation to the watershed areas is further prejudiced by the adaptive response to prolonged partial asphyxia seen in the mature fetus. In the presence of persistent asphyxia and acidosis, redistribution of cerebral blood flow is seen. Perfusion is preferentially maintained to the brain stem and central structures within the CNS (eg the respiratory centre) as these are essential to maintain life after birth. This results in cortical hypoperfusion, exacerbating the watershed effect, and explaining why parasagittal injury is seen classically after prolonged partial asphyxia, and why it is usually not associated with basal ganglia damage.

The consequence is that the subcortical white matter in the parasagittal watershed is most likely to be damaged during the asphyxial insult of prolonged partial asphyxia. The importance of hypotension in parasagittal injury is clear. In a feline model, if central blood pressure is maintained artificially during hypoxia, cerebral damage is ameliorated markedly.[164] The local haemodynamic effect has been shown in fetal sheep, where infarction in the parasagittal areas is produced if cuffs are inflated around the carotid arteries, which in the sheep reduces perfusion to the whole brain.[165] Parasagittal neuronal cell death is a pattern that is well recognized in the human infant.[166–168]

Brief total asphyxia

This term refers to a period of anoxia or near-total hypoxia of lethal severity where damage occurs after about 10 minutes.

Brief total asphyxia is more easily produced in the experimental model. Complete occlusion of the iliac arteries or umbilical cord leads rapidly to fetal anoxia or near total hypoxia. Again, Myers' group first defined the pattern of change and its consequences for the monkey fetus,[169] and similar changes have been seen in other species.[170] After a brief rise in blood pressure, bradycardia occurs within 90 seconds and is promptly followed by hypotension. In the face of severe hypoxia and hypercarbia, anaerobic metabolism generates a lactic-acid load, and metabolic acidosis builds up rapidly over the first 10 minutes. At about 10 minutes, fetal blood shows a pH value of <7.0 and a marked base deficit, with high lactate levels. Between 10 and 20 minutes, the risk of cerebral injury increased and in Myers' model, neuronal damage was first seen at 12–13 minutes and became increasingly more severe. If brief total asphyxia persists beyond 20 minutes, risk of fetal death increases and beyond 30–35 minutes, death is almost inevitable.

The parallel in clinical practice is complete cord obstruction with cord prolapse or sudden cessation of uterine perfusion – for example, uterine rupture. Brief total cerebral anoxia–ischaemia may also occur when a critical degree of fetal acidaemia leads to circulatory arrest.

The pattern of damage following brief total asphyxia is different from that seen in prolonged partial asphyxia. The precise areas of brain damage differ between species and may include the cerebellum[169] and hippocampus.[162] The common factor is damage to the basal ganglia, a collective name for the deep grey matter structures which are arranged around the internal capsule. The basal ganglia comprise the caudate nucleus, the lentiform nucleus and the amygdala. The lentiform nucleus has two components: the globus pallidus and the putamen.

The basal ganglia are structures with high metabolic requirements, demonstrable on positron emission studies of glucose metabolism,[171] in an area of the brain which is well myelinated[172] and has a high density of glutaminergic neurons. These factors predispose the basal ganglia to damage in brief total asphyxia.

In contrast, the cortex is relatively resistant to damage in brief total asphyxia and is an area more richly innervated by GABAergic neurons.[170] If brief total asphyxia persists, damage may be more widespread but does not affect the cortex in the parasagittal areas as seen in prolonged partial asphyxia. In brief total asphyxia (see Figures 14.5 and 14.6), cortical damage, following injury to the basal ganglia, typically affects the pre- and post-central gyri (also known as the perirolandic area) which includes the primary motor cortex, a pattern that can be seen on MRI.[150,168,173,174]

The models of prolonged partial asphyxia and brief total asphyxia are useful in considering cerebral damage and its pathogenesis. Like all pure models, their application to clinical medicine is not precise. If fetal hypoxia progresses, the fetus may first suffer a sub-lethal degree of hypoxia followed by a period of brief total asphyxia. Neither is the response of the brain to hypoxia stereotypic. A diverse number of clinical outcomes are recognized and do not always relate as one might anticipate to the areas of damage defined on detailed brain imaging.

Neurodevelopmental outcome

Cerebral palsy

CP is classified clinically by the combination of neurological findings and their distribution in the four limbs (see Figure 14.7).[175]

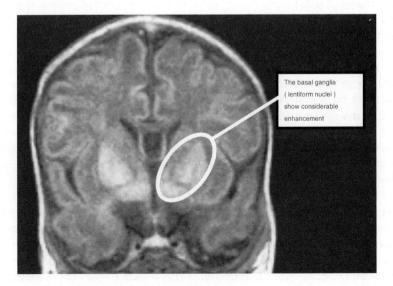

The basal ganglia (lentiform nuclei) show considerable enhancement

Fig. 14.5. Bilateral basal ganglia injury following uterine rupture and brief total asphyxia.

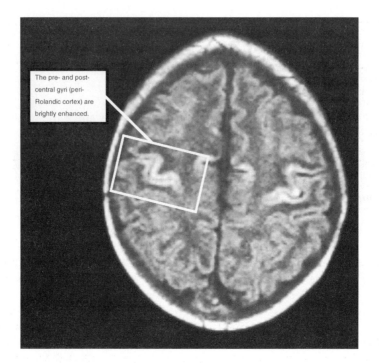

The pre- and post-central gyri (peri-Rolandic cortex) are brightly enhanced.

Fig. 14.6.   Cortical injury following brief total asphyxia.

Spastic quadriplegia

Spastic quadriplegia is the most common form of CP secondary to perinatal hypoxic ischaemic damage.[168,176–178] All four limbs are affected by the motor defect, and children with spastic quadriplegia face major problems. This group of children includes those who are totally dependent, requiring help with feeding and all bodily functions and for whom therapy aims at reducing complications and contractures and increasing comfort. The first signs of CP are usually apparent within the first year of life, although spasticity may not be evident at this stage and caution must be taken in interpreting studies where follow-up is limited to infancy.[179]

Spastic quadriplegia is associated frequently with other neurodevelopmental problems. Severe learning difficulty (mental retardation) is common[176] and many children are microcephalic.[178] Cortical blindness is seen frequently and is not always related to the severity of CP,[180] but deafness is relatively uncommon.

In a retrospective study of children with CP, those with or without a neonatal encephalopathy were compared. Spastic quadriplegia was the only form of CP to show a statistically significant association with neonatal encephalopathy as a marker of perinatal asphyxia.[181] Spastic quadriplegia is more common after severe neonatal encephalopathy.[182] In the Albertan follow-up studies,[183] the grade of neonatal encephalopathy was classified according to the infants' worst neurological status

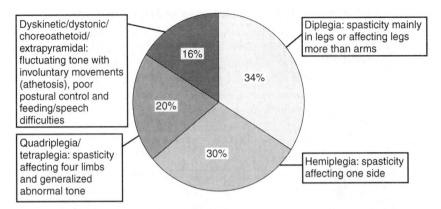

Fig. 14.7. Distribution of different types of cerebral palsy.[175]

between one hour and seven days of age. The tight definitions of encephalopathy used in Alberta[182] resulted in a clear relationship between neonatal illness and outcome. In the severe form of HIE – marked by the presence of flaccidity, stupor and the absence of primitive reflexes – all surviving infants developed spastic quadriplegia. By comparison, amongst the group with moderate HIE, 12% had CP, of which a quarter were classified as spastic quadriplegia. Other studies have demonstrated a less clear correlation between staging of HIE and spastic quadriplegia, although the prognostic value of the grading of HIE is seen in almost all publications.[184]

The pathological corollary of spastic quadriplegia was known from postmortem studies and is now confirmed with the use of detailed brain imaging techniques.[185] Changes in signal intensity of an MR scan are seen in the subcortical white matter in the parasagittal areas, changes which persist and which are predictive of adverse outcome and spastic quadriplegia.[150,168,186,187] In the presence of parasagittal damage, the basal ganglia are characteristically normal on early scanning.[149]

The conditions necessary for parasagittal brain injury will exist in the presence of prolonged partial asphyxia (see above), where periods of fetal bradycardia, lack of cardiac compensation, redistribution of cerebral blood flow away from the cortex, and loss of cerebral blood flow autoregulation conspire to deprive these areas of the brain of blood.[188,189]

The timing of injury during prolonged partial asphyxia is difficult to address. It is intuitive that the effects of hypoxia must be dependent upon its severity and duration. The duration of prolonged partial asphyxia that can be survived without damage is not known. The narrow margin between asphyxia that is harmless and that which is rapidly lethal has been discussed elsewhere.[160] Prolonged partial asphyxia occurs in the hinterland between these two states. In the animal model of prolonged partial asphyxia leading to parasagittal damage, rapid changes may be seen within minutes of the onset of asphyxia, which, if sustained for only 10 minutes, is followed by rapid resolution and some selective neuronal loss.[165] If asphyxia is present for 30 minutes, the parasagittal region shows a biphasic time course, with two peaks of cerebral oedema at seven and 28 hours, akin to the clinical picture seen in babies. Prolonged partial asphyxia produced by partial obstruction to flow through the cord, results in watershed damage after one to two hours, and is followed by an encephalopathy.[161] In contrast, if partial cord occlusion is maintained for three to fours hours in laboratory animals, blood lactate levels rise to over 14 mmol/l, and over half the animals die.[190]

It is generally held that the human fetus may survive prolonged partial asphyxia for a period of around one hour before compensatory mechanisms are overcome, leading to marked acidosis, hypotension and possible damage. In our clinical practice, we see infants with observations suggesting prolonged partial asphyxia for less than one hour who develop watershed injury, and many others with prolonged abnormalities on CTG consistent with prolonged partial asphyxia in whom outcome is normal. Partial asphyxia may last many hours and it has been suggested that the duration may extend to days. The maximum duration of partial asphyxia is not known and clearly would depend upon the exact degree of hypoxia. In general, however, the notion of prolonged partial asphyxia lasting at least one hour in infants who suffer parasagittal damage seems to marry well with our experience and with the limited evidence available.

Dyskinetic cerebral palsy

The term 'dyskinetic CP' is largely used synonymously with 'chorioathetoid CP' and marks the presence of extrapyramidal symptoms. Previously, this has been known as 'dystonic CP', although this term is less useful in that it simply implies that muscle tone is abnormal – a feature shared with spasticity.

The typical picture of dyskinetic CP is characteristic and well recognized. Muscle tone varies from spastic to hypotonic and is reduced at rest. Increased muscle tone is seen particularly when purposeful movements are attempted. These movements may be prevented by the presence of chorioathetosis, a movement disorder characterized by writhing, sinuous movements of the limbs particularly marked during attempts to perform tasks requiring coordination. The child or adult affected by dyskinetic CP may be severely disabled by this. Day-to-day life is made more difficult by the coincidental problems with swallowing, feeding and oromotor function. Dysarthria is often present and words may be articulated so poorly that very few people can understand the child's speech. In typical dyskinetic CP, head growth is preserved and there is relative or complete preservation of intellectual function. The devastating combination of normal intelligence and an inability to speak, feed oneself or perform relatively simple motor tasks means that dyskinetic CP can be a particularly difficult disorder to live with.

Diagnosis is difficult. If dyskinetic movements are less marked, recognition may require skill and experience. Confusion with cerebellar ataxia may occur. Certainly, dyskinesia is seldom diagnosed in the first year of life and usually becomes apparent with the evolving picture of CP.[191] In a study based on a survey at an adult neurology centre, dyskinesia was found in 10 patients in whom it was secondary to perinatal cerebral damage.[192] IQs were largely in the normal range. The mean age of onset of dyskinesia was 12.9 years (range: 5–21 years) emphasizing the need for follow-up into the school years if dyskinesia is to be detected.

Dyskinetic CP represents an unusual form of the disease. In a Liverpool study, 1.6% of the 1056 children with CP were found to have a combination of dyskinesia, normal IQ and delivery at term.[193] Amongst infants in the Albertan study,[183] none of the children with severe HIE developed dyskinetic CP, whilst this neurological outcome was seen in 5% of the children with a history of a moderate HIE.

There is now a combination of animal experiments, clinical observations and imaging evidence which indicates that dyskinetic CP is caused by damage to the basal ganglia (see above). When movement is initiated by the cerebral cortex, impulses pass through the corticospinal and corticobulbar pathways and also into the corticostriatal projection. The basal ganglia in combination with the substantia nigra exercise a largely inhibitory effect upon these motor signals, modifying them and improving the quality and control of movement and function. The importance of the basal ganglia in control of movement and posture can be seen in patients suffering conditions such as Parkinson's disease and Huntingdon's chorea.

In children with dyskinetic CP, the pathology in the basal ganglia is well recognized.[194] The original pathological descriptions of basal ganglia damage referred to the diagnosis of *status marmoratus*, alluding to the marble-like appearance of the basal ganglia due to abnormal patterns of myelination after injury.[195] Such damage may now be seen on MR scan even in the first days of life.[150,168,196] The long-term prognosis of MR appearances in the neonatal period are difficult to determine in view of the late appearance of dyskinesia in children with CP.[192] Care must be taken in interpreting the available data, many of which include follow-up of infants after neonatal MRI for a period of only one year.[168,197] Upon early follow-up, basal ganglia damage leading to dyskinesia may be apparent only in the most severely damaged infants.

Basal ganglia damage is the pathological corollary of brief total asphyxia. The predilection for damage in certain areas of the brain has been demonstrated well in a number of animal species, as discussed above. In the human fetus, damage during brief total asphyxia is concentrated on the most metabolically active parts of the brain, including the basal ganglia, and may extend to the pre- and post-central gyri, the so-called 'perirolandic cortex', while sparing the parasagittal cortex.[149] The changes may be seen early on an MR scan, although they may not be as visible as damage to the white matter without the use of special enhancing techniques.[198]

In 1994, Rosenbloom reported on a group of children from Liverpool.[105] Amongst 17 children with dyskinetic CP, two had severe jaundice, one a metabolic defect, and in four, no cause was apparent. In 10 children (1% of all CP patients in the region), there was a history suggestive of late fetal hypoxia of short duration. This period of brief total hypoxia was the result of events such as cord occlusion, severe antepartum haemorrhage and undiagnosed breech. Only one of the children developed a severe HIE requiring ventilation for seven days. Neonatal encephalopathy was less severe in the others. The children had a typical picture of dyskinetic motor impairment and had normal intellect. In the Boston study of late-onset dyskinesia,[192] the evidence for perinatal brain insult was noted but was less clearly presented. Two children developed dyskinetic CP after episodes of acute hypoxia at three years and at 13 months, secondary to a choking episode and collapse following a scald, respectively.[191] In a follow-up study[168] at one year of age, some of the infants with neonatal MR evidence of basal ganglia damage showed evidence of dyskinetic CP, whilst the main observation was that basal ganglia damage was associated with more severe forms of CP. This might reflect the early follow-up, however. In a study of early MR performed in the first 10 days after birth complicated by intrapartum hypoxia,[150] seven of the 20 infants studied had changes limited to the basal ganglia and the perirolandic cortex, without evidence of watershed infarction. All of these had a history of acute, severe hypoxia due to cord accident, placental abruption, uterine rupture or acute cardiocirculatory arrest.

Hemiplegia

Hemiplegia accounts for about a third of all CP cases and is more common than spastic quadriplegia.[7-9,16,32,176,178] It appears less often to be due to intrapartum asphyxia than to either the spastic quadriplegic or dyskinetic forms of CP.

The child with hemiplegia typically has increased tone and reflexes on one side. Spasticity is usually more apparent in the upper limb. Children cope well with hemiplegia and often intellectual function is preserved and the interference with normal life is less than one might anticipate.

The cerebral abnormality responsible for hemiplegic CP may result either from a focal lesion confined to one hemisphere or from asymmetrically distributed lesions involving both hemispheres (Figure 14.8). The focal lesions are mainly arterial infarctions secondary to vascular thrombosis or embolization and the bilateral lesions mainly the result of hypoxia and reduced cerebral blood flow such as occur during asphyxia. Why a generalized reduction in the flow of blood and oxygen to the brain

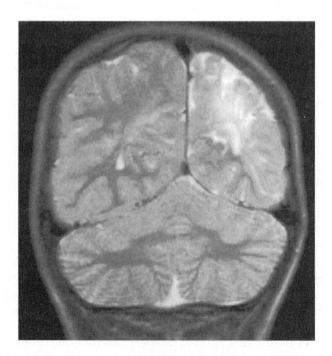

Fig. 14.8. Asymmetric distribution of cerebral injury in a child with hemiplegia secondary to birth asphyxia.

sometimes results in almost unilateral injury is not understood, although an obvious explanation is asymmetry of the cerebral vasculature.

Cerebral artery embolism is probably rare. It is well recognized in twin pregnancy, in the twin-to-twin transfusion syndrome, and is an important part of the explanation of the neurodevelopmental problems seen in the surviving twin after intra-uterine death of the co-twin.[199] Embolic disease is also seen in infants who have congenital heart disease, in those with severe neonatal illness associated with coagulation abnormalities, and following cannulation of central vessels, notably in infants receiving extracorporeal membrane oxygenation (ECMO).[200]

Pure thrombosis occurs in association with large germinal matrix/intraventricular bleed, a condition much more typically seen in the pre-term infant.[149] It may also be recognized at term, although not in association with intrapartum asphyxia.[201] Focal lesions are also well recognized in the infants of mothers addicted to cocaine, especially the pure base, crack.[202]

Focal ischaemic lesions occurring in the region supplied by one of the main cerebral arteries, and often associated with secondary haemorrhage into the infarcted brain, are often called 'neonatal strokes'. This has been estimated to occur in one in 5000 newborn infants. The brain supplied by the middle cerebral artery is affected most commonly, and three to four times more commonly on the left rather than the right.[203] In these infants, the clinical course is characterized by seizures in the neonatal period, which may be focal or generalized, and the absence of severe systemic illness.[204] In a study in 1979,[205] radionuclide scanning demonstrated unilateral middle cerebral artery region abnormalities in six of 56 infants with perinatal hypoxia–ischaemia. In one of the six infants, the neonatal abnormalities resolved and a normal outcome was seen; whilst in the other five, hemiplegia resulted. More recent data suggest that any association with peripartum asphyxia is weak, and asphyxia appears to be an uncommon cause of focal arterial infarction.[206]

With regard to asymmetrical bilateral lesions secondary to hypoxia and ischaemia, there is no doubt that hemiplegia may follow intrapartum asphyxia.[168,179,205,207–210] It is equally clear that in most children with hemiplegia, a perinatal aetiology cannot be determined from the history. In two-thirds of children with hemiplegia, no history of perinatal hypoxia is found, reflecting a wide variety of conditions that may lead to focal cerebral damage.[211] Perinatal cerebral damage, however, remains an important – and the single most common – cause of hemiplegia.[212]

In a prospective study in one health region,[213] asymmetrical CP was found to have a positive association with a history suggestive of perinatal asphyxia. However, in that study, the majority of asymmetrical CP was diplegic and thus likely to be the result of asymmetric PVL and to have its origins before 34 weeks gestation. In most studies following-up children with a history of perinatal hypoxia and neonatal encephalopathy, a small number of children have hemiplegia. MR scanning shows asymmetric brain swelling in the neonatal period, suggesting an acute aetiology in association with a grade II encephalopathy and consequent hemiparesis with a near normal optimality score (a system for grading overall disability).[168] Two earlier studies showed hemiplegia occurring in around 10% of children with a history of intrapartum asphyxia and neonatal encephalopathy. In a further study,[178] a similar proportion developed hemiparesis – including children with and without intellectual delay. In only one of these children was microcephaly noticed.[208]

It appears that an asymmetric CP may result from intrapartum hypoxia but that this association is much less strong that seen in spastic quadriplegia or dyskinetic CP. In the analysis of perinatal history amongst children with CP, hemiplegia was less likely to be associated with a history suggestive of intrapartum hypoxia (odds ratio: 0.3 [95% confidence interval of 0.1–0.8]).[181]

The Hammersmith group have prospectively followed infants with focal abnormalities on MR scan in the newborn period.[209,210] The focal abnormalities may be seen in the newborn infant presenting with seizures in the absence of a more marked systemic illness and without a history of intrapartum hypoxia. The precise aetiology of this focal abnormality is not clear but the changes on MR scan suggest that the events leading to focal infarction are acute and perinatal. This study of 24 infants provides compelling evidence of the predictive value of MR. Focal changes were seen in the cerebral hemisphere, basal ganglia and posterior limb of the internal capsule. Adverse outcome, upon follow-up for at least one year, was only seen in infants in whom damage was seen in all three of these areas. Amongst these eight children, seven had asymmetric CP and one a normal outcome. Abnormalities of neonatal EEG were also predictive of hemiplegia. Focal cerebral damage was positively associated with subsequent visual impairment.[180]

There seems little doubt that focal brain lesions may occur in the perinatal period. There is good circumstantial evidence that focal neurological disability may result from a global hypoxic–ischaemic cerebral insult. Future studies using MR scans may prove extremely helpful in unraveling the relationship between the insult, the brain pathology and the outcome. At present, only if there is compelling evidence of severe fetal asphyxia, combined with the absence of other explanation for focal cerebral injury on imaging and full paediatric investigation, should one consider attributing hemiplegic CP to an intrapartum cause.

Ataxic cerebral palsy

Ataxia is an unusual feature, seen in only about 1% of children with CP. Careful neurological assessment is essential to differentiate the problems with coordination, postural control, gait and speech from those seen in dyskinetic CP. In animals, as discussed above, the cerebellum may be particularly predisposed towards hypoxic–ischaemic damage. In humans, however, ataxic CP is associated with a large number of inherited and congenital abnormalities.[210] Detailed paediatric neurological assessment and investigation is necessary in such children. If damage to the cerebellum sufficient to lead to ataxic CP can occur in association with intrapartum hypoxia, the coincidence is rare – as testified by the presence of ataxic CP in less than 1% of school age children followed up after neonatal encephalopathy in the Albertan study.[176]

Isolated mental impairment as an outcome of intrapartum asphyxia

The conventional view is that when intrapartum asphyxia causes brain injury, there is always motor impairment and that isolated mental impairment is not a form of disability that can be attributed to intrapartum asphyxia. Some of the difficulties associated with trying to establish the full spectrum of disability arising from intrapartum asphyxia have been discussed earlier in this chapter. In order to establish a significant association between intrapartum asphyxia and any adverse outcome that is uncommon relative to CP, it is necessary to follow a large cohort of asphyxiated babies for a very long time. The most informative study of this kind has been conducted in the Neonatal Follow-up Clinic in Alberta, Canada, by Dr Charlene Robertson.[29,30,214,215] In this study, 253 term infants who had suffered from moderate or severe HIE associated with birth asphyxia were followed into their school years. Data were available on 192 of them, and they were compared with appropriately selected peer groups for a variety of outcome measures. Not surprisingly, the children in the asphyxia group who developed CP had markedly lower IQ scores than the children in the control groups. However, the children in the asphyxia group who showed no signs of CP also had significantly lower scores than the controls for full-scale, verbal and performance IQ tests. The differences in mean scores were less marked than in the case of the children with CP but were sufficient to lead to considerably poorer school performance. In the worst comparison, 39% of the study children achieved more than one grade below the expected level in arithmetic, compared with 9% of the control group.[29] A few of the asphyxiated children who did not have CP were severely intellectually retarded (Charlene Robertson, personal communication). These data demonstrate that perinatal asphyxia can cause impaired intellectual function without causing impaired motor function.

Other studies provide some evidence of mental impairment in children with a convincing history of perinatal asphyxia. In children with a history of intrapartum hypoxia and neonatal encephalopathy, positron emission tomography was used to assess cerebral blood flow – an increase in cerebral blood flow was associated with lower IQs in the 4–12-year-old age group. Two infants had markedly high cerebral blood flow but did not develop CP on follow-up; one of these had a low IQ.[216] In a follow-up study amongst children with CP,[217] abnormalities of cerebral oxidative metabolism with low levels of high-energy phosphates in the neonatal period relate closely to mental retardation in association with motor problems. In the same studies,[217] low neonatal phosphocreatine levels were associated with poor subsequent head growth.

In the medico-legal context, the burden of proof should be set higher for uncommon adverse outcomes of intrapartum asphyxia than for those that are common. This is because the lower the prior probability of a causal link, the more evidence is required to establish probable causation. In the case of isolated intellectual impairment, we would suggest that, as well as convincing evidence of intrapartum asphyxia of potentially damaging severity (as outlined earlier), there should be imaging evidence of hypoxic–ischaemic brain injury. Moreover, other causes of impaired intellect should have been excluded as far as possible by appropriate investigation. It is also important to look for evidence of deafness[29] and minor motor abnormalities which may be apparent when intellectual impairment is due to perinatal asphyxia.[218,219] It is also worth looking back at the history for evidence of a transient motor problem in early life.[220]

References

1 Mutch L, Alberman E, Hagberg B, Kodama K, Perat MV. Cerebral palsy epidemiology: where are we now and where are we going? *Developmental Medicine & Child Neurology* 1992; 34: 547–551.

2 Pharoah PO. The epidemiology of chronic disability in childhood. *International Rehabilitation Medicine* 1985; 7: 11–17.

3 Stanley F, Alberman E (eds.) *The Epidemiology of the Cerebral Palsies*. Oxford: Blackwell Scientific Publications, 1984.

4 Newacheck PW, Taylor WR. Childhood chronic illness: prevalence, severity and impact. *American Journal of Public Health* 1992; 82: 364–371.

5 Colver AF, Gibson M, Hey EN, Jarvis SN, Mackie PC, Richmond S. Increasing rates of cerebral palsy across the severity spectrum in north-east England. *Archives of Disease in Childhood* 2000; 83: F7–F12.

6 Pharoah PO, Cooke T, Johnson MA, King R, Mutch L. Epidemiology of cerebral palsy in England and Scotland, 1984-9. *Archives of Disease in Childhood (Fetal Neonatal Edition)* 1998; 79: F21–F25.

7 Jarvis SN, Holloway JS, Hey EN. Increase in cerebral palsy in normal birthweight babies. *Archives of Disease in Childhood* 1985; 60: 113–121.

8 Hagberg B, Hagberg G, Olow I, von Wendt L. The changing panorama of cerebral palsy in Sweden. V. The birth year period 1979–82. *Acta Paediatrica Scandanavica* 1989; 78: 283–290.

9 Dowding VM, Barry C. Cerebral palsy: changing patterns of birthweight and gestational age. *Irish Medical Journal* 1988; 81: 25–28.

10 Stanley F, Watson L. The cerebral palsies in Western Australia: trends, 1968–1981. *American Journal of Obstetrics & Gynecology* 1988; 158: 89–93.

11 Riikonen RS, Raumavirta S, Sinivouri E, Seppala T. Changing pattern of cerebral palsy in the southwest region of Finland. *Acta Paediatrica Scandanavica* 1989; 78: 581–587.

12 Torfs CP, van den BB, Oechsli FW, Cummins S. Prenatal and perinatal factors in the etiology of cerebral palsy. *Journal of Pediatrics* 1990; 116: 615–619.

13 Meberg A. Declining incidence of low birth weight - impact on perinatal mortality and incidence of cerebral palsy. *Journal of Perinatal Medicine* 1990; 18: 195–200.

14 Nelson KB, Ellenberg JH. Antecedents of cerebral palsy. Multivariate analysis of risk. *New England Journal of Medicine* 1986; 315: 81–86.

15 Pharoah PO, Cooke RW, Cooke T, Rosenbloom L. Birthweight-specific trends in cerebral palsy. *Archives of Disease in Childhood* 1990; 65: 602–606.

16 Pharoah PO, Platt MJ, Cooke T. The changing epidemiology of cerebral palsy. *Archives of Disease in Childhood (Fetal Neonatal Edition)* 1996; 75: F169–F173.

17 Little WJ. On the influence of abnormal parturition, difficult labours, premature birth and asphyxia neonatorum on the mental and physical condition of the child. *Transactions of the Obstetric Society of London* 1862; 3: 293–344.

18 Freud S, Russin LAT. Infantile cerebral paralysis. Corla Gables, Florida: University of Miami Press, 1968.

19 Perlstein MA. Infantile cerebral palsy – classification and clinical correlations. *JAMA* 1952; 149: 30–34.

20 O'Reilly DE, Walentynowicz JE. Etiological factors in cerebral palsy: an historical review. *Developmental Medicine & Childhood Neurology* 1981; 23: 633–642.

21 Paneth N, Fox HE. The relationship of Apgar score to neurologic handicap: a survey of clinicians. *Obstetrics & Gynecology* 1983; 61: 547–550.

22 Blair E, Stanley FJ. Intrapartum asphyxia: a rare cause of cerebral palsy. *Journal of Pediatrics* 1988; 112: 515–519. [Published erratum appears in *J Pediatr* 1988; 113(2): 420].

23 Naeye RL, Peters EC, Bartholomew M, Landis JR. Origins of cerebral palsy. *American Journal of Disease in Childhood* 1989; 143: 1154–1161.

24 Nelson KB, Ellenberg JH. Antecedents of cerebral palsy. Multivariate analysis of risk. *New England Journal Medicine* 1986; 315: 81–86.

25 Gaffney G, Flavell V, Johnson A, Squier MV, Sellers S. Model to identify potentially preventable cerebral palsy of intrapartum origin. *Archives of Disease in Childhood (Fetal Neonatal Edition)* 1995; 73: F106–F108.

26 Fenn P, Diacon S, Gray A, Hodges R, Rickman N. Current cost of medical negligence in NHS hospitals: analysis of claims database. *BMJ* 2000; 320: 1567–1571.

27 Fenn P, Hermans D, Dingwall R. Estimating the cost of compensating victims of medical negligence. *BMJ* 1994; 309: 389–391.

28 Pharoah PO. Epidemiology of cerebral palsy. *Journal of the Royal Society of Medicine* 1981; 74: 516–520.

29 Robertson CM, Finer NN. Long-term follow-up of term neonates with perinatal asphyxia. *Clinical Perinatology* 1993; 20: 483–500.

30 Robertson CM, Finer NN, Grace MG. School performance of survivors of neonatal encephalopathy associated with birth asphyxia at term. *Journal of Pediatrics* 1989; 114: 753–760.

31 Nelson KB, Ellenberg JH. Antecedents of CP: multivariate analysis of risk. *New England Journal of Medicine* 1986; 315: 81–86.

32 Nelson KB, Ellenberg JH. Epidemiology of cerebral palsy. *Advances in Neurology* 1978; 19: 421–435.

33 Nelson KB, Ellenberg JH. Obstetric complications as risk factors for cerebral palsy or seizure disorders. *JAMA* 1984; 251: 1843–1848.

34 Ellenberg JH, Nelson KB. Early recognition of infants at high risk for cerebral palsy: examination at age four months. *Developmental Medicine & Child Neurology* 1981; 23: 705–716.

35 Drage JS, Kennedy C, Berendes H, Schwarz BK, Weiss W. The Apgar score as an index of infant morbidity. A report from the collaborative study of cerebral palsy. *Developmental Medicine & Child Neurology* 1966; 8: 141–148.

36 Dite GS, Bell R, Reddihough DS, Bessell C, Brennecke S, Sheedy M. Antenatal and perinatal antecedents of moderate and severe spastic cerebral palsy. *Australian & New Zealand Journal of Obstetrics & Gynaecology* 1998; 38: 377–383.

37 MacLennan A. A template for defining a causal relation between acute intrapartum events and cerebral palsy: international consensus statement. *BMJ* 1999; 319: 1054–1059.

38 Rosso IM, Cannon TD, Huttunen T, Huttunen MO, Lonnqvist J, Gasperoni TL. Obstetric risk factors for early-onset schizophrenia in a Finnish birth cohort. *American Journal of Psychiatry* 2000; 157: 801–807.

39 Borell U, Fernstrom I, Ohlson L, Wiqvist N. Influence of uterine contractions on the uteroplacental blood flow at term. *American Journal of Obstetrics & Gynecology* 1965; 93: 44–57.

40 Fendel H, Fettweis P, Billet P *et al.* Doppler studies of arterial utero-fetoplacental blood flow before and during labour. *Zeitschrift Geburtshilfe Perinatologie* 1987; 191: 121–129.

41 Olofsson P, Thuring-Jonsson A, Marsal K. Uterine and umbilical circulation during the oxytocin challenge test. *Ultrasound Obstetrics & Gynecology* 1996; 8: 247–251.

42 Huch R, Huch A, Rooth G. *Laboratory Investigation of Fetal Disease* (AJ Barson [eds.]) Bristol: John Wright & Sons, 1981.

43 Hooper SB, Walker DW, Harding R. Oxygen, glucose, and lactate uptake by fetus and placenta during prolonged hypoxemia. *American Journal of Physiology* 1995; 268: R303–R309.

44 Carter BS, Moores RR Jr, Teng C, Meschia G, Battaglia FC. Main routes of plasma lactate carbon disposal in the midgestation fetal lamb. *Biology of the Neonate* 1995; 67: 295–300.

45 Carter BS, Moores RR Jr., Battaglia FC, Meschia G. Ovine fetal placental lactate exchange and decarboxylation at midgestation. *American Journal of Physiology* 1993; 264: E221–E225.

46 Piquard F, Schaefer A, Dellenbach P, Haberey P. Lactate movements in the term human placenta *in situ*. *Biology of the Neonate* 1990; 58: 61–68.

47 Engle WD, Laptook AR, Perlman JM. Acute changes in arterial carbon dioxide tension and acid-base status and early neurologic characteristics in term infants following perinatal asphyxia. *Resuscitation* 1999; 42: 11–17.

48 MacLennan A. A template for defining a causal relation between acute intrapartum events and cerebral: international consensus statement. *BMJ* 1999; 319: 1054–1059.

49 Sehdev HM, Stamilio DM, Macones GA, Graham E, Morgan MA. Predictive factors for neonatal morbidity in neonates with an umbilical arterial cord pH less than 7.00. *American Journal of Obstetrics & Gynecology* 1997; 177: 1030–1034.

50 Goldaber KG, Gilstrap LC, Leveno KJ, Dax JS, McIntire DD. Pathologic fetal acidemia. *Obstetrics & Gynecology* 1991; 78: 1103–1107.

51 Helwig JT, Parer JT, Kilpatrick SJ, Laros RK Jr. Umbilical cord blood acid-base state: what is normal? *American Journal of Obstetrics & Gynecology* 1996; 174: 1807–1812.

52 Eskes TK, Jongsma HW, Houx PC. Percentiles for gas values in human umbilical cord blood. *European Journal of Obstetrics, Gynaecology & Reproductive Biology* 1983; 14: 341–346.

53 Yeomans ER, Hauth JC, Gilstrap LC, III, Strickland DM. Umbilical cord pH, pCO_2, and bicarbonate following uncomplicated term vaginal deliveries. *American Journal of Obstetrics & Gynecology* 1985; 151: 798–800.

54 Thorp JA, Sampson JE, Parisi VM, Creasy RK. Routine umbilical cord blood gas determinations? *American Journal of Obstetrics & Gynecology* 1989; 161: 600–605.

55 Vandenbussche FP, Oepkes D, Keirse MJ. The merit of routine cord blood pH measurement at birth. *Journal of Perinatal Medicine* 1999; 27: 158–165.

56 Johnson JWC, Riley W. Cord blood gas studies: a survey. *Clinical Obstetrics & Gynecology* 1993; 36: 99–101.

57 Josten BE, Johnson TR, Nelson JP. Umbilical cord blood pH and Apgar scores as an index of neonatal health. *American Journal of Obstetrics & Gynecology* 1987; 157: 843–848.

58   Khan SN, Ahmed GS, Abutaleb AM, Hathal MA. Is the determination of umbilical cord arterial blood gases necessary in all deliveries? Analysis in a high-risk population. *Journal of Perinatology* 1995; 15: 39–42.

59   Riley RJ, Johnson JWC. Collecting and analyzing cord blood gases. *Clinical Obstetrics & Gynecology* 1993; 36: 13–23.

60   Gordon A, Johnson JWC. Value of umbilical blood acid-base studies in fetal assessment. *Journal of Reproductive Medicine* 1985; 30: 329–333.

61   Egan JFX, Vintzileos AM, Campbell WA. Arteriovenous cord blood pH discordancy in a high risk population and its significance. *Journal of Maternal & Fetal Medicine* 1992; 1: 39–42.

62   Boesel RR, Olson AE, Johnson JWC. Umbilical cord blood studies help assess fetal respiratory status. *Contemporary Obstetrics & Gynaecology* 1986; 28: 63–67.

63   Brar HS, Wong MK, Kirschbaum TH, Paul RH. Umbilical cord acid base changes associated with perinatal cardiac failure. *American Journal of Obstetrics & Gynecology* 1988; 158: 511–518.

64   Westgate J, Garibaldi JM, Greene KR. Umbilical cord blood gas analysis at delivery: a time for quality data. *British Journal of Obstetrics & Gynecology* 1994; 101: 1054–1063.

65   Belai Y, Goodwin TM, Durand M, Greenspoon JS, Paul RH, Walther FJ. Umbilical arteriovenous pO_2 and pCO_2 differences and neonatal morbidity in term infants with severe acidosis. *American Journal of Obstetrics & Gynecology* 1998; 178: 13–19.

66   Vandenbussche FP, Griever GE, Oepkes D, Postuma MC, Le Cessie S, Keirse MJ. Reliability of individual umbilical artery pH measurements. *Journal of Perinatal Medicine* 1997; 25: 340–346.

67   Sykes GS, Molloy PM. Effect of delays in collection or analysis on the results of umbilical cord blood measurements. *British Journal of Obstetrics & Gynaecology* 1984; 91: 989–992.

68   Strickland DM, Gilstrap LC, III, Hauth JC, Widmer K. Umbilical cord pH and pCO_2: effect of interval from delivery to determination. *American Journal of Obstetrics & Gynecology* 1984; 148: 191–194.

69   Kirshon B, Moishe KJ. Effect of heparin on umbilical arterial blood gases. *Journal of Reproductive Medicine* 1989; 34: 267–271.

70   Apgar V. A proposal for a new method of evaluation of the newborn infant. *Anesthetics & Analgesia* 1953; 32: 260–267.

71   Dawes GS. Fetal and neonatal physiology. Chicago: Year Book Medical Publishers Inc, 1968.

72   Myers RE. Two patterns of perinatal brain damage and their conditions of occurrence. *American Journal of Obstetrics & Gynecology* 1972; 112: 246–276.

73   Myers R. Four patterns of perinatal brain damage and their conditions of occurrence in primates. *Advances in Neurology* 1975; 10: 223–234.

74   Duffy T, Cavazzuti M, Cruz N. Local cerebral glucose metabolism in newborn dogs: effects of hypoxia and halothane anaesthesia. *Annals of Neurology* 1982; 11: 233–247.

75   Szymonowicz W, Walker AM, Cussen L, Cannata J, Yu VY. Developmental changes in regional cerebral blood flow in fetal and newborn lambs. *American Journal of Physiology* 1988; 254: H52–H58.

76   Abrams RM, Ito M, Frisinger JE, Patlak CS, Pettigrew KD, Kennedy C. Local cerebral glucose utilization in fetal and neonatal sheep. *American Journal of Physiology* 1984; 246: R608–R618.

77   Abrams RM, Cooper RJ. Effect of ketamine on local cerebral glucose utilization in fetal sheep. *American Journal of Obstetrics & Gynecology* 1987; 156: 1018–1023.

78   Chugani HT, Phelps ME. Maturational changes in cerebral function in infants determined by 18FDG positron emission tomography. *Science* 1986; 231: 840–843.

79   Haddad GG, Donnelly DF, Getting PA. Biophysical properties of hypoglossal neurons in vitro: intracellular studies in adult and neonatal rats. *Journal of Applied Physiology* 1990; 69: 1509–1517.

80   Ashwal S, Dale PS, Longo LD. Regional cerebral blood flow: studies in the fetal lamb during hypoxia, hypercapnoea, acidosis and hypotension. *Pediatric Research* 1984; 18: 1309–1311.

81   Behrman RE, Lees MH. Organ blood flows of the fetal, newborn and adult rhesus monkey: a comparative study. *Biology of the Neonate* 1971; 18: 330–340.

82   Behrman RE, Lees MH, Peterson EN, De Lannoy CW, Seeds AE. Distribution of the circulation in the normal and asphyxiated fetal primate. *American Journal of Obstetrics & Gynecology* 1970; 108: 956–969.

83   Szymonowicz W, Walker AM, Yu VY, Stewart ML, Cannata J, Cussen L. Regional cerebral blood flow after hemorrhagic hypotension in the preterm, near-term, and newborn lamb. *Pediatric Research* 1990; 28: 361–366.

84   Ashwal S, Majcher JS, Longo LD. Patterns of fetal lamb regional cerebral blood flow during and after prolonged hypoxia: studies during the posthypoxic recovery period. *American Journal of Obstetrics & Gynecology* 1981; 139: 365–372.

85   Groenendaal F, van der GJ, van Haastert IC, Eken P, Mali WP, De Vries LS. Findings in cerebral proton spin resonance spectroscopy in newborn infants with asphyxia, and psychomotor development. *Nederlands Tijdschrift Geneeskunde* 1996; 140: 255–259.

86 Penrice J, Cady EB, Lorek A *et al*. Proton magnetic resonance spectroscopy of the brain in normal preterm and term infants, and early changes after perinatal hypoxia-ischemia. *Pediatric Research* 1996; 40: 6–14.

87 Penrice J, Lorek A, Cady EB *et al*. Proton magnetic resonance spectroscopy of the brain during acute hypoxia-ischemia and delayed cerebral energy failure in the newborn piglet. *Pediatric Research* 1997; 41: 795–802.

88 Roth SC, Edwards AD, Cady EB *et al*. Relation between cerebral oxidative metabolism following birth asphyxia, and neurodevelopmental outcome and brain growth at one year. *Developmental Medicine & Child Neurology* 1992; 34: 285–295.

89 Taylor DL, Edwards AD, Mehmet H. Oxidative metabolism, apoptosis and perinatal brain injury. *Brain Pathology* 1999; 9: 93–117.

90 Amess PN, Penrice J, Cady EB *et al*. Mild hypothermia after severe transient hypoxia-ischemia reduces the delayed rise in cerebral lactate in the newborn piglet. *Pediatric Research* 1997; 41: 803–808.

91 van Cappellen AM, Heerschap A, Nijhuis JG, Oeseburg B, Jongsma HW. Hypoxia, the subsequent systemic metabolic acidosis, and their relationship with cerebral metabolite concentrations: an *in vivo* study in fetal lambs with proton magnetic resonance spectroscopy. *American Journal of Obstetrics & Gynecology* 1999; 181: 1537–1545.

92 Robertson NJ, Cox IJ, Cowan FM, Counsell SJ, Azzopardi D, Edwards AD. Cerebral intracellular lactic alkalosis persisting months after neonatal encephalopathy measured by magnetic resonance spectroscopy. *Pediatric Research* 1999; 46: 287–296.

93 Hanrahan JD, Cox IJ, Azzopardi D *et al*. Relation between proton magnetic resonance spectroscopy within 18 hours of birth asphyxia and neurodevelopment at 1 year of age. *Developmental Medicine & Child Neurology* 1999; 41: 76–82.

94 Constantinou JE, Gillis J, Ouvrier RA, Rahilly PM. Hypoxic-ischaemic encephalopathy after near miss sudden infant death syndrome. *Archives of Disease in Childhood (London)* 1989; 64: 703–708.

95 Ahn MO, Korst LM, Phelan JP, Martin GI. Does the onset of neonatal seizures correlate with the timing of fetal neurologic injury? *Clinical Pediatrics (Philadelphia)* 1998; 37: 673–676.

96 Mehmet H, Edwards AD. Hypoxia, ischaemia and apoptosis. *Archives of Disease in Childhood* 1996; 75: F73–F75.

97 Mehmet H, Yue X, Penrice J *et al*. Relation of impaired energy metabolism to apoptosis and necrosis following transient cerebral hypoxia-ischaemia. *Cell Death & Differentiation* 1998; 5: 321–329.

98 Yue X, Mehmet H, Penrice J *et al*. Apoptosis and necrosis in the newborn piglet brain following transient cerebral hypoxia-ischaemia. *Neuropathology & Applied Neurobiology* 1997; 23: 16–25.

99 Felderhoff-Mueser U, Taylor DL, Greenwood K *et al*. Fas/CD95/APO-1 can function as a death receptor for neuronal cells *in vitro* and *in vivo* and is upregulated following cerebral hypoxic-ischemic injury to the developing rat brain. *Brain Pathology* 2000; 10: 17–29.

100 Sarnat HB, Sarnat MS. Neonatal encephalopathy following fetal distress: a clinical and encephalographic study. *Archives of Disease in Childhood (London)* 1976; 33: 696–705.

101 Levene MI, Grindulis H, Sands C, Moore J. Comparison of two methods of predicting outcome in perinatal asphyxia. *Lancet* 1986; 67–69.

102 Robertson CM, Finer NN. Term infants with hypoxic-ischaemic encephalopathy: outcome at 3.5 years. *Developmental Medicine & Child Neurology* 1985; 27: 473–484.

103 Hill A. Current concepts of hypoxic-ischemic cerebral injury in the term newborn. *Pediatric Neurology* 1991; 7: 317–325.

104 Funayama CA, Moura-Ribeiro MV, Goncalves AL. Hypoxic-ischemic encephalopathy in newborn infants. Acute period and outcome. *Arquivosde Neuropsiquiatria* 1997; 55: 771–779.

105 Rosenbloom L. Dyskinetic cerebral palsy and birth asphyxia. *Developmental Medicine & Child Neurology* 1994; 36: 285–289.

106 Pasternak JF, Gorey MT. The syndrome of acute near-total intrauterine asphyxia in the term infant. *Pediatric Neurology* 1998;18:391-8.

107 Bocking AD, Gagnon R, White SE, Homan J, Milne KM, Richardson BS. Circulatory responses to prolonged hypoxemia in fetal sheep. *American Journal of Obstetrics & Gynecology* 1988; 159: 1418–1424.

108 Roca Gonzalez AM, Lopez Santiveri A, de la Rosa de los Rios C, Rodriguez Miguelez JM, Figueras Aloy J, Jimenez Gonzalez R. Manifestaciones extraneurologicas de la enfermedad hipoxico-isquemica en el recien nacido. [Non-neurologic manifestations in hypoxic-ischemic disease in newborn infants.] *Anales Espanoles de Pediatria* 1992; 36: 201–203.

109 Wayenberg JL, Vermeylen D, Damis E. Definition of asphyxia neonatorum and incidence of neurologic and systemic complications in the full-term newborn. *Archives de Pediatrie*1998; 5: 1065–1071.

110 Miltenyi M, Pohlandt F, Boka G, Kun E. Tubular proteinuria after perinatal hypoxia. *Acta Paediatrica Scandanavica* 1981; 70: 399–403.

111 Karlowicz MG, Adelman RD. Nonoliguric and oliguric acute renal failure in asphyxiated term neonates. *Pediatrics & Nephrology* 1995; 9: 718–722.

112 Jayashree G, Dutta AK, Sarna MS, Saili A. Acute renal failure in asphyxiated newborns. *Indian Pediatrics* 1991; 28: 19–23.

113 Martin Ancel A, Garcia Alix A, Gaya F, Cabanas F, Burgueros M, Quero J. Multiple organ involvement in perinatal asphyxia. *Journal of Pediatrics* 1995; 127: 786–793.

114 Luciano R, Gallini F, Romagnoli C, Papacci P, Tortorolo G. Doppler evaluation of renal blood flow velocity as a predictive index of acute renal failure in perinatal asphyxia. *European Journal of Pediatrics* 1998; 157: 656–660.

115 Lopez DO, Rodriguez-Alarcon GJ, Oliveros PR, Martin VL, Linares UA, Cotero LA. Acute renal failure in perinatal asphyxia. *Anales Espanoles de Pediatria* 1983; 19: 475–480.

116 Perlman JM, Tack ED. Renal injury in the asphyxiated newborn infant: relationship to neurologic outcome. *Journal of Pediatrics* 1988; 113: 875–879.

117 Saili A, Sarna MS, Gathwala G, Kumari S, Dutta AK. Liver dysfunction in severe birth asphyxia. *Indian Pediatrics* 1990; 27: 1291–1294.

118 Phelan JP, Ahn MO, Korst L, Martin GI, Wang YM. Intrapartum fetal asphyxial brain injury with absent multiorgan system dysfunction. *Journal of Maternal Fetal Medicine* 1998; 7: 19–22.

119 Lamblin MD, André M, Challamel MJ *et al*. Electroencephalography of the premature and term newborn. Maturational aspects and glossary. *Neurophysiologie Clinique* 1999; 29: 123–129.

120 Mizrahi EM, Kellaway P. Characterization and classification of neonatal seizures. *Neurology* 1987; 37: 1837–1844.

121 Boylan GB, Pressler RM, Rennie JM *et al*. Outcome of electroclinical, electrographic, and clinical seizures in the newborn infant. *Developmental Medicine & Child Neurology* 1999; 41: 819–825.

122 al Naqeeb N, Edwards AD, Cowan FM, Azzopardi D. Assessment of neonatal encephalopathy by amplitude-integrated electroencephalography. *Pediatrics* 1999; 103: 1263–1271.

123 Azzopardi D, Guarino I, Brayshaw C *et al*. Prediction of neurological outcome after birth asphyxia from early continuous two-channel electroencephalography. *Early Human Development* 1999; 55: 113–123.

124 Gire C, Nicaise C, Roussel M *et al*. Hypoxic–ischemic encephalopathy in the full-term newborn. Contribution of electroencephalography and MRI or computed tomography to its prognostic evaluation. Apropos of 26 cases. *Neurophysiologie Clinique* 2000; 30: 97–107.

125 Holmes G, Rowe J, Hafford J, Schmidt R, Testa M, Zimmerman A. Prognostic value of the electroencephalogram in neonatal asphyxia. *Electroencephalography & Clinical Neurophysiology* 1982; 53: 60–72.

126 Sinclair DB, Campbell M, Byrne P, Prasertsom W, Robertson CM. EEG and long-term outcome of term infants with neonatal hypoxic-ischemic encephalopathy. *Clinical Neurophysiology* 1999; 110: 655–659.

127 Toet MC, Hellstrom-Westas L, Groenendaal F, Eken P, De Vries LS. Amplitude integrated EEG 3 and 6 hours after birth in full term neonates with hypoxic-ischaemic encephalopathy. *Archives of Disease in Childhood (Fetal Neonatal Edition)* 1999; 81: F19–F23.

128 Biagioni E, Bartalena L, Boldrini A, Pieri R, Cioni G. Constantly discontinuous EEG patterns in full-term neonates with hypoxic-ischaemic encephalopathy. *Clinical Neurophysiology* 1999; 110: 1510–1515.

129 Peden CJ, Cowan FM, Bryant DJ *et al*. Proton MR spectroscopy of the brain in infants. *Journal of Computer-Assisted Tomography* 1990; 14: 886–894.

130 Hanrahan JD, Sargentoni J, Azzopardi D *et al*. Cerebral metabolism within 18 hours of birth asphyxia: a proton magnetic resonance spectroscopy study. *Pediatrics Research* 1996; 39: 584–590.

131 Cowan F. Outcome after intrapartum asphyxia in term infants. *Seminars Neonatology* 2000; 5: 127–140.

132 Rutherford MA, Pennock JM, Schwieso JE, Cowan FM, Dubowitz LM. Hypoxic ischaemic encephalopathy: early magnetic resonance imaging findings and their evolution. *Neuropediatrics* 1995; 26: 183–191.

133 Rutherford MA, Pennock JM, Counsell SJ *et al*. Abnormal magnetic resonance signal in the internal capsule predicts poor neurodevelopmental outcome in infants with hypoxic-ischemic encephalopathy. *Pediatrics* 1998; 102: 323–328.

134 Oatridge A, Hajnal JV, Cowan FM, Baudouin CJ, Young IR, Bydder GM. MRI diffusion-weighted imaging of the brain: contributions to image contrast from CSF signal reduction, use of a long echo time and diffusion effects. *Clinical Radiology* 1993; 47: 82–90.

135 Cowan FM, Pennock JM, Hanrahan JD, Manji KP, Edwards AD. Early detection of cerebral infarction and hypoxic ischemic encephalopathy in neonates using diffusion-weighted magnetic resonance imaging. *Neuropediatrics* 1994; 25: 172–175.

136 Mercuri E, Guzzetta A, Haataja L *et al*. Neonatal neurological examination in infants with hypoxic ischaemic encephalopathy: correlation with MRI findings. *Neuropediatrics* 1999; 30: 83–89.

137 Mercuri E, Cowan F, Rutherford M, Acolet D, Pennock J, Dubowitz L. Ischaemic and haemorrhagic brain lesions in newborns with seizures and normal Apgar scores. *Archives of Disease in Childhood (Fetal Neonatal Edition)* 1995; 73: F67–F74.

138 de Haan HH, Gunn AJ, Gluckman PD. Experiments in perinatal brain injury: what have we learnt? *Perinatal & Neonatal Medicine* 1996; 1: 16–25.

139 Dobbing J, Sands J. Comparative aspects of the brain growth spurt. *Early Human Development* 1979; 3: 79–83.

140 Painter MJ. Animal models of perinatal asphyxia: contributions, contradictions, clinical relevance. *Seminars in Pediatric Neurology* 1995; 2: 37–56.

141 Boyle R. New pneumatical experiments about respiration. *Philosophical Transactions of the Royal Society of London* 1670; 62: 2011–2031.

142 LeGallois. *Experiments on the Principle of Life.* Philadelphia: 1813.

143 Bert P. *Lecons sur la Comparee de la Respiration.* Paris, 1870.

144 Fazekas JF, Alexander FAD, Himwich HE. Tolerance of the newborn to anoxia. *American Journal of Physiology* 1940; 134: 281–298.

145 Stafford A, Weatherall JAC. The survival of young rats in nitrogen. *Journal of Physiology* 1960; 153: 457–472.

146 Krageloh-Mann I, Petersen D, Hagberg G, Vollmer B, Hagberg B, Michaelis R. Bilateral spastic cerebral palsy — MRI pathology and origin. Analysis from a representative series of 56 cases. *Developmental Medicine & Child Neurology* 1995; 37: 379–397.

147 Pharoah PO, Cooke T, Johnson MA, King R, Mutch L. Epidemiology of cerebral palsy in England and Scotland, 1984–9. *Archives of Disease in Childhood (Fetal Neonatal Edition)* 1998; 79: F21–F25.

148 Wood NS, Marlow N, Costeloe K, Gibson AT, Wilkinson AR, for the EPIcure study group. Neurologic and developmental disability after extremely preterm birth. *New England Journal of Medicine* 2000; 343: 378–384.

149 de Vries LS, Rennie JM. Preterm brain injury. In: JM Rennie, NRC Roberton (eds.) *Textbook of Neonatology.* Edinburgh: Churchill Livingstone, 1999: 1252–1271.

150 Barkovich AJ, Westmark K, Partridge C, Sola A, Ferriero DM. Perinatal asphyxia: MR findings in the first 10 days. *American Journal of Neuroradiology* 1995; 16: 427–438.

151 Badawi N, Kurinczuk JJ, Keogh JM et al. Intrapartum risk factors for newborn encephalopathy: the Western Australian case-control study. *BMJ* 1998; 317: 1554–1558.

152 Badawi N, Kurinczuk JJ, Keogh JM et al. Antepartum risk factors for newborn encephalopathy: the Western Australian case-control study. *BMJ* 1998; 317: 1549–1553.

153 Ellis M, Manandhar N, Manandhar DS, Costello AM. Risk factors for neonatal encephalopathy in Kathmandu, Nepal, a developing country: unmatched case-control study. *BMJ* 2000; 320: 1229–1236.

154 Gaffney G, Squier MV, Johnson A., Flavell V, Sellers S. Clinical associations of prenatal ischaemic white matter injury. *Archives of Disease in Childhood* 1994; 70: F101–F106.

155 Dobson PC, Abell DA, Beisher NA. Mortality and morbidity of fetal growth retardation. *Australian & New Zealand Journal of Obstetrics & Gynecology* 1981; 21: 69–72.

156 Kjellmer I, Thordstein M, Wennergren M. Cerebral function in the growth-retarded fetus and neonate. *Biology of the Neonate* 1992; 62: 265–270.

157 Williams K, Hennessy E, Alberman E. Cerebral palsy: effects of twinning, birthweight, and gestational age. *Archives of Disease in Childhood (Fetal Neonatal Edition)* 1996; 75: F178–F182.

158 Pharoah PO, Cooke T. Cerebral palsy and multiple births. *Archives of Disease in Childhood (Fetal Neonatal Edition)* 1996; 75: F174–F177.

159 Petterson B, Nelson KB, Watson L, Stanley F. Twins, triplets, and cerebral palsy in births in Western Australia in the 1980s. *BMJ* 1993; 307: 1239–1243.

160 Myers RE. Threshold values of oxygen deficiency leading to cardiovascular and brain pathological changes in term monkey fetuses. *Advances in Experimental Medical Biology* 1973; 37: 1047–1053.

161 Brann AW Jr, Myers RE. Central nervous system findings in the newborn monkey following severe *in utero* partial asphyxia. *Neurology* 1975; 25: 327–338.

162 Gunn AJ, Parer JT, Mallard EC, Williams CE, Gluckman PD. Cerebral histologic and electrocorticographic changes after asphyxia in fetal sheep. *Pediatrics Research* 1992; 31: 486–491.

163 Ball RH, Parer JT, Caldwell LE, Johnson J. Regional blood flow and metabolism in ovine fetuses during severe cord occlusion. *American Journal of Obstetrics & Gynecology* 1994; 171: 1549–1155.

164 Courten-Myers GM, Kleinholz M, Wagner KR, Myers RE. Fatal strokes in hyperglycemic cats. *Stroke* 1989; 20: 1707–1715.

165 Williams CE, Gunn A, Gluckman PD. Time course of intracellular edema and epileptiform activity following prenatal cerebral ischemia in sheep. *Stroke* 1991; 22: 516–521.

166 Hill A, Volpe JJ. Seizures, hypoxic-ischemic brain injury, and intraventricular hemorrhage in the newborn. *Annals of Neurology* 1981; 10: 109–121.

167 Williams CE, Gunn AJ, Mallard C, Gluckman PD. Outcome after ischemia in the developing sheep brain: an electroencephalographic and histological study. *Annals of Neurology* 1992; 31: 14–21.

168 Rutherford M, Pennock J, Schwieso J, Cowan F, Dubowitz L. Hypoxic-ischaemic encephalopathy: early and late magnetic resonance imaging findings in relation to outcome. *Archives of Disease in Childhood (Fetal Neonatal Edition)* 1996; 75: F145–F151.

169 Myers RE. Two patterns of perinatal brain damage and their conditions of occurrence. *American Journal of Obstetrics & Gynecology* 1972; 112: 246–276.

170 Mallard EC, Waldvogel HJ, Williams CE, Faull RL, Gluckman PD. Repeated asphyxia causes loss of striatal projection neurons in the fetal sheep brain. *Neuroscience* 1995; 65: 827–836.

171 Chugani HT, Phelps ME, Mazziotta JC. Positron emission tomography study of human brain functional development. *Annals of Neurology* 1987; 22: 487–497.

172 Hasegawa M, Houdou S, Mito T, Takashima S, Asanuma K, Ohno T. Development of myelination in the human fetal and infant cerebrum: a myelin basic protein immunohistochemical study. *Brain Development* 1992; 14: 1–6.

173 Barkovich AJ. MR and CT evaluation of profound neonatal and infantile asphyxia. *American Journal of Neuroradiology* 1992; 13: 959–972.

174 Rutherford MA, Pennock JM, Murdoch-Eaton DM, Cowan FM, Dubowitz LM. Athetoid cerebral palsy with cysts in the putamen after hypoxic–ischaemic encephalopathy. *Archives of Disease in Childhood* 1992; 67: 846–850.

175 Rosen MG, Dickinson JC. The incidence of cerebral palsy. *American Journal of Obstetrics & Gynecology* 1992; 167: 417–423.

176 Robertson CM, Finer NN, Grace MG. School performance of survivors of neonatal encephalopathy associated with birth asphyxia at term. *Journal of Pediatrics* 1989; 114: 753–760.

177 Robertson CM, Finer NN. Long-term follow-up of term neonates with perinatal asphyxia. *Clinical Perinatology* 1993; 20: 483–500.

178 Shankaran S, Woldt E, Koepke T, Bedard MP, Nandyal R. Acute neonatal morbidity and long-term central nervous system sequelae of perinatal asphyxia in term infants. *Early Human Development* 1991; 25: 135–148.

179 Low JA, Galbraith RS, Muir DW, Killen HL, Pater EA, Karchmar EJ. Motor and cognitive deficits after intrapartum asphyxia in the mature fetus. *American Journal of Obstetrics & Gynecology* 1988; 158: 356–361.

180 Mercuri E, Atkinson J, Braddick O et al. Visual function and perinatal focal cerebral infarction. *Archives of Disease in Childhood (Fetal Neonatal Edition)* 1996; 75: F76–F81.

181 Gaffney G, Flavell V, Johnson A, Squier M, Sellers S. Cerebral palsy and neonatal encephalopathy. *Archives of Disease in Childhood (Fetal Neonatal Edition)* 1994; 70: F195–F200.

182 Sarnat HB, Sarnat MS. Neonatal encephalopathy following fetal distress. A clinical and electroencephalographic study. *Archives of Neurology* 1976; 33: 696–705.

183 Robertson CM. Long-term follow-up of term infants with perinatal asphyxia. In: DK Stevenson, P Sunshine (eds.) *Fetal and Neonatal Brain Injury.* Oxford: Oxford University Press, 1997: 613–630.

184 Peliowski A, Finer NN. Birth asphyxia in the term infant. In: JC Sinclair, MB Bracken (eds.) *Effective Care of the Newborn Infant.* Oxford: Oxford University Press, 1992: 249–280.

185 Rivkin MJ, Volpe JJ. Hypoxic-ischemic brain injury in the newborn. *Seminars in Neurology* 1993; 13: 30–39.

186 Rutherford MA, Pennock JM, Counsell SJ et al. Abnormal magnetic resonance signal in the internal capsule predicts poor neurodevelopmental outcome in infants with hypoxic–ischemic encephalopathy. *Pediatrics* 1998; 102: 323–328.

187 Barkovich AJ, Hajnal BL, Vigneron D et al. Prediction of neuromotor outcome in perinatal asphyxia: evaluation of MR scoring systems. *American Journal of Neuroradiology* 1998; 19: 143–149.

188 Lou HC, Lassen NA, Friis-Hansen B. Impaired autoregulation of cerebral blood flow in the distressed newborn infant. *Journal of Pediatrics* 1979; 94: 118–121.

189 Boylan GB, Young K, Panerai RB, Rennie JM, Evans DH. Dynamic cerebral autoregulation in sick newborn infants. *Pediatric Research* 2000; 48: 12–17.

190 de Haan HH, Van Reempts JL, Vles JS, de Haan J, Hasaart TH. Effects of asphyxia on the fetal lamb brain. *American Journal of Obstetrics & Gynecology* 1993; 169: 1493–1501.

191 Amiel-Tison C, Stewart A. Follow up studies during the first five years of life: a pervasive assessment of neurological function. *Archives in Disease of Childhood* 1989; 64: 496–502.

192 Saint Hilaire MH, Burke RE, Bressman SB, Brin MF, Fahn S. Delayed-onset dystonia due to perinatal or early childhood asphyxia. *Neurology* 1991; 41: 216–222.

193 Rosenbloom L. Dyskinetic cerebral palsy and birth asphyxia. *Developmental Medicine & Child Neurology* 1994; 36: 285–289.

194 Brun A, Kyllerman M. Clinical, pathogenetic and neuropathological correlates in dystonic cerebral palsy. *European Journal of Paediatrics* 1979; 131: 93–104.

195 Carpenter MB. Athetosis and the basal ganglia. *Archives of Neurology & Psychology* 1977; 63: 875–901.

196   Westmark KD, Barkovich AJ, Sola A, Ferriero D, Partridge JC. Patterns and implications of MR contrast enhancement in perinatal asphyxia: a preliminary report. *American Journal of Neuroradiology* 1995; 16: 685–692.

197   Cowan F. Outcome after intrapartum asphyxia in term infants. *Seminars in Neonatology* 2000; 5: 127–140.

198   Robertson RL, Ben Sira L, Barnes PD *et al*. MR line-scan diffusion-weighted imaging of term neonates with perinatal brain ischemia. *American Journal of Neuroradiology* 1999; 20: 1658–1670.

199   West CR, Adi Y, Pharoah PO. Fetal and infant death in mono- and dizygotic twins in England and Wales 1982-91. *Archives of Disease in Childhood (Fetal Neonatal Edition)* 1999; 80: F217–F220.

200   Cilley RE, Zwischenberger JB, Andrews AF, Bowerman RA, Roloff DW, Bartlett RH. Intracranial hemorrhage during extracorporeal membrane oxygenation in neonates. *Pediatrics* 1986; 78: 699–704.

201   Levene MI. Intracranial haemorrhage at term. In: JM Rennie, NRC Roberton (eds.) *Textbook of Neonatology*. Edinburgh: Churchill Livingstone, 1999: 1223–1231.

202   Heier LA, Carpanzano CR, Mast J, Brill PW, Winchester P, Deck MD. Maternal cocaine abuse: the spectrum of radiologic abnormalities in the neonatal CNS. *American Journal of Neuroradiology* 1991; 12: 951–956.

203   de Vries LS, Levene MI. Cerebral ischaemic lesions. In: MI Levene, RJ Lilford (eds.) *Fetal and Neonatal Neurology and Neurosurgery*. Edinburgh: Churchill Livingstone, 1995: 367–386.

204   Fujimoto S, Yokochi K, Togari H *et al*. Neonatal cerebral infarction: symptoms, CT findings and prognosis. *Brain Development* 1992; 14: 48–52.

205   O'Brien MJ, Ash JM, Gilday DL. Radionuclide brain-scanning in perinatal hypoxia/ischaemia. *Developmental Medicine & Child Neurology* 1979;21:161-73.

206   Govaert P, Matthys E, Zecic A, Roelens F, Oostra A, Vanzieleghem B. Perinatal cortical infarction within middle cerebral artery trunks. *Archives of Disease in Childhood (Fetal Neonatal Edition)* 2000; 82: F59–F63.

207   Voorhies TM, Ehrlich ME, Frayer W, Lee BC, Vannucci RC. Occlusive vascular disease in perinatal cerebral hypoxia-ischemia. *American Journal of Perinatology* 1983; 1: 1–5.

208   Fitzhardinge PM, Flodmark O, Fitz CR, Ashby S. The prognostic value of computed tomography as an adjunct to assessment of the term infant with postasphyxial encephalopathy. *Journal of Pediatrics* 1981; 99: 777–781.

209   Mercuri E, Cowan F, Rutherford M, Acolet D, Pennock J, Dubowitz L. Ischaemic and haemorrhagic brain lesions in newborns with seizures and normal Apgar scores. *Archives of Disease in Childhood (Fetal Neonatal Edition)* 1995; 73: F67–F74.

210   Mercuri E, Rutherford M, Cowan F *et al*. Early prognostic indicators of outcome in infants with neonatal cerebral infarction: a clinical, electroencephalogram, and magnetic resonance imaging study. *Pediatrics* 1999; 103: 39–46.

211   Brown JK, Lin JP, Minns RA. Disorders of movement: cerebral palsy. In Campbell AGM, McIntosh N (eds.) *Forfar and Arneil's Textbook of Pediatrics*. Edinburgh: Churchill Livingstone, 1998: 738–762.

212   Evans DJ, Levene MI. Hypoxic-ischaemic injury. In: JM Rennie, NRC Roberton (eds.) *Textbook of Neonatology*. Edinburgh: Churchill Livingstone, 1999: 1231–1251.

213   Cooke RW. Cerebral palsy in very low birthweight infants. *Archives of Disease in Childhood* 1990; 65: 201–206.

214   Robertson CM, Etches PC, Goldson E, Kyle JM. Eight-year school performance, neurodevelopmental, and growth outcome of neonates with bronchopulmonary dysplasia: a comparative study. *Pediatrics* 1992; 89: 365–372.

215   Robertson CM, Finer NN. Educational readiness of survivors of neonatal encephalopathy associated with birth asphyxia at term. *Journal of Developmental and Behavioural Pediatrics* 1988; 9: 298–306.

216   Rosenbaum JL, Almli CR, Yundt KD, Altman DI, Powers WJ. Higher neonatal cerebral blood flow correlates with worse childhood neurologic outcome. *Neurology* 1997; 49: 1035–1041.

217   Roth SC, Baudin J, Cady E *et al*. Relation of deranged neonatal cerebral oxidative metabolism with neurodevelopmental outcome and head circumference at 4 years. *Developmental Medicine & Child Neurology* 1997; 39: 718–725.

218   Tandon A, Ramji S, Kumari S, Goyal A, Chandra D, Nigam VR. Cognitive abilities of asphyxiated survivors beyond 5 years of age. *Indian Pediatrics* 1998; 35: 605–612.

219   Hagberg B. Pre- and perinatal environmental origin in mild mental retardation. *Upsala Journal of Medical Science* 1987; 44: 178–182.

220   Rosenbloom L. Perinatal asphyxial injury: clinical sequelae. *Clinical Risk* 1996; 2: 43–46.

Part IV
Gynaecology

15

Gynaecological Surgery and Oncology

Pat Soutter

Part 1. Gynaecological surgery

Introduction

This chapter will discuss what can go wrong during gynaecological surgery, why complications occur, how to reduce the risk, and how to deal with the problems that arise. Complications associated with endoscopy, surgical sterilization, abortion and urogynaecology are all dealt with elsewhere. This chapter will consider open laparotomy and major vaginal surgery.

Not only are the depths of the female pelvis a considerable distance from the abdominal wound through which the gynaecological surgeon operates but it is also one of the more congested parts of the human body, where the urinary tract, the intestinal tract and the genital tract all jostle together to reach the outside world. Each brings its own luxuriant blood supply to which are added the large vessels that supply the legs and the buttocks. Hard against the pelvic sidewall, seldom seen by most gynaecologists, are the lumbo-sacral nerves and their many branches. Running alongside the structural supports of the pelvis is the autonomic nerve supply to bowel and bladder. A veritable minefield for the unwary or the unfortunate. As if this were not enough, the pelvic veins are both bereft of valves to prevent back flow from the huge vena cava and are notorious for their anatomical inconsistency. Add to this the distortion of disease or previous surgery and the stage is set for challenging surgery where even the most careful and experienced may encounter desperate situations.

Pre-operative preparation

Explanation and consent

It is fundamental that the patient should have as clear an understanding as possible about the procedure she is about to undergo so that she may give her consent in the full knowledge of what the risks may be. No surgeon wants to frighten his patient unduly – especially if surgery is unavoidable and the serious risks are rare. One view is that the patient with cancer has more than enough to worry about without being given a detailed account of all the possible complications. Telling her all about what might go wrong puts the surgeon 'in the clear' but increases to almost intolerable levels the patient's fear. On the other hand, most patients are aware that operations can go wrong and find it helpful to have a discussion about the potential hazards that puts these into perspective. It is useful to talk about the following: the problems that are likely to arise; the complications that might happen; and those that are unlikely. Ideally, each discussion should be documented, although some conversations take place when the notes are not available. The main purpose of the documentation is to ensure that other members of the team know what has already been discussed.

If consent is conditional, the terms of these conditions need to be written down to avoid future misunderstandings. The surgeon also must make clear what will *not* be done at this procedure – even if it seems obvious that a second laparotomy will be required. The exception to this is when the surgery is urgent and lifesaving. Resection of damaged bowel should obviously be undertaken but anterior resection for diverticulosis should not. Removal of malignant ovaries might be correct practice if the surgeon involved is qualified to do so but removal without consent of ovaries apparently affected by endometriosis would not.

Identify factors that alter risk

Previous pelvic surgery can turn a routine operation into a nightmare. A careful history of surgical intervention will alert the gynaecologist to possible problems. The bladder may be firmly adherent to the uterus after a Caesarean section and loops of bowel may be fastened firmly in the pelvis after an appendicectomy.

Medical problems will all require careful assessment and consultation with the relevant medical specialist. This is not the place for a litany of the disorders that can impinge upon the safety of pelvic surgery, but some examples may serve to illustrate the importance of this point. Diabetic women seldom have problems if their glucose control is good and kept within acceptable levels after the operation but wound infection and poor healing will result if control is inadequate. Rarely, the highly fatal necrotizing fasciitis may supervene with terrifying suddenness.[1] Patients with Systemic Lupus Erythematosus may have a severe vasculitis that makes them more prone to haemorrhage and impairs wound healing. Their immunosuppressive treatment will make them more susceptible to infection. Neurological assessment of the patient with multiple sclerosis or assessment of joint mobility in the patient with rheumatoid arthritis is of particular importance if leg stirrups are to be employed. Whatever the medical problem, complications may be avoided most readily by close collaboration with the physicians who normally look after her.

Obesity is an increasingly common risk factor. This not only makes the operation technically more difficult but increases the risk of postoperative respiratory insufficiency and of thromboembolic disease. Pelvic haematoma, wound infection and dehiscence are all more common in the obese patient.

Many patients are taking drugs that impair their fitness for surgery. The most commonest of these is tobacco. This will affect the patient's lungs and substantially increase the risk of postoperative chest infection, which will impair mobility and heighten the risk of thromboembolic disease. Coughing will add to the risk of wound disruption. Corticosteroids such as prednisolone make infection and poor wound healing more likely. Women taking the oral contraceptive pill or hormone replacement therapy have a slightly greater risk of thromboembolic disease but there is no need to ask them to stop these unless there is some other risk factor.[2]

Prepare the patient for surgery

Thromboembolic disease is one of the main causes of death after major surgery.[3] This is particularly true for women undergoing surgery for cancer, partly because these women often have an increased tendency to thrombosis, partly because the surgery is more prolonged and partly because the tumour may compress the pelvic veins, causing an undetected preoperative clot. This clot can detach when the tumour is removed and migrate to the lung, causing a pulmonary embolism. These risks can be mitigated substantially by the correct use of anti-embolism stockings and low-dose heparin.[4] If the patient has a relatively recent thrombus in the leg or pelvic veins, a filter may be placed in the inferior vena cava percutaneously via the neck veins before the operation. If it is judged safe to do so, some of these filters can be removed a few days later before they have become embedded in the vein walls.

Prophylactic antibiotics remain relatively controversial prior to routine abdominal hysterectomy but are probably beneficial in vaginal hysterectomy and in complex abdominal hysterectomy.[5] In most cases, a single dose of antibiotics is as effective as multiple-dose regimens.

Bowel preparation is not strictly necessary for most gynaecological surgery but a disposable enema or suppositories the night before surgery will ensure that the rectum is empty and does not limit access to the pelvis. The women will also be more comfortable in the first couple of days after her operation.

Pre-operative physiotherapy is very valuable for patients with respiratory problems. It ensures that their chest is as clear as possible before the operation and teaches them the exercises they will need to perform after surgery. In the same vein, smokers should always be advised to stop smoking and the overweight encouraged to lose weight. Unfortunately, this advice usually falls on deaf ears.

Intra-operative management

The route

The provisional decision whether to use an abdominal or a vaginal approach for hysterectomy should be made before theatre but the final assessment of suitability for vaginal hysterectomy is performed under anaesthesia. Each surgeon has personal criteria for attempting vaginal hysterectomy that are based upon training and experience. While some advocate the vaginal removal of large fibroid uteri, most gynaecologists adopt a more cautious approach. Some also describe the removal of the ovaries with or without the Fallopian tubes by a vaginal approach but this requires both special training and instruments. In the event of difficulty, the surgeon should not hesitate to change to an abdominal approach.

The incision

The choice and placing of the incision is important in order to provide adequate access. However, vertical wounds heal less well than transverse incisions and are more likely to dehisce or herniate. A vertical wound that extends into the upper abdomen will interfere with respiration after the operation. Even in operations for malignant disease, a transverse incision is usually preferable unless access to the abdomen above the pelvic brim is required. My colleagues and I very rarely use a vertical incision when performing a radical hysterectomy for cervical cancer and generally limit its use to women with ovarian cancer or other large masses that could not be removed through a transverse incision.

Ideally, the incision should not be placed in a skin crease that will become a moist sulcus when the patient is sitting up. In benign surgery, it is usual to place the incision about 4 cm cephalad of the symphysis pubis. When more access is required, it is helpful to move the incision a further 2–4 cm cephalad so that the aperture in the abdominal wall becomes more diamond-shaped than triangular. To increase the aperture still further, the rectus muscles may be dislocated from their insertion on the pubic rami. In women with a massive pendulous apron of fat, care is required in the siting of the incision. No attempt should be made to pull the apron back because that is tiring for the assistants and the surgeon and ensures that the incision is placed in moist skin beneath the apron where healing will be slow. Instead, the apron should be left to hang naturally and a transverse incision made through the apron into the abdomen. Care is required to ensure that the incision is placed sufficiently cephalad and directed vertically downward to arrive in the abdominal cavity at an appropriate position. It is usually best to view the patient from the side on the theatre table after she has been anaesthetized and to identify the site of the incision with an indelible marker pen before preparing the skin and positioning the drapes.

Vascular damage

Haemorrhage is the complication that every surgeon fears most. It may result from damage to a large vessel but is often due to bleeding from many small vessels. Reducing the risk of haemorrhage begins with careful, gentle packing of the bowel out of the pelvis. The bowel must be kept out of the pelvis as much as possible but the packs should not compress the inferior vena cava and obstruct the flow of blood out of the pelvis. Excessively tight packing results in distended pelvic veins and excessive venous bleeding. In the same way, a modest head down tilt lowers the venous pressure in the pelvis and reduces blood loss.

Bleeding may occur from the main uterine or ovarian vessels while they are being identified, clamped and ligated. This is especially likely when the anatomy is distorted by pathology or previous surgery. Careful identification of the anatomy and good surgical technique will reduce but not eliminate this risk. The proximity of the ureter to these vessels at the pelvic brim and lateral to the cervix is an added problem. Ligation of the descending vaginal branch of the uterine artery and the accompanying vein can be especially challenging. I use a figure-of-eight suture in the angle of the vagina to ensure that the heel of the pedicle that contains these vessels does not slip out of the ligature. If bleeding from these vessels occurs, it will usually be controlled temporarily with pressure while appropriate instruments and ligatures are readied. The swab can then be removed gradually, exposing more of the field bit by bit until the bleeding point is revealed. Suction may be needed to keep the operative field clear.

The location of the ureter must be determined by palpation or inspection before attending to the bleeding vessel. It is usually best to stop the bleeding by grasping the vessel gently with fine, long-handled artery forceps or with the diathermy dissecting forceps. If the haemorrhage is arrested, the vessel may be permanently sealed with diathermy if it is small enough; alternatively, a ligature or suture will be required.

Damage to the large iliac vessels usually occurs only during surgery for cancer when lymph nodes or tumour are being removed from the surface of the vessels. However, deeply infiltrating endometriosis may become adherent to the internal iliac vessels and any retroperitoneal tumour or postoperative adhesions may distort the anatomy so that the iliac vessels are exposed to trauma. In most cases, tears in the common and external iliac veins can be repaired by suturing with fine vicryl. Damage to the arteries is usually less of a problem because the muscular vessel wall constricts and contains the haemorrhage. Local pressure, sometimes supplemented by sutures, usually gives a very satisfactory result. The real danger comes from damage to the internal iliac veins and their branches, the superior gluteal vein or large ragged tears removing parts of the wall of the external or common iliac veins. The deeply placed veins retract into the muscles on the pelvic sidewall where they become relatively inaccessible. Deeply placed mattress sutures are required to control the haemorrhage. Unfortunately, such sutures may involve one of the large pelvic nerves. This will only become apparent after the operation when the patient wakes up. It may prove impossible to control bleeding from these veins completely. Opinion is divided on the value of ligation of the internal iliac artery in this setting. My own experience is disappointing. Firm packing may prove to be the only alternative.

More common than either of the two dramatic scenarios above but equally dangerous is a steady ooze from many small venules and arterioles. This usually follows an extensive dissection such as may be required to remove an endometrioma, or to mobilize an adherent bladder. This often happens at the end of a long operation during which there has been a slow but steady blood loss which, because it has not been particularly dramatic, has not been fully replaced. A consumptive coagulopathy results as the clotting factors are exhausted. The first step therefore is to hold a hot pack firmly on the bleeding area for 10 minutes. The second is to commence the prompt replacement of blood and clotting factors. When the pack is removed gently, all may be well or no more than two or three bleeders may persist. These may be controlled with judicious use of diathermy. If there is still significant generalized blood loss not obviously coming from a single significant vessel, a hot pack should be reinserted and kept firmly in place until the blood volume and clotting factors have been replaced adequately. This may take more than an hour during which there is much merit in the surgical team taking a break. If necessary, the abdomen may be closed with the packs in place. Antibiotics are given and the packs removed gently the following day.

Urinary tract

Damage to the ureters occurs most commonly close to the cervix. Occasionally, the ureter may be injured at the pelvic brim when the ovarian vessels are being ligated.

The ureters may be cut, crushed or ligated but devascularization in a pelvic haematoma is common. The ureter is damaged most often when the surgeon is trying to control haemorrhage or when postoperative bleeding occurs. The injury usually becomes apparent after the operation, either when a uretero-vaginal fistula develops and the patient begins to leak urine constantly or when she complains of loin pain.

Damage to the bladder that is recognized during the operation is easily repaired in two layers. The bladder is drained by catheter for five to seven days to allow the repair to heal. Injury that goes unrecognized may result in a vesico-vaginal fistula – a hole that connects the bladder and the vagina. This results in constant leakage of urine. If the bladder had been damaged directly during the operation, the fistula becomes apparent soon after the operation. On the other hand if, as is more common, the fistula is due to the effects of a pelvic haematoma, it may not develop until several days after the operation.

The risks of urinary tract damage can be mitigated by good surgical technique. It is usually easy to identify the ovarian vessels and the ureter at the pelvic brim if the peritoneal incision through the round ligaments has been extended cranially. The ureter can be seen and felt attached to the underside of the peritoneum. The peritoneum between the vessels and the ureter is opened and enlarged gently, and the vessels clamped and ligated safely. The vesico-uterine fold of peritoneum should be divided carefully and the bladder lifted anteriorly to help define the plane between it and the uterus. When the correct plane has been entered, the bladder may be safely displaced caudally by gentle dissection with a single layer of a swab over one finger. This dissection should begin in the midline but must extend laterally to displace the bladder and lower ureter off the front of the cervix. This may provoke bleeding from the bladder pillars, which can be controlled with careful diathermy. If the bladder is adherent and resistant to this gentle manoeuvre, careful sharp dissection will be required to mobilize the bladder from the front of the cervix.

The ureter may be palpated between thumb and forefinger in the leaf of peritoneum just postero-lateral to the uterine cervix before the uterine clamps are applied. To avoid injury to the ureter in difficult cases, the uterine artery may be clamped, divided and ligated at the level of the internal os. A second, straight clamp is placed medial to this pedicle and as close to the uterus as possible but not attempting to include the vaginal angle. When this pedicle is divided and ligated, the ureter is displaced laterally and the angle of the vagina exposed safely. It is important to tie these ligatures close to the clamp rather than more laterally, where the ureter may become incorporated. Once the uterus has been removed safely, it is important to suture the vaginal vault with a technique that ensures good haemostasis to reduce the risk of vault haematoma. For the same reason, the anterior wall of the vagina and the base of the bladder should be inspected carefully before closing the abdomen. Some surgeons report excellent results with a vaginal 'T' tube drain on gentle suction.[6]

Intestinal tract

Injury to small bowel usually results from dissecting adhesions caused by previous surgery, infection, endometriosis or cancer. In most cases, provided the mesentery of the bowel is undamaged, small holes can be repaired in two layers, taking care not to narrow the lumen. More extensive damage will require assessment by a gastrointestinal surgeon. The rectum is more susceptible to damage during pelvic surgery because of its intimate relations with the vagina. When the Pouch of Douglas behind the uterus is obliterated by adhesions or endometriosis, the risk of damage increases exponentially. Damage to the rectum recognized during the operation will require careful repair in two layers. If the damage is anything more than a small hole, it is usually safer to cover the repair with a sigmoid colostomy. The advice of a colorectal surgeon is invaluable.

Neurological damage

Numbness of the abdominal skin following a transverse incision is very common indeed. It is due to the unavoidable division of the many small nerves supplying the area. This usually resolves over a period of one to two years. Occasionally, a retractor will compress the ileo-inguinal or genitofemoral nerves, giving numbness over the mons pubis and anterior vulva or the upper thigh and labium majus. Radical hysterectomy will almost invariably disrupt the nerve supply to both bladder and rectum. This results in varying degrees of bladder and bowel hypotonia and lack of sensation. Fortunately, these usually improve substantially in the first few weeks after the operation and continue to do so for up to two years.

When dealing with intra-operative complications of any sort, the surgeon should not hesitate to ask for the help of another experienced colleague. Not only is such a person likely to be a much better assistant during a difficult operation but he or she will provide both practical and moral support at a time of very considerable stress.

Vaginal surgery

The problem of access that is such a feature of pelvic surgery is nowhere more acute than in vaginal surgery. However, reduced morbidity and more rapid recovery make the vaginal approach the route of choice whenever possible.

The more difficult the operation, the greater the potential for complications. The uterus must be mobile. While hysterectomy can be achieved without significant uterine descent, most surgeons would prefer to be able to reach the uterosacral ligaments comfortably before undertaking a vaginal hysterectomy. Similarly, most would not attempt to remove a uterus greater than the size of a 12-week pregnancy.

As with abdominal hysterectomy, it is important to identify the plane between the bladder and the cervix and to mobilize gently and displace the bladder thoroughly so that it and the ureters are moved out of harm's way. This is particularly important and often more difficult when the uterus has prolapsed completely through the vaginal entrance – a complete procidentia. If a hole is made in the bladder, it is repaired in two layers. Because this hole is more likely to be in the base of the bladder, care is needed not to damage or kink the ureter. The vascular pedicles need to be clamped and ligated with especial care because the vessels will retract into the pelvis if they slip out and can be very difficult to retrieve. Some surgeons put a second ligature around the pedicles and tie the uterosacral and the tubovarian pedicles together at the end of the operation, sometimes also incorporating the vaginal vault in this ligature. The aim of this is to reduce the risk of subsequent prolapse of the bowel into the vagina. The risk is of damage to the pedicles and of fixing the ovaries close to the vaginal vault, where they may cause dyspareunia. There is no advantage in closing the peritoneum because it provides no support and will cover the defect in 48 hours. During a posterior repair, the rectum may be entered inadvertently. Provided that a satisfactory two-layer repair can be achieved, it is not usually necessary to cover this with a colostomy because the repair is retroperitoneal and will discharge through the vagina – and not into the peritoneal cavity – if it breaks down. After suturing together the levator muscles, a digital rectal examination should be performed to ensure that the sutures have not entered the rectum.

Postoperative management

Thromboembolic disease

Pulmonary embolism is the most feared of postoperative complications. It may present anywhere on a spectrum that extends from sudden death to mild chest pain and breathlessness. Indeed, it is quite likely that many remain undiagnosed and quite silent.

Prevention with the assiduous use of anti-embolism stockings, low-dose heparin, physiotherapy and early mobilization offer the best protection. Careful inspection of the legs for signs of deep venous thrombosis is good practice but probably of very little value in the prevention of pulmonary embolism. A high index of suspicion and prompt investigation of those with worrying signs or symptoms are essential. Ventilation perfusion scans can do no more than indicate the likelihood of embolism but a spiral CT (computed tomography scan) may be able to demonstrate thrombus in a pulmonary vessel. Prompt heparinization is probably safer than observation in cases of uncertainty.

Haemorrhage

Concealed postoperative haemorrhage is signalled first by a rising pulse rate and a reduction in urinary output. The hands and feet become cold due to constriction of the peripheral vessels in an attempt to maintain the blood pressure. Finally, when all the compensatory mechanisms have been exhausted, the blood pressure will fall. Hopefully, the warning signs will have been spotted before the fall in blood pressure becomes profound. Replacement of blood lost with blood substitutes and then blood products is essential. If the surgery has been confined to the pelvis, the most effective way of dealing with postoperative haemorrhage is angiography and embolization of the bleeding vessels. This usually avoids the need for further surgery. If angiography is not available, or other pathology is also suspected, a repeat laparotomy will be required.

Wound

Wound infection is one of the common postoperative complications. This is usually very mild and superficial but can be very serious. Necrotizing fasciitis has already been mentioned. Wound dehiscence is a complication confined almost exclusively to vertical incisions. This can be made less likely by closing the abdominal wall in one layer apart from the skin.

Infection

Urinary-tract infection and chest infection are the other common problems. The latter can be particularly serious, especially in those whose respiratory function is already compromised. A particular problem after both abdominal and vaginal hysterectomy is an infected vault haematoma. Vault haematomata are very common and usually asymptomatic. However, when the haematoma becomes infected it will give rise to pelvic pain and pyrexia. This is treated with antibiotics and the haematoma usually discharges into the vagina with what can be a very frightening gush of fresh and altered blood. Sometimes, if there is a large collection in the pelvis it is prudent to incise and drain this under general anaesthesia. The discharge usually settles down in a week or so with few sequelae. Some women do continue to have pelvic pain for many months while the inflammatory process resolves.

Fistula

Urinary and faecal fistulae into the vagina have been discussed above. Faecal fistulae may develop through the abdominal wound.

Later complications

Problems of micturition and defecation have already been mentioned. These are usually problems associated with radical hysterectomy but may also follow vaginal surgery for prolapse or urinary incontinence. There is some evidence to suggest that urinary incontinence is slightly more common in the years after abdominal surgery. Painful intercourse may follow any vaginal operation but is uncommon after an abdominal hysterectomy. If adhesions have formed after the operation, abdominal pain and even bowel obstruction may result, sometimes many years later. Among women who have undergone pelvic or groin node dissection, lymphoedema of the leg or mons pubis affects about 23%.[7] The degree of swelling is very variable and depends upon the extent of the dissection. The risk is increased very sharply if postoperative radiotherapy is administered.

Part 2. Gynaecological oncology

The management of women with gynaecological cancer has gradually evolved into a separate subspecialty. It is now widely recognized that women with any of these cancers should be treated by a dedicated multidisciplinary team, in a designated regional centre. The objective is to enable a rapid evaluation by all the relevant experts in a centre equipped to perform all the necessary investigations and able to offer the full range of treatment options. Unfortunately, it is also becoming an area in which medico-legal issues are appearing with ever-increasing frequency.

Pre-invasive disease

Cervical intra-epithelial neoplasia

Pre-invasive disease of the cervix is by far the commonest of pre-invasive conditions. Cervical cytology was first introduced to detect pre-invasive squamous cell lesions, now called cervical intra-epithelial neoplasia (CIN). The aim was to reduce the incidence of squamous-cell cancer of the cervix. It has been spectacularly successful in achieving that objective. However, unsurprisingly, it has been largely unsuccessful in affecting the incidence of adenocarcinoma of the cervix, which now represents 25% of all invasive cervical cancers – having previously been only 4% of the total.[8] This change is due to the massive reduction in the number of squamous-cell carcinomas, achieved through cytology screening.

Colposcopy and treatment of CIN

Women with abnormal smears, suspicious symptoms or a clinically suspicious cervix are referred for colposcopy. The cervix is inspected through an instrument like a pair of binoculars and a dilute solution of acetic acid is applied to the cervix. This turns areas of CIN white. Unfortunately, other benign and normal conditions also turn white, so the magnification provided by the colposcope is needed to attempt to distinguish between them. A biopsy is performed for confirmation. If the whole lesion is visible, a small biopsy may be taken with punch biopsy forceps but this can be misleading if an unrepresentative sample has been taken. A larger conization or cone biopsy may be taken by any one of several instruments. Conization is not only diagnostic but is also usually therapeutic. An alternative approach to lesions that are fully visible and which the colposcopist is confident are not invasive is to ablate the area of abnormality with diathermy, cryocautery, laser vaporization or 'cold' coagulation. This requires a diagnostic punch biopsy first. Treatment of CIN by these outpatient procedures is highly successful in good hands. The cumulative incidence of recurrent CIN is 10% by 10 years and of invasive cancer is only 0.58% by eight years.[9]

One of the problem areas is failing to recognize invasion and treating with ablation or an inadequate, superficial, fragmented conization. It is important not to use ablative treatment if there is any risk of invasion. This includes women with what seem to be large, severe CIN III lesions. If the whole of the lesion is visible on the ectocervix, the conization must be at least 7 mm long to include lesions that extend into deep cervical glands. My own experience has led me to aim for 10 mm.

The biggest problems in colposcopy relate to those women in whom the squamocolumnar junction lies in the canal. It is all too easy to underestimate the extent to which a lesion involves the endocervical canal and if the whole lesion cannot be seen clearly, invasion cannot be excluded. Even if the ultimate intention is to treat the woman with hysterectomy, a diagnostic cone biopsy is mandatory to exclude invasive cancer. If a prior cone biopsy shows CIN II–III extending to the upper, endocervical margins, residual invasive disease has not been excluded. A second cone biopsy may be a prudent investigation before hysterectomy. If there are good reasons for not doing this, they must be documented clearly and the potential risk discussed with the patient.

Conization may rarely result in torrential haemorrhage for which an emergency hysterectomy is required. This is more likely if the cervix has been treated before. Stenosis of the cervix is not uncommon following conization but it is very uncommon for it to give rise to problems with menstruation or subsequent pregnancy. The opposite extreme of cervical incompetence leading to premature delivery is even more uncommon and is only seen after a very long biopsy of the cervix which removes a large amount of tissue.[10]

Vulval intra-epithelial neoplasia

Vulval intra-epithelial neoplasia (VIN) is very much less common than CIN, the risk of progression to invasion is less well documented and the treatment is both less effective and more mutilating.[11]

Most women with VIN present with itching or soreness of the vulva but only a small minority of women with these symptoms have VIN. It can usually be recognized by naked-eye inspection if the observer is experienced but is best seen under low magnification and good illumination. Many people use the colposcope for this purpose. Dilute acetic acid will help to delineate areas of VIN but the colour changes take far longer to develop on the vulva than on the cervix or vagina.

The diagnosis may be confirmed by small, punch biopsies but these are more likely to be unrepresentative than cervical biopsies because of the larger size and multifocal nature of most VIN. There are essentially two schools of thought about the management of VIN. One school advocates early excision biopsy of *all* visible lesions – sometimes preceded by multiple 'mapping' punch biopsies. In women with large, widespread lesions, this may necessitate superficial vulvectomy. The argument for this is that the future risk of invasive disease will be reduced. The other school adopts a conservative approach, excising lesions only if they are causing symptoms that cannot be controlled by topical steroids or if invasive disease is suspected. The reasoning behind this approach is that some of these lesions will regress, and that excision is followed by a very high rate of recurrence and can be mutilating.

Endometrial hyperplasia

There is much confusion about the terminology used and the risk of malignancy associated with endometrial hyperplasia.[12] Cystic hyperplasia is found commonly in postmenopausal women, is not premalignant and requires no further treatment or follow-up. Atypical hyperplasia contains glands that show nuclear atypia and may coexist with endometrial cancer in 20–50% of cases. Progression to invasion may occur in up to 89%. Hysterectomy and bilateral salpingo-oophorectomy is recommended for these women. Those who hope for further children may be treated with progestins but they then require long-term follow-up. The prospects for fertility may well remain poor and the recurrence rate is high. Complex or adenomatous hyperplasia is often found in association with atypical hyperplasia, in which case it should be treated in the same way as an atypical lesion. When adenomatous hyperplasia occurs without atypia, the risk of malignancy is probably low, and further management can be based upon subsequent symptoms.

Cervical cancer

Cervical cancer is increasingly often diagnosed by cervical screening. Such women have a better prognosis than those who present to their doctor with symptoms. Postcoital bleeding is the classical symptom associated with cervical cancer, but this is a common complaint and only 4% will have a malignancy.[13] In most cases, these tumours are clinically obvious to gynaecologists at least, although it would probably be unreasonable to expect a general practitioner to recognize cervical cancer. Intermenstrual bleeding and heavy periods may also be due to cervical cancer but these are even more common complaints and are very rarely caused by cancer. The same may be said of abdominal pain or backache which, when associated with cervical cancer, usually reflect very advanced disease with a poor prognosis.

The investigation of a woman with cervical cancer should include a biopsy confirming the diagnosis, an examination under anaesthesia to assess the size and location of the tumour clinically, a chest X-ray or CT of the chest to identify pulmonary metastases, and an intravenous urogram (or some similar imaging investigation of the urinary tract). We tend to rely upon an abdominal CT scan performed to identify enlarged para-aortic nodes. CT imaging in the pelvis is unreliable for the most part. Magnetic resonance imaging (MRI) is undoubtedly the investigation of choice when looking at the size of the tumour and identifying enlarged pelvic lymph nodes. However, the interpretation of these images requires a radiologist with experience of cervical cancer. The quality of MRI images of the cervix is improved beyond all recognition by the use of an endovaginal receiver coil.[14]

Younger women have most to gain from radical surgery for early tumours. For the remainder, concurrent chemoradiotherapy has become the treatment of choice.[15] The complications associated with radical hysterectomy have been described above. Clearly, all of these complications are more likely in association with radical surgery.

Endometrial cancer

Endometrial cancer is most common after the menopause and most women present with postmenopausal or perimenopausal bleeding. However, in younger women, it may cause irregular or heavy periods. There is no effective screening test for endometrial cancer. Transvaginal ultrasound, so useful in the triage of symptomatic women with postmenopausal bleeding, is unhelpful in asymptomatic women because of the very high false-positive rate.

Investigation includes confirmation of the diagnosis by biopsy or review of previous biopsies, and chest X-ray to identify pulmonary metastases. Examination under anaesthesia is helpful to identify vaginal metastases and the rare case with infiltration into the parametria. It may also identify adnexal spread but that is usually recognized on ultrasound. Hysteroscopy is used to identify spread to the cervix. Concerns that this may result in dissemination of the tumour are misplaced. MRI can be used to identify those with deep invasion of the myometrium and to recognize enlarged pelvic lymph nodes.

The standard treatment of endometrial cancer is a 'simple' total abdominal hysterectomy and bilateral salpingo-oophorectomy. There is no benefit from radical excision of the parametria or upper vagina. The role of lymphadenectomy is controversial. If the tumour invades deeply into the myometrium or if the histology is high grade, pelvic radiotherapy is usually offered. However, recent data from a controlled trial in Holland[16] suggests that it is equally effective to wait and treat only those who develop a recurrence.

Ovarian cancer

There are two main varieties of ovarian cancer. Epithelial ovarian cancer is the commoner variety, is found predominantly in older women and carries a high mortality. The non-epithelial group is relatively rare and found mainly in children and young women. On the whole, these are very sensitive to chemotherapy and have a good prognosis.

Epithelial ovarian cancer usually presents at an advanced stage with widespread disease throughout the abdomen. This is probably because is grows silently in the pelvis and does not cause symptoms until it is already very large. However, there is some evidence that at least some ovarian cancers grow very quickly. The symptoms most often associated with ovarian cancer are abdominal pain, discomfort and distension. These are very non-specific and could be due to any one of a myriad of other conditions. There is considerable interest in developing a screening strategy for ovarian cancer but no effective method has emerged as yet. Ultrasound and testing for the tumour marker CA125 in blood samples both give high false-positive rates, leading to unnecessary operations.[17] Pre-operative confirmation of the diagnosis is not possible. A chest X-ray is taken to identify lung metastases. If there is concern about the possibility of colorectal cancer, endoscopy or a barium enema may be appropriate.

The surgical treatment of ovarian cancer involves a total abdominal hysterectomy and bilateral salpingo-oophorectomy with removal of the oementum and any other foci of resectable tumour. The aim, of course, is to remove all of the tumour if possible. This is followed by chemotherapy with platinum- and taxane-based chemotherapy. Radiotherapy has little to offer.

Vulval cancer

Vulval cancer is largely a disease of older women. Most present with sympto-matic ulcers.

Investigation consists of a biopsy to confirm the diagnosis, chest X-ray to identify pulmonary metastases, careful palpation of the groins to detect enlarged lymph nodes and examination under anaesthesia to identify urethral or rectal involvement. Ultrasound of the groin combined with cytological examination of fine needle aspirates of suspicious nodes may assist in identifying groin node disease preoperatively but cannot exclude metastatic disease.

The treatment is surgical. Radical removal of the primary tumour is combined with groin node dissection through separate incisions unless the nodes are obviously clinically enlarged. If the tumour is situated on one side away from the midline, dissection of the opposite groin may be omitted unless the ipsilateral groin contains metastatic disease. Postoperative pelvic radiotherapy is given if more than two lymph nodes are involved with tumour. In some cases, pre-operative radiotherapy may be given to the vulva to shrink the tumour before surgery.

The effects of delays in diagnosis and treatment

Delays in instituting treatment are endemic in the NHS due to lack of resources. Not only is this distressing for patients and their relatives but also the deleterious effect of delay upon prognosis is becoming more widely appreciated. Not infrequently, delays in treatment result in operable tumours becoming inoperable. Squamous-cell tumours double in volume every seven weeks on average,[18] so a cervical cancer 2.5 cm in diameter would double in volume from 8.2 cm^3 to 16.4 cm^3 in only seven weeks and, in the process, would have crossed the threshold into a group with a poorer prognosis. This knowledge must spur us all on to shorten the gap between diagnosis and treatment as far as remains consistent with appropriate assessment and treatment. Better to wait a week than to offer suboptimal treatment but better still to see referred patients promptly, complete the investigations efficiently and be able to offer appropriate treatment within 20 working days of the first appointment.

Conclusion

As in every field of medicine, there is in gynaecology the opportunity for great good or great harm. The more difficult the task attempted, the greater the risk involved. In closing, I can do no better than to quote the words of Professor Chris Hudson to those who offer professional opinions on medico-legal matters – that 'maloccurrence is not *ipso facto* malpractice'.

References

1   Addison WA, Livengood CH, Hill GB, Sutton GP, Fortier KJ. Necrotising faciitis of vulvar origin in diabetic patients. *Obstetrics and Gynecology* 1984; 63: 473–479.
2   Royal College of Obstetricians and Gynaecologists. *Report of the Working Party on Prophylaxis Against Thromboembolism in Obstetrics and Gynaecology.* London, 1995.
3   National Confidential Enquiry into Perioperative Deaths (NCEPOD). *The Report of the National Confidential Enquiry into Perioperative Deaths 1991/2.* London, 1993.
4   Thromboembolic Risk Factors (THRIFT) Consensus Group. Risk of and prophylaxis for venous thromboembolism in hospital patients. *BMJ* 1992; 305: 567–574.
5   Mittendorf R, Aronson MP, Berry RE. Avoiding serious infections associated with abdominal hysterectomy: a meta-analysis of antibiotic prophylaxis. *American Journal of Obstetrics and Gynecology* 1993; 169: 1119–1124.

6   Swartz WH, Tanaree P. T-tube suction drainage and/or prophylactic antibiotics: a randomised study of 451 hysterectomies. *Obstetrics and Gynecology* 1976; 47: 665–670.

7   Grimshaw RN, Murdoch JB, Monaghan JM. Radical vulvectomy and bilateral inguino-femoral lymphadenectomy through separate incisions – experience with 100 cases. *International Journal of Gynaecological Cancer* 1993; 3: 18–23.

8   Bergstrom R, Sparen P, Adami H-O. Trends in cancer of the cervix uteri in Sweden following cytology screening. *British Journal of Cancer* 1999; 81: 159–166.

9   Soutter WP, de Barros Lopes A, Fletcher A, Monaghan JM, Duncan ID, Kitchener HC. Invasive cervical cancer after conservative therapy for cervical intraepithelial neoplasia. *Lancet* 1997; 349: 978–980.

10   Raio L, Ghezzi F, di Naro E, Gomez R, Luscher KP. Duration of pregnancy after carbon dioxide laser conisation of the cervix: influence of cone height. *American Journal of Obstetrics and Gynecology* 1997; 90: 978–982.

11   Acheson N, Ganesan R, Chan KK. Premalignant vulvar disorders. *Current Obstetrics and Gynaecology* 2000; 10: 12–17.

12   Soutter WP. Premalignant disease of the lower genital tract. In: R Shaw, WP Soutter, S Stanton (eds.) *Gynaecology*, 2nd edn. London: Churchill Livingstone, 1997: 521–540.

13   Rosenthal AN, Panoskaltsis T, Smith T, Soutter WP. The frequency of significant pathology in women attending a general gynaecological service who complain of post-coital bleeding. *British Journal of Obstetrics and Gynaecology* 2001; 108: 103–106.

14   deSouza NM, McIndoe GAJ, Soutter WP, Krausz T, Chui M, Hughes C, Mason WP. Value of magnetic resonance imaging with an endovaginal receiver coil in the preoperative assessment of stage I and IIa cervical neoplasia. *British Journal of Obstetrics and Gynaecology* 1998; 105: 500–507.

15   Monaghan JM. Time to add chemotherapy to radiotherapy for cervical cancer. *Lancet* 1999; 353: 1288–1289.

16   Creutzberg CL, van Putten WLJ, Koper PCM *et al.* Surgery and postoperative radiotherapy versus surgery alone for patients with stage-7 endometrial carcinoma: multicentre randomised trial. *Lancet* 2000; 355: 1404.

17   Urban N. Screening for ovarian cancer – time for a randomised trial. *BMJ* 1999; 319: 1317–1318.

18   Steel GG. *Growth Kinetics of Tumours*. Oxford: Clarendon Press, 1977.

▶16

Endoscopy

Peter C Buchan

Introduction

Over the past 20 years, the diagnostic and therapeutic applications of laparoscopic and hysteroscopic surgical techniques have increased dramatically. Consumer enthusiasm for these techniques, fuelled by the media, led to a considerable pressure on consultants in both NHS and private practice to be able to perform these new techniques. Initially, many of the new procedures were attempted with minimal training and the results – in terms of both excessive morbidity and mortality – were impressive.

Until the early 1990s, there were very few British training centres where laboratory simulation and hands-on clinical teaching and training could be given, although there were centres in mainland Europe and the United States. By the mid-1990s, a number of British gynaecological endoscopy units were offering training, and in 1994 the Royal College of Obstetricians and Gynaecologists produced the report of the Working Party on training in gynaecological endoscopic surgery; its implementation document[1] highlighted the need for structured training prior to unsupervised clinical practice.

The 1990s have seen a realistic appraisal of many endoscopic techniques, and endometrial ablation has not replaced hysterectomy, nor has laparoscopically assisted hysterectomy replaced the abdominal and vaginal procedures.

The turbulent introduction of endoscopic techniques in the early 1990s has been replaced by a more tranquil environment – where training, case selection and an increased awareness of the potential dangers of endoscopic surgery give a considerably greater degree of confidence in the application of these techniques, which are now becoming an established and high-quality part of gynaecological practice.

Patient expectations need to be informed not by the tabloid newspapers. Instead, information should be imparted principally in question-and-answer sessions with a medical adviser who is aware of the techniques, the advantages, disadvantages and complication rates, backed up by written information. This allows the patient time to reconsider the matter away from the often amnesiac tension of a hospital consulting room. GPs also need to be informed of the indications for and complication rates of endoscopic procedures in the hands of their local hospital colleagues. Transparency and honesty have to be built into the counselling environment. The General Medical Council document *Changing Times, Changing Culture*[2] states, 'People want doctors who are up to date and skilful who will treat them with kindness and consideration and respect their views. They want doctors they can trust.' This is also the wish of the vast majority of the medical profession. When it comes to endoscopic surgery, being up to date and skilful is of paramount importance before unsupervised clinical practice is offered.

Patient's consent for surgical training

Special consent is required when a patient is admitted to a centre of excellence in the expectation of being dealt with by an experienced and skilful surgeon and may have her operation conducted by a visiting trainee surgeon who may have little, if any, practical experience of clinical endoscopic surgery. Frequently, patients are exceedingly generous in their agreement to allow their surgical procedure to be used in a teaching or training exercise; but their consent for this should be sought and assurance given that the appropriately skilled trainer will – at all times – remain in overall control of and in attendance at their operation.

Stratification of endoscopic procedures by levels of training

In recognition of the need for endoscopic surgery to be stratified by level of difficulty and for the training requirements to be defined, the Royal College of Obstetricians and Gynaecologists Working Party in gynaecological endoscopic surgery published its implementation report.[1]

This document divided laparoscopic procedures into four levels:

▶ Level one covers diagnostic laparoscopy.

▶ Level two includes minor laparoscopic procedures, such as sterilization, linear salpingostomy and/or salpingectomy for ectopic pregnancy and diathermy of early (revised AFS [American Fertility Society] stage one) endometriosis.

▶ Level three includes more extensive procedures requiring additional training such as laser/diathermy to more advanced (revised AFS stages two and three) endometriosis, laparoscopic uterosacral nerve ablation, salpingo-oophorectomy, adhesiolysis of moderate bowel adhesions and laparoscopically assisted vaginal/subtotal hysterectomy (without significant associated pathology).

▶ Level four requires subspecialist or advanced/tertiary level endoscopic skills, including laparoscopic hysterectomy with associated pathology, total hysterectomy, myomectomy, pelvic lymphadenectomy, pre-sacral neurectomy, laparoscopic surgery for advanced (revised AFS stage three and four) endometriosis and laparoscopic incontinence and suspension procedures.

Hysteroscopic procedures were divided into three levels:

▶ Level one: simple procedures such as diagnostic hysteroscopy and removal of polyps and intra-uterine contraceptive devices.

▶ Level two: minor operative procedures such as removal of pedunculated fibroids and large polyps and division of adhesions in minor Asherman's syndrome.

▶ Level three: more complex operative procedures requiring additional training, including division/resection of uterine septum, endometrial resection or ablation, resection of submucous fibroids and endoscopic surgery for major degrees of Asherman's syndrome.

This document gave a structure to the levels of training and expertise that gynaecologists should demonstrate before being accredited, in either the NHS or private practice. These documents carry the power of 'recommendations' only – there is no binding requirement. However, there is real pressure from the general public, Government and the litigation departments of NHS Trusts and private hospitals for a more regulated system of accreditation for and audit of surgical training and competence. These recommendations should serve to improve the quality of care for patients and the quality of training for the next generation of endoscopic surgeons.

Hysteroscopic surgery

Hysteroscopic surgery has a wide and ever-increasing number of applications from diagnostic hysteroscopy through endometrial resection, myomectomy, tubal occlusion, to uterine reconstruction. Training courses are available throughout the UK in accredited centres of excellence where laboratory and theoretical instruction are complemented by hands-on clinical sessions under expert supervision.

Complications and competent responses

Uterine perforation and visceral damage

The most common occasion when perforation occurs is during the initial instrumentation of the cervix and uterine cavity. The position and size of the uterus must be ascertained by a careful examination before dilatation of the cervix. Failure to ascertain whether the uterus is anteverted or retroverted still remains a common cause of accidental and avoidable perforation (Figure 16.1). Gentle, slow dilatation of the cervix and insertion of the hysteroscope under video inspection of the cervical canal will help the operator to avoid perforation in the vast majority of cases. The uterus whose cavity is distorted by fibroids or is weakened by post-menopausal atrophy or endometrial cancer is the most likely to suffer perforation despite routine precautions.

When perforation occurs while using a dilator, 5 mm hysteroscope, curette or polyp forceps, the patient usually needs little more than explanation, the administration of antibiotics and observation for three to four hours for signs of continued bleeding or the development of infection. Explanation should include a description of the injury,

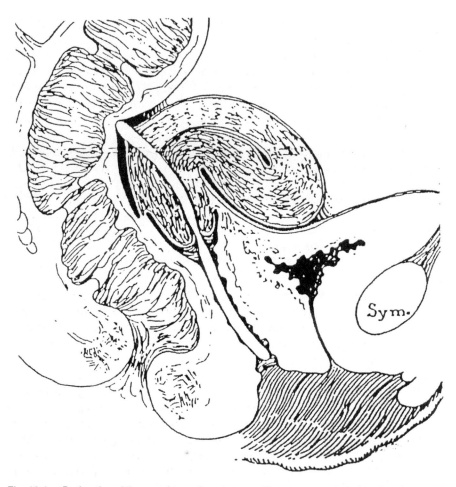

Fig. 16.1. Perforation of the acutely anteflexed uterus. The uterus was thought to be retroverted, and the dilator was erroneously directed posteriorly. Reproduced, with permission, from *Operative Gynaecology*, 6th edition. RF Mattingly and JD Thompson (eds.) Dilatation of the cervix and curettage of the uterus. Philadelphia: JB Lippincott Co., p. 502. Sym, symphysis pubis.

why it occurred, the possible complications, the associated signs and symptoms and the actions to be taken. Good communication with the GP is important.

If perforation occurs with a large-diameter instrument, if tissue has been grasped and avulsion has been attempted or if there is significant revealed bleeding, laparoscopy can be helpful in defining the extent of any injury and in dealing with bleeding from the uterine tear. During operative hysteroscopy, perforation should be suspected if there is a large deficit of distension media or if there is a sudden loss of vision due to collapse of the uterus and bleeding. If the perforation is made while using an activated resection loop or laser fibre, in almost all cases a laparotomy should be performed, as bowel injury may be very difficult – if not impossible – to exclude by laparoscopy. A laparotomy and oversewing a diathermy injury to the bowel will give the patient a nasty surprise if she has not been warned of this possibility in her pre-operative counselling and consenting. However, the trauma will be immensely less than if she is admitted with faecal peritonitis requiring colostomy and repeated surgery over several months to deal with a diathermy burn to the transverse colon.

Radiofrequency-induced endometrial ablation has been evaluated and with further technical refinements may have a place in the clinical management of menorrhagia. Considerable damage can be caused to adjacent viscera, vagina, bowel and bladder, unless these techniques are carefully controlled and vulnerable structures shielded. Despite some encouraging reports, this technique remains experimental and patients to whom this technique is offered should be made aware of the experimental nature and not-inconsiderable risks of this procedure.

Haemorrhage

This is not a common complication of hysteroscopic surgery but is recognized to occur after endometrial resection, particularly if the loop cuts deeply or repeatedly at the level of the internal os, where the large perforating branches of the uterine artery descend through the cervix to reach the upper vagina. Care should be taken, particularly when using the long single strip technique for endometrial resection, not to cut too deeply at this point. This is especially important in patients who have had a previous cone biopsy. Immediate postoperative haemorrhage is much less common after laser or roller-ball ablation. Hysteroscopic myomectomy has particular dangers of haemorrhage both early and late; pre-operative treatment with gonadotrophin releasing hormone (GnRH) agonists may reduce this risk. Primary postoperative haemorrhage is usually controlled with the use of a balloon catheter inserted in the uterine cavity and kept inflated for about four hours. Delayed haemorrhage is rare and most commonly associated with infection, treatment of which, along with balloon catheter tamponade, usually resolves the problem.

Uterine distension media problems

The dangers of CO_2 and air embolism are well recognized and easily avoided. Anaphylaxis as a result of exposure to high molecular weight dextran occurs in 0.01% of cases. Because of these risks, outpatient hysteroscopy should be carried out only where appropriate monitoring and resuscitation facilities are available.

Glycine is the commonest distension fluid used in operative hysteroscopy. The dangers of excess glycine absorption resulting in TURP (TransUrethral Resection of the Prostate) Syndrome or cardiorespiratory overload are well recognized and are generally avoidable with competent fluid balance accounting and diuretic therapy.

Use of normal saline solution as a distension fluid does not carry the risks of the TURP Syndrome, but the risks of overload are still present. Saline cannot be used for electrosurgical procedures, however, and its use is restricted to diagnostic and laser procedures.

Laparoscopic surgery

I do not intend to deal with standard laparoscopic techniques – these are dealt with extensively in textbooks such as *Textbook of Laparoscopy*.[3] Rather, I will seek to discuss issues of particular medico-legal interest.

Appropriateness of laparoscopic versus open route for surgery

Hysterectomy

The considerable morbidity associated with the learning curve in the introduction of laparoscopically assisted hysterectomy is emphasized by Garry.[4] He quotes a Finish series[5] in which 1165 cases produced 14 vascular complications (1.2%) 17 bladder lesions (1.5%), 15 ureteric lesions (1.2%) and 5 electrosurgical burns of the bowel (0.4%). A study into the incidence of ureteric complications following different hysterectomy techniques[6] reported an overall incidence of ureteric damage after hysterectomy of 0.1%, but following abdominal hysterectomy it was 0.04%, after vaginal hysterectomy, 0.02% but after laparoscopic hysterectomy, 1.39%. Many publications attest to the extreme rarity of ureteric damage following abdominal and vaginal hysterectomy and to the continuing higher incidence following laparoscopic hysterectomy. This is attributed frequently to learning-curve problems. But as both vaginal and abdominal hysterectomy have a learning curve for the trainee, the most reasonable conclusion is that laparoscopic hysterectomy is more difficult, has less margin for error and is particularly vulnerable to technical inadequacy on behalf of the operator or his equipment. Unless the problems of 'learning curve morbidity' can be overcome by laboratory training and before clinical practice, I seriously question the need for and safety of laparoscopically assisted vaginal hysterectomy. In the hands of a small number of experienced surgeons, it may be safe but any perceived advantages of the technique are far outweighed by the very real increase in risk of serious complications. A complication rate higher than that of traditional vaginal or abdominal hysterectomy would surely make this procedure medically, as well as medico-legally, inadvisable.

Tubal ectopic pregnancy

In most medico-legal cases involving ectopic pregnancy, the alleged breach of duty relates to delay in diagnosis. If standard clinical guidelines (concerning listening to the patient's history, undertaking and recognizing the significance of a physical examination of the patient and arranging the appropriate tests [eg human chorionic gonadotrophin, ultrasound and laparoscopy] and responding appropriately to the results) were followed, most of these cases would not arise.

The next most common cause of complaint relates to the use of laparotomy instead of laparoscopy in the treatment of the ectopic pregnancy, once diagnosed.

A postal survey of 1420 practising British consultant gynaecologists[7] showed that hysteroscopic surgery was available in only 43% of the respondent's hospitals and hysteroscopic surgery was performed routinely for ectopic pregnancy in only 13%. The conclusion drawn by these investigators was that 'Laparoscopic surgery for ectopic pregnancy is still not available to the majority of British women. The development of training programmes in the technique is a priority'. Even if it *were* available, there is little evidence to show that tubal conservation by salpingotomy or methotrexate injection confers any future reproductive advantage when compared with salpingectomy – either laparoscopic or open. In patients who have previously lost the other Fallopian tube there is advantage in conserving the tube with the ectopic, but one in five of these women will have a subsequent repeat ectopic. The principal advantage of endoscopic management is in the shorter duration of hospitalization, the more rapid return to work and the reduced risk of post-surgical adhesions.

There are two clinical circumstances in which open surgical treatment is preferable; the first is in the presence of haemodynamically compromising haemorrhage and the second where there is complex associated pathology, usually with chronic pelvic inflammatory disease.

Endoscopic management of ectopic pregnancy is, in the majority of cases, in the patient's best interest, but it is not yet available generally. That lack of availability is a sad reflection on the availability of training and the junior-doctor-based service offered by the threadbare British National Health Service.

Complications of laparoscopic surgery

Surgical risk assessment

The risk to the patient with previous laparotomy or history of peritonitis is due to their raised incidence of intra-abdominal adhesions, with the omentum or bowel being adherent to the scarred peritoneum. The obese patient is at risk because of difficulty in assessing the distance of travel of the trocar for entry into the peritoneum and the inability to transilluminate the abdominal wall for subsequent portal entry. The very thin generally have a short travel distance between the anterior abdominal wall and the abdominal viscera and the major blood vessels and also may have low resistance in their anterior-wall tissues, tending to allow over-travel of the Veress needle or trocar at insertion.

While these risk factors do not preclude laparoscopy, there is need for careful pre-operative counselling, with a written record of the points covered in the discussion with the patient, and particularly careful attention to the safety procedures aimed at reducing visceral and vascular injury should be followed and noted.

Abdominal entry injuries

This is when almost 50% of laparoscopic injuries occur – injury to the bowel or to the large retroperitoneal blood vessels being the most serious.

In the majority of cases in UK gynaecological practice, the Veress needle and initial trocar are inserted 'blindly' through the traditional subumbilical point. The standard techniques and siting for Veress needle and trocar insertion are well described in standard texts on operative laparoscopy,[3] as are the safety measures to avoid the dangers of bowel and vascular injury. Volume 8[6] of *Gynaecological Endoscopy* (1999)[8] was dedicated to questions of technique and safety at laparoscopic entry and gives a comprehensive review of the world literature on the complications and a detailed discussion of the appropriate safety measures.

A review of 357,257 laparoscopies using the closed technique showed entry-related bowel complications in 103 (0.03%) and 69 (0.02%) of blood vessel injury and using the open laparoscopic entry technique, the incidence of bowel injury was 0.04% and there were no vessel injuries. Open entry therefore eliminates vascular injury but still permits bowel damage when there are bowel adhesions present.

Currently, there is a robust debate about the safest method of laparoscopic entry. The Royal College of Surgeons of England's formal basic surgical skills course states quite definitely that the 'open Hasson approach' should be preferred in all circumstances. Semm and Semm[8] conclude that 'Blind puncture should be proscribed in the next millennium'.

Nevertheless, it must be recognised that the majority of UK gynaecologists continue to use 'blind entry' techniques for both the Veress needle and the initial trocar. As vessel injuries and type 1 bowel injury are almost completely eliminated by 'open entry' techniques, if 'blind' techniques are still to be used then the well-recorded safety measures must be applied rigorously in each case. The guidelines for patient selection and the range of safety procedures required for 'closed entry' techniques are well described in the standard texts.[3,8] The conclusion drawn by the editor of *Gynaecological Endoscopy*[8] is that 'With good techniques and appropriate case selection, the risk of such complications occurring is less than 1 per 1000 laparoscopies'. This is still worse than the 0.4 per 1000 complication rate with 'open' entry techniques. Because of the increased safety of the open-entry technique in low-risk cases, bowel injury occurring during blind-entry laparoscopy and posterior vessel injury in all cases represent unacceptable practice because there is a safer alternative – open entry – available. Gynaecologists will need to learn this technique and use it in all cases if the rash of laparoscopic litigation is not to become confluent.

Electrosurgical injury

Where electrodiathermy is used, particular care must be taken with the choice of and use of equipment. A detailed description of the dangers and precautions associated with both monopolar and bipolar diathermy is beyond the scope of this text, but every surgeon who practises endoscopic surgery must be aware of the dangers of arcing and capacitance coupling, as well as the more obvious ways in which skin, bowel, ureter and bladder may be damaged by avoidable electrothermal insult. Theatre technical and nursing staff have to be competent with the equipment used in theatre, the positioning and supervision of electrode sites and the avoidance of hybridization of metal and plastic instruments.

The use of faulty electrosurgical equipment and the repeat use of single-use disposables is almost always indefensible. If diathermy has been used and a patient's postoperative recovery pattern is unusual, visceral electrodiathermy burn must be considered.

Competent response to vascular damage

Figures 16.2 and 16.3 show the relationship between the standard laparoscopy portal sites and the major blood vessels of the abdominal wall and cavity that are vulnerable to injury.

Injury to the inferior epigastric artery may only be identified once an additional portal trocar is removed. The laparoscope should be left in place and the removal of all additional portal trocars made under direct vision. Suturing under direct vision is required and if that is not possible then exploration of the puncture down from the skin may be required. With this type of bleeding it is important to leave the laparoscope in place until the artery has been sutured so that continuing internal bleeding can be excluded once the skin has been closed.

Injury to the aorta, vena cava or iliac vessels may occur if the trocar is advanced too far within the abdominal cavity. Such injuries should not occur; they are usually caused by failure to observe the standard insertion procedures, by inserting the needle

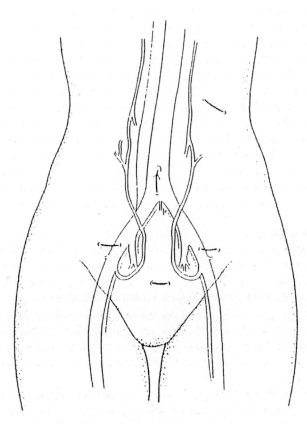

Fig 16.2. The relationship of the standard laparoscopy portal sites and the inferior epigastric arteries in the anterior abdominal wall and the major vessels of the abdominal cavity.

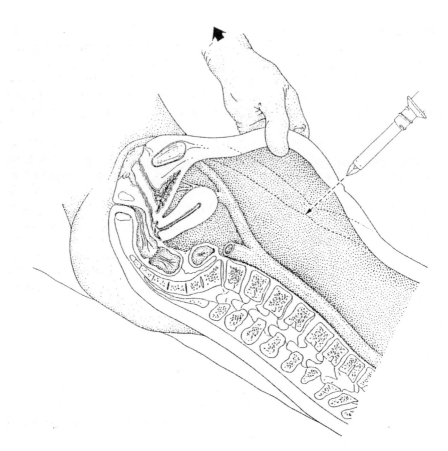

Fig. 16.3. The relationship between the trocar entry point and the abdominal viscera and vessels.

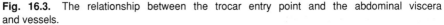

or trocar at the wrong angle or advancing it too far. Immediate midline laparotomy and vascular surgical assistance are required. These injuries will be avoided by the use of 'open' entry techniques.

Competent response to suspected bowel damage

'As endoscopic procedures are becoming more popular we are seeing an increasing number of severe and sometimes fatal complications arising from inadvertent damage to the gastro-intestinal tract.'[9] Bowel injury can be caused during any laparoscopic procedure and an awareness of this should be at the front of every endoscopic surgeon's mind.

The bowel may be damaged by the Veress needle, although a single needle puncture usually will not lead to any significant morbidity. Damage by the trocar may tear the bowel wall, allowing significant peritoneal contamination. It is important to note that small-bowel contents are bacteriologically sterile and initially there is a chemical peritonitis with pain, distension, continuing bowel sounds and no pyrexia. Bacterial peritonitis ensues after about 48 hours when the patient's condition rapidly deteriorates. Colonic damage will present much more rapidly with faecal peritonitis and severe systemic illness. Diathermy burns usually take a few days to perforate, and re-admission 48 hours after laparoscopic electrosurgery requires a high level of suspicion. Injury with scissors or a YAG or CO_2 laser give immediate signs and symptoms.

If bowel injury is suspected, an early laparotomy is likely to minimize morbidity, and delay is almost certain to maximize it. Any patient with persistent postoperative pain requires urgent investigation – laparotomy is an early diagnostic procedure. Persistent pain combined with abdominal distension continuing for more than 24 hours after laparoscopy almost always has a serious cause – vascular or visceral damage. The postoperative recovery after an extensive endometriosis dissection is different from that after a laparoscopic sterilization. For that reason, among others, those giving the aftercare to patients recovering from endoscopic surgery must be acquainted with the normal recovery patterns from the different procedures. Variation from normal recovery patterns requires experienced senior review or general surgical opinion at an early stage.

Post-complication risk management

There are several levels at which risk management is practised. At each level, the primary objective is to reduce the adverse consequences for the individual and to ensure a minimum repetition risk. It is also important to reduce the adverse effects on medical and nursing staff and on the hospital.

Post-accident counselling

When there is an adverse outcome, a full and honest account of why it happened and what is being done to put things right must be given to the patient and her relatives. Any attempt to avoid explanation will have adverse consequences for both patient and hospital. Clearly, if the patient has been counselled pre-operatively of the risks of a particular procedure so as to give consent, she will be likely to accept the explanation given when a recognized complication occurs. Post-accident counselling must be recorded thoroughly without apportioning blame. This is particularly important with endoscopic surgery, where short stay, minimal discomfort and effective outcomes are expected. The statement by the surgeon that he is sorry for the bad outcome is not an admission of liability but common courtesy.

Personal, surgical unit and national audit

In order to assess complication and success rates on an individual and unit level, it is necessary to keep an audit of all surgical procedures. This is of particular importance when new techniques are being developed. Repeated complications will be noted and the surgeons involved will have an early opportunity to revise their skills, techniques or equipment. Adverse-event reporting has to be seen as good practice and must be made non-threatening.

The same arguments apply to national audit. The Medical Research Council and the Royal Colleges have carried out valuable work improving standards for patients and surgeons by multicentre audit of new (and even old) surgical procedures. These have proved of considerable value in assessing the appropriate introduction of procedures such as hysteroscopic endometrial resection and ablation. It is of the first importance that surgical audit should be extended to cover both NHS and private hospital practice. The lack of peer review that may exist in the private sector might allow unsafe practice to go on and may even allow surgeons with inadequate training to carry out inappropriate procedures in the private sector. Health insurers, as well as NHS management, have a duty of care to audit the quality of surgical service.

Conclusions

Minimal-access surgery has become an established part of gynaecological practice in many but not all British Hospitals. Training of the coming generation of gynaecological specialists must include a thorough grounding in these techniques. For the next ten years, there will be units where endoscopic surgery is not offered widely because the consultants in post have not been trained. In many cases, they will be just too busy to take the time to learn. This is a problem for regional NHS managers to overcome, with cross-referral services being facilitated so that patients can receive the most appropriate treatment as near to home as possible.

The complications of both hysteroscopic and laparoscopic surgery are well recognized. Most can be avoided by careful adherence to safe-practice guidelines. Many of the complications are due to learning-curve inexperience, and training in recognized centres of excellence is required. This presents ethical problems for surgeons in the training centres, and the counselling and consenting of patients who are 'used' as training models needs to be handled with honesty.

Minimal-access surgery requires – for the patient – maximal access to information. With the expectations of effective treatment, relative lack of pain and rapid recovery, patients need to be made aware of the real risks and benefits of endoscopic surgery and of the consequences if and when things go wrong. Complication-free surgery is the desire of every patient and the aspiration of every surgeon, but reality has not yet got the message. In endoscopic surgery, the reality is that the margin of error is small, and unless meticulous attention is paid to training, technique and technology then accidents will continue to occur and only rigorous personal, hospital and national audit will be able to identify the extent of the problem. To wait until medico-legal pressure and bad publicity become the goads to action is bad for patients, surgeons and hospitals.

References

1   Royal College Of Obstetricians and Gynaecologists. *Implementation of the Recommendations of the Working Party on Training in Gynaecological Endoscopic Surgery.* London, December 1994.

2   General Medical Council. *Changing Times, Changing Culture*. London, June 2000.
3   Hulka JF, Reich H. Abdominal entry. In: *Textbook of Laparoscopy*. London: WB Saunders & Co., 1994: Chapter 8.
4   Garry R. Towards evidenced-based hysterectomy. *Gynaecological Endoscopy* 1998; 7: 225–233.
5   Harkki-Siren P, Sjoberg J, Tiitinen A. Urinary tract injuries after hysterectomy. *Obstetrics and Gynaecology* 1998; 92: 113–118.
6   Harkki-Siren P, Sjoberg J, Makinen J *et al*. Finnish national register of laparoscopic hysterectomies: a review and complications of 1165 operations. *American Journal of Obstetrics and Gynecology* 1997: 176: 118–122.
7   Saidi SA, Butler-Manuel SA and Powell MC. Use of laparoscopic surgery for the treatment of ectopic pregnancy in the UK: a national survey. *Gynaecological Endoscopy* 1999; 8: 81–84.
8   Multiple authors. *Gynaecological Endoscopy* 1999; 8: 315–403.
9   Garry R. The Achilles heel of minimal access surgery. *Gynaecological Endoscopy* 1994; 3: 201–202.

▶17 ;

Contraception and Sterilization

Peter Bowen-Simpkins and James Owen Drife

Introduction

Contraception and sterilization accounted for over one-third of all gynaecology claims notified to the Medical Defence Union in the early 1990s.[1] Most contraception claims concerned general practitioners, rather than gynaecologists or family planning doctors, and a limited review[2] has suggested that relatively more problems involve the intra-uterine contraceptive device (IUCD) than other forms of contraception. Up-to-date data are awaited from the NHS Litigation Authority (NHSLA).

Sterilization has become very popular in the UK over the past 30 years. Today, over 30% of women and 25% of men over the age of 35 have been sterilized. These procedures can fail (the failure rate of female sterilization is discussed later in this chapter), and with such a large number of people being sterilized it is not surprising, perhaps, that failure gives rise to a large number of medico-legal claims. Early claims based on breach of contract failed; but the doctor has a duty to carry out the operation correctly and if he/she does not, a claim will be successful.[3]

Failure is not the only reason for litigation. If complications occur with contraception or sterilization, the woman may allege that she was inadequately counselled, that inadequate notice was taken of contraindications or – in the case of contraceptive devices or sterilization operations – that the doctor lacked technical skill or training.

Most of the women who ask for advice on contraception or sterilization are healthy. This means that the question of balancing the effects of disease against the effect of treatment does not arise. The woman must be fully counselled about the risks and side effects of the method she is contemplating, but that is not to say that she must be confronted with an exhaustive list of rare problems. Common sense and clinical judgement are required when counselling women on this subject, as with others. The standard at present in English law is that of the responsible doctor, not that of the prudent patient. In other jurisdictions outside the British Isles, the prudent patient test is referred to as 'informed consent' but there is no such doctrine in English law. In other words, the doctor giving information so as to obtain consent is judged by the standard of his peers.

Oral contraception

The combined oral contraceptive pill

The combined oral contraceptive pill became available in the United States in June 1960 and one year later in the UK. It remains the most popular form of contraception in both countries, particularly for women under the age of 35 – a Royal College of General Practitioners study[4] showed that 95% of sexually active women in the UK under the age of 30 reported the use of oral contraceptives at some time in their life.

The pill must be prescribed by a doctor and comes under schedule IV of the Poisons Act 1972. Nevertheless, it is probably one of the safest forms of medication. The associated annual death rate, per 100,000 non-smoking women under the age of 35, is less than for home accidents or road-traffic accidents. Despite this, it still receives considerable media attention in terms of associated morbidity and mortality.

Allegations about oral contraception are likely to relate to inadequate advice about drug interactions or about the correct method of using the contraceptive, or to prescription of the wrong drug. Patient recall of instructions given prior to prescribing is frequently incomplete and therefore it is essential that the medical advisor uses information leaflets wherever possible and records precisely what advice was given.

It is essential that a careful medical history be taken so that a reasonable decision can be made as to the most appropriate form of contraception. There are a number of absolute and relative contraindications to the combined oral contraceptive. Most important of these are a personal history of venous or arterial thrombosis, severe or multiple risk factors for arterial disease, heart disease with pulmonary hypertension or risk of embolus, transient cerebral ischaemia and various forms of severe migraine. Other rarer contraindications specifically related to liver disease are all listed in the manufacturer's data sheet.

Relative contraindications to its use include:

▶ a family history of venous thromboembolism (VTE) in a first-degree relative or a family history of a thrombophilia such as Factor V Leiden;

▶ obesity (ie a body mass index of above 30 kg/m^2);

▶ long-term immobilization; and

▶ severe varicose veins.

Risk factors for arterial disease include the following factors, which should be considered as relative contraindications:

▶ A family history of arterial disease in a first-degree relative

▶ Diabetes mellitus

▶ Hypertension with a systolic above 140 mmHg and diastolic above 90 mmHg

▶ Smoking

▶ Age over 35 years

▶ Obesity

▶ History of migraine.

Where a practitioner has doubts about the safety of prescribing a combined oral contraceptive, help can be obtained readily from the medical department of a relevant pharmaceutical company or, if the doctor is a member or diplomat, from the Faculty of Family Planning and Reproductive Health Care of the Royal College of Obstetricians and Gynaecologists (RCOG).

Choice of preparation

The oestrogen content ranges from 20–50 μg and the progestogens vary from the so-called 'second-generation' progestogens, such as norethisterone, levonorgestrel and medroxyprogesterone acetate, to 'third-generation' progestogens such as desogestrel and gestodene. In general, the preparation with the lowest oestrogen and progestogen content that gives good cycle control and minimal side effects should be chosen.

The third-generation progestogens have been reported to have less adverse effects on lipids and are probably best suited for women who experience side effects such as acne, headache, depression or weight gain with other progestogens. However, women should be advised that third-generation progestogens have been associated with an increased risk of VTE.

The incidence of VTE in healthy non-pregnant women who are not taking an oral contraceptive is about five cases per 100,000 women per year. The mortality is about one in 1,000,000. The risk in pregnancy is 60 cases per 100,000 women. In 1995, the UK government publicised figures suggesting that the risk of VTE in those taking second-generation progestogens was approximately 15 per 100,000, whereas in those using third-generation progestogens, it was doubled to 30 per 100,000. This resulted in a massive change over from third- to second-generation progestogens. In the ensuing five years, there has not been the expected decrease in the incidence of VTE in pill users for multifactorial reasons associated with the original figures. Subsequently, the estimated risk has been revised to 25 per 100,000 women per year.[5]

It must be stressed to patients that the absolute risk remains very small and well below the risk associated with pregnancy. Provided that women are informed and accept the relative risk of VTE, the choice of oral contraceptive is for the woman, together with the prescriber, jointly to decide in the light of her individual medical history and any contra-indications.[6]

Drug interactions

The effectiveness of combined and progestogen-only contraceptives may be reduced considerably by interaction with drugs that induce hepatic enzyme activity. The anti-epileptic drugs (except sodium valproate) are the most commonly used enzyme-inducers, and patients must be advised that if they are taking anti-epileptic therapy then a preparation containing 50 μg ethinyloestradiol is necessary to provide full contraception.

The enzyme-inducers rifampicin and rifabutin are so potent that an alternative method of contraception is always recommended.

Broad-spectrum antibiotics may reduce the efficiency of the combined oral contraceptive pill by altering the bacterial flora of the gut, thus impairing the absorption of the pill.[7]

Similarly, diarrhoea and vomiting can interfere with the absorption of the pill and additional precautions should be used during gastrointestinal upsets and for seven days after recovery. All such points are indicated clearly in the manufacturer's instructions contained within the packets of the pill, but they should be discussed with the woman before the initial prescription so that she is fully aware of such interactions.

The risk of teratogenesis from the combined preparations is close to nil. Bracken found a risk ratio of 0.99 for all important malformations in a meta analysis of 12 prospective studies.[8]

Dianette® (Schering) is a combined oestrogen/anti-androgen preparation containing ethinyl oestradiol and cyproterone acetate. It should be considered primarily as a treatment for acne and hirsuitism although it acts as an effective contraceptive in the same way as other combined pills. Long-term use seems to be safe, although the makers do recommend tests of liver function every three years. If taken accidentally in pregnancy there is a risk of feminization of the male fetus.

Follow up

Check visits are usually carried out at three-monthly intervals for the first two visits and then six-monthly afterwards if all is normal. The two most important aspects are checks on the woman's weight and blood pressure. New risk factors such as the occurrence of migraine need to be looked for and the visit offers the opportunity to perform cervical cytology and breast examination if indicated.

Screening for thrombophilic tendencies, sugar levels and lipids need only be performed in an 'at risk' population.

Progestogen-only pills

These preparations offer a suitable alternative when oestrogens are contra-indicated (see above). However, they have a higher failure rate than the combined preparation and must be taken more accurately. The contraindications are considerably fewer than for the combined preparations. They include pregnancy, undiagnosed vaginal bleeding, severe arterial disease and various liver problems. The interactions with drugs and antibiotics are similar to those of the combined oral contraceptive pill.

The major problem with the progestogen-only pills (POPs) is that they lead to menstrual irregularities. The bleeding pattern may initially be chaotic but after a time may settle down to a regular cycle or, in up to 15% of users, amenorrhoea. A small number of women develop symptomatic functional ovarian cysts and women must be warned about these. Pregnancies that arise in POP users are more likely to be ectopic than pregnancies occurring in the general population, although the overall risk of pregnancy remains very low. Other side effects include nausea, vomiting, headaches, dizziness, breast discomfort, depression, skin disorders and weight change. All these factors must be discussed with the woman before commencing therapy.

The most important difference between the combined oral contraceptive pill and the POP is the accuracy with which the preparation must be taken. With the former, there is a 12-hour leeway, should a pill be missed, for efficacy to continue. With the POP, this is reduced to three hours, and if it is taken outside this time additional methods of contraception must be used for the next seven days.

Injectable steroid contraceptives

Injectable steroid contraceptives are used widely in developing countries and depomedroxyprogesterone acetate (DMPA) has been used widely in the UK since its licence was extended in 1984.

DMPA is given as a deep intra-muscular injection, usually into the gluteal muscles, every twelve weeks. The dose is 150 mg per injection. Its advantages are as follows:

▶ It is highly effective

▶ It has a long action following a single injection

▶ It is simple to administer

▶ There is a freedom from the fear of forgetting

▶ It is independent of coitus.

In addition, there is no suppression of lactation, there is minimal gastrointestinal disturbance and the continuation rate is high.

Amenorrhoea is a common side effect and this can be a major advantage in developing countries where iron-deficiency anaemia is a problem. Another advantage is that there is regular contact with health personnel because of the three-monthly duration of each injection.

The potential for toxicity of DMPA appears to extremely low in animal studies. Studies in the beagle bitch suggested an association between the use of high doses of DMPA and the development of breast lumps; however, after careful evaluation of these findings, it was concluded that the animal model was not appropriate for assessing the carcinogenic risks associated with the drug.[9]

A World Health Organization (WHO) collaborative study of neoplasia and steroid contraceptives concluded that DMPA does not increase the risk of endometrial, ovarian, liver, breast or cervical cancer.[10,11] There is no association with an increased risk of cardiovascular disease, changes in blood pressure or changes in blood coagulation. As it does not cross into breast milk, it can be used safely by lactating mothers.

A major disadvantage of DMPA is that once that it has been given, its effects are irreversible and will continue for some time. There is a high incidence of amenorrhoea with less than 30% of women experiencing even one normal cycle throughout treatment. The incidence of amenorrhoea increases with the duration of treatment. It is essential that a woman is told at the beginning of treatment that irregular and unpredictable bleeding or spotting are normal but usually decrease as treatment continues. In the event of excessive or prolonged bleeding, cyclical administration of oral oestrogen will usually solve the problem but this should not be used for more than one or two cycles.

Weight gain has been regularly observed in users and varies between 0.5 and 2 kg after one year's use. In a clinical trial evaluating the efficacy of DMPA in 3905 women, 46% reported side effects.[12] Headaches occurred in 17.5%, abdominal distension or discomfort in nearly 12% and nervousness in 11%. Mood changes, particularly depression, are reported and the drug should be avoided in women with a history of depression.

There are few contraindications to the use of the drug, but these include a sensitivity to medroxyprogesterone acetate, undiagnosed vaginal bleeding, undiagnosed breast pathology and pre-existing pregnancy. In the infrequent event of the drug being given and pregnancy developing, the woman will be concerned about possible teratogenicity. Certain progestogens have been associated with masculinization of the external genitalia of the female fetus but this has not been shown with DMPA at doses as high as 400 mg.

Prolonged use of DMPA usually induces amenorrhoea and this is associated with low levels of circulating oestrogens. This in turn may lead to a greater chance of developing osteoporosis but the effects of amenorrhoea on bone mass in the short-term seem to be reversible.[13] In general, and particularly for women over the age of 40, it is probably advisable that the drug be discontinued if she has persistently low oestrogen levels.

A major problem associated with DMPA is its long-term effect on fertility and the menstrual cycle. The average duration to conception after the last injection is nine months. Data from several investigations indicate that regular menstruation is re-established in about 50% of subjects by six months after the last injection, in 75% by one year and 85% by 18 months (compared with almost immediately after cessation of POPs and COCs). After two years, pregnancy rates are comparable to those among previous users of the oral contraceptive pills. There is some evidence to suggest that the longer the preparation is used, the slower the return of fertility, but this may relate to the age of the patient. The return of fertility is similar to the figures quoted above for menses.

Deficiencies in counselling appear to be the main area of contention in the medico-legal field. Of all forms of contraception, counselling is probably the most important with this particular drug, and careful note-taking is essential. The issue of consent and understanding is particularly important with DMPA. Like all contraceptives, it is a drug given to healthy women, so the normal balancing of risks of treatment against the risk from an untreated disease cannot be applied.

It is a long-acting drug, so once the injection has been given the woman has to live with any side effects and accept that she cannot conceive until the effects of the injection wear off. Also, it appears that of the women for whom the drug has been prescribed in the UK, a considerable proportion are those who are least able, for reasons of social background or personal characteristics, to understand and decide upon the complex issues of risk and benefit. Because of its long and often unpleasant side effects, its use is only acceptable if consent is obtained from the recipient. The most important points that must be made and understood by the woman are:

▶ the irreversibility of its use for at least 12 weeks and possibly longer;

▶ its effect on the menstrual cycle in almost all cases; and

▶ the delay in return of a normal menstrual cycle, and with it fertility, which may extend for up to two years.

An information leaflet should be used and the written consent obtained from the woman wherever possible.

Two other areas of concern are:

▶ The timing of the injection, which should be in the first seven days of the cycle, or within six weeks of childbirth. This will avoid giving the injection where there is already a pre-existing pregnancy.

▶ The site of the injection must be deep intramuscular – injections into the upper arm may not be efficient.

Contraceptive implants

Implanon®

Implanon® (Organon) is a single flexible rod measuring 40 mm × 2 mm. It contains etonorgestrel (68 mg), which is the active metabolite of desogestrel and which is released from Implanon® in a controlled fashion over three years. Within one day of insertion of the device, blood levels of etonorgestrel are achieved which inhibit ovulation. After removal of the device, 90% of women begin ovulating within the first 30 days. Its contraceptive efficacy is unsurpassed and in 73,429 cycles, no pregnancies have been reported.[14]

Etonorgestrel's main action appears to be inhibition of luteinising hormone. This means that pre-ovulatory follicles continue to produce oestradiol and this may have important implications in the terms of bone-mineral density. The bleeding pattern with Implanon® is similar to other progestogen-only preparations but it is worth noting that the incidence of infrequent, frequent and prolonged bleeding reaches a plateau after about three months of use.

Adverse experiences such as acne, breast pain, headache, weight increase and emotional lability are similar to those seen with other progestogen-only preparations.[15]

Doctors wishing to use Implanon® must be fully trained in both the insertion technique and the removal technique, and are advised to obtain a letter of competence in these techniques from the Faculty of Family Planning and Reproductive Healthcare of the RCOG.

The correct timing for the insertion should be within seven days of the start of a menstrual period or within six weeks of parturition. Counselling of the patient is paramount and it is important to stress the changes in bleeding pattern as with other progestogen-only preparations. Its immediate efficacy and the return to normality afterwards should be explained, and the insertion and removal techniques need to be discussed.

Supportive information should be given and the manufacturer supplies this.

Norplant®

Norplant® (Wyeth–Ayerst) is a long-acting implant releasing levonorgestrel. It consists of six identical flexible rods that are inserted subdermally into the lower part of the non-dominant upper arm of the woman. It lasts for five years and the problems associated with it are similar to other long-acting progestogen only contraceptives.

Its distribution has recently been discontinued (November 1999) amid concerns over side effects (eg disruption of the menstrual cycle, hair loss, eye disorders and headaches) but some women may have the system in place until 2004.

The effects of Norplant® are almost immediately reversible on removal. The doctor removing the system should be fully trained in the technique and have a letter of competence.

Emergency contraception

Emergency contraception is defined as the use of a drug or device as an emergency measure to prevent pregnancy after unprotected intercourse. It implies something not to be used routinely but which can still prevent pregnancy if other options have failed or regular contraception was not used. Although the terms 'morning-after pill' and 'post-coital contraception' are also used to describe the same approach, these can cause confusion regarding the timing and purpose, and are best avoided.[16]

Hormonal methods can be used up to 72 hours after the first act of unprotected intercourse. The post-coital insertion of an IUCD is an option that can be used up to five days after the estimated time of ovulation and can be left in the uterus as a long-term regular contraceptive method.[17]

The Yuzpe regimen for emergency contraception involves the use of two tablets of a high-dose combined oral contraceptive (each tablet containing ethinyl oestradiol [50 µg] and levonorgestrel [250 µg]); the second tablet is taken 12 hours after the first. Pregnancy rates vary between 0.2% and 3%. Recently, levonorgestrel (0.75 mg per dose, given twice 12 hours apart) has been shown[18] to have an effectiveness superior to the Yuzpe regimen with significantly fewer side effects. This year (2001), the UK Government deregulated emergency contraception in the form of the levonorgestrel pill, and this is now available over the counter. It remains unclear, however, who will be legally responsible if, for instance, a woman suffers from a catastrophic event following over-the-counter prescribing of the post-coital pill.

The principal indications for emergency contraception are:

▶ unprotected sex

▶ barrier method failure

▶ potential pill failure when alternative methods are not used within seven days after two or more combined pills are missed from the first seven pills; or four or more pills mid-packet; or one or more POPs are missed or taken more than three hours after the usual time

▶ potential IUCD failures.

Counselling must cover the main side effects, which are very few. They are most commonly reported as nausea or vomiting or occasional headaches and breast tenderness. Food should be taken shortly after ingesting the tablets to minimize the side effects. There may be an enhanced anticoagulant effect of warfarin after giving levonorgestrel for emergency contraception.[19]

To increase the efficacy of the method, the woman should be advised not to have intercourse again until the onset of menstruation or, alternatively, to use safe methods of contraception in the intervening time. There should be no delay in the onset of menses and it is very important that the doctor prescribing the method should ensure that there is adequate follow-up within three weeks of treatment so that an ongoing pregnancy can be excluded and future contraception discussed. The risks of teratogenicity to a fetus are extremely small and, as yet, have not been determined.

The modes of contraceptive action of levonorgestrel are believed to be primarily prevention of ovulation, interference with fertilization by altering the tubal transport of sperm and ova, and inhibition of implantation by altering the endometrium.

The use of the IUCD as a form of post-coital contraception requires the same counselling as described for the intra-uterine contraception under other circumstances (discussed below).

The under-age girl

The Family Law Reform Act 1969 allows teenagers over the age of 16 to consent to their own medical treatment. However, the law in England and Wales relating to girls under the age of 16 has been somewhat altered after the *Gillick* case.[20] In 1985, the House of Lords overturned an Appeal Court judgment in the case brought by Mrs Victoria Gillick; and Lord Fraser issued the following guidelines:

It is reasonable to prescribe contraception without parental knowledge and consent if:

1. the girl, although under 16 years of age, is able to understand the doctor's advice;
2. she cannot be persuaded to inform her parents or allow the doctor to inform them;
3. she is very likely to begin or continue having sexual intercourse regardless of contraceptive treatment;
4. the girl's physical or mental health, or both, are likely to suffer unless she receives contraceptive advice to treatment;
5. the value of parental support has been discussed and she cannot be persuaded to inform her parents.

At all times, the young girl must have 100% assurance of confidentiality. Consent given in such a way is valid for all methods of contraception except sterilization. The decision in the *Gillick* case applies equally in Northern Ireland. In Scotland, girls younger than 16 can give their own consent to contraceptive treatment, provided they are capable of understanding the proposed treatment.[21]

Intra-uterine contraceptive devices

The insertion of an IUCD is a minor surgical procedure. The practitioner performing such a procedure must have been trained adequately and ideally should have a letter of competence confirming this. Most complaints concerning the IUCD relate to perforation of the uterus with the device. In the past, infection also played a major part but this has now become less of a problem.

Mode of action

- All types of IUCDs lead to a marked increase in the number of leukocytes both in the endometrium and in uterine and tubal fluids. These seem to have a direct effect against sperm.

- Inert and copper devices lead to elevated levels of many prostaglandins.

- Copper enhances the foreign body reaction and leads to a range of biochemical changes in the endometrium.

- Copper ions are toxic to sperm and blastocyst.

The main effect is believed to be by preventing fertilization and not by preventing implantation of a fertilized egg.

Problems associated with the IUCD

The overall failure rate is between 0.3 and 2 per 100 woman-years but this is considerably lowered with the use of the levonorgestrel-releasing system (Mirena® [Schering]). Reference has already been made to the problems of infection and uterine perforation, but other problems that may arise are:

- intra-uterine pregnancy with an increased risk of miscarriage

- extra-uterine pregnancy

- expulsion with a risk of pregnancy

- malposition of the device leading to lost threads

- pain and abnormal bleeding, particularly an increase in duration and heaviness.

The risk of pelvic inflammatory disease (PID) varies enormously according to the background rate of PID in the population studied. The WHO's IUD Clinical Trial data show that the overall rate of PID amongst 22,908 patients undergoing IUCD insertions and during 51,399 women-years of follow-up was 1.6 cases per 1000 woman-years of use.[22,23] After adjustment for confounding factors, PID risk was more than six times higher during the 20 days after insertion than during later times. The risk was low and constant for up to eight years of follow-up. The rates varied according to geographical area (highest in Africa and lowest in China) and were inversely associated with age. These findings indicate that PID amongst IUCD users was most strongly related to the insertion process and to the background risk of sexually transmissible disease. Also, because PID is an infrequent event beyond the first 20 days after insertion, an IUCD should be left in place up to its maximum life span and not be replaced routinely at an earlier date unless there are other indications.[20,21]

The risk of infection at the time of insertion can be minimized by screening all patients for sexually transmitted diseases, particularly chlamydia, at the first visit. At the time of insertion, the cervix needs to be carefully examined for the presence of a purulent discharge and, in its absence, careful cleaning with an antiseptic solution should be performed. At present, routine full antibiotic cover for insertion is not considered to be appropriate.

Patients should be warned that, particularly in the three weeks after insertion, should they develop pelvic pain, an increased vaginal discharge, offensive discharge or a raised temperature, they must report back to a doctor as soon as possible – preferably the doctor who performed the procedure – so that appropriate antibiotic therapy can be instituted. In general, the device should be removed, although this is not mandatory.

Actinomyces-like organisms (ALOs) are often found in the cervical smears of IUCD users. Their presence is directly proportional to the years that the device has been in position and after five years over 20% of patients carry the infection. In the presence of an ALO on a cervical smear, the patient should be re-called without delay and carefully questioned about the occurrence of pain, dyspareunia or excessive discharge. Endocervical swabs should be taken and if there are any symptoms – such as tenderness on examination – the device should be removed and sent for culture. The latter procedure, with replacement of the device after a short period of time, is often all that is necessary for the disappearance of the ALO.[7]

Perforation

Most perforations first present as a pregnancy with lost threads. Alternatively, pain and bleeding may occur immediately after the insertion, indicating that the device has been passed through the uterine wall. Occasionally, patients present with lost threads and abdominal pain due to adhesion formation associated with the copper or progestogen on the device. The rate of perforation is quoted commonly as one per 1000 insertions but it is probably lower for 'T'-shaped devices.

The factors that affect perforation are as follows:

 Recent pregnancy – the uterus in this circumstance is very soft and perforation is therefore much easier.

 linear devices inserted by the 'push' technique – these are more likely to perforate than newer devices, which are inserted using a withdrawal technique.

 the experience of the practitioner – this is the most important factor.

It is essential for a full bimanual pelvic examination to be carried out before the insertion of the device and the axis of the uterus ascertained (ie whether it is anteverted or retroverted). A holding forceps or tenaculum should be affixed to the anterior lip of the cervix and then a uterine sound passed along the axis to determine the depth of the uterus. This should be a relatively painless and simple procedure. Once these necessary steps have been undertaken, the device can be inserted along the axis already determined.

In the very occasional case where perforation does occur, the device should be removed. If the strings are no longer visible, it is usually necessary to ascertain the position of the device by using ultrasound and, possibly, abdominal X-ray. If the latter is used, a radio-opaque instrument such as a uterine sound should be placed in the uterine cavity. Once the position of the device has been ascertained, laparoscopy should be undertaken. If a device has been within the pelvic or abdominal cavity for some time, adhesion formation may have taken place – usually involving the omentum but occasionally involving the bowel. In these circumstances, laparotomy may be necessary to remove the device.[24]

Other problems related to IUCDs

Other problems include an increase in menstrual loss and associated dysmenorrhoea. These problems are common and the patient should be counselled concerning them. Simple non-hormonal treatments such as the use of tranexamic acid are often all that is required.

A surprisingly common litigation issue is failure of removal of a device, either at the time of sterilization or for other reasons. In one such case (unreported), a doctor failed to inform a patient that he had not removed a device because he felt that her risks of pregnancy were very great and that she was likely to be non-compliant with the pill. Some 15 years later, when she was in a stable relationship, she received prolonged investigations for infertility and it was not until she had an ultrasound scan, prior to *in vitro* fertilization, that the device was found. A settlement was reached out of court and a substantial sum of money paid to the patient.

The levonorgestrel-containing intra-uterine system (Mirena®)

This intra-uterine system (IUS) releases 20 µg of levonorgestrel per day into the uterine cavity. The pregnancy rate is lower than with the standard IUCD (Pearl Index 0.05 cf. 1–4).[25] It is associated with a lower incidence of PID (perhaps because of the thick cervical mucus plug that is formed), a marked reduction in menstrual flow (75–100% after six months),[26] and a reduction in dysmenorrhoea. Its profile therefore is totally dissimilar to that of the conventional IUCD. The major problem associated with its use is the unscheduled bleeding that can occur for at least the first three months after fitting and women must be carefully counselled about this before insertion. Other problems, particularly of perforation, are the same as with the normal device.

The levonorgestrel IUS is being used increasingly for the control of menorrhagia in the older woman and for uterine protection in the peri- and post-menopause. Once it is fitted in the post-menopausal woman, an oestrogen – by whichever route the patient chooses – can be administered on a continuous basis; and in over 79% of patients, amenorrhoea will occur.[27] The IUS needs changing every five years.

Whatever device is chosen, the technical ability of the doctor fitting it is paramount, and proper counselling before insertion of a device must take place and be recorded in the notes.

Other methods of contraception

Occlusive caps or diaphragms need to be fitted carefully by a doctor or nurse who is correctly trained in the technique. These methods require considerable motivation on the part of the woman. It is vital that detailed training in the fitting of the device is given and that adequate follow-up is provided before the method is used for contraception.

It should be noted that a number of lubricants and other topical vaginal preparations might accelerate the deterioration of the latex. They are predominantly oil-based substances and, most importantly, many of the anti-fungal vaginal preparations fall within this group. Patients must be advised about this.

Condoms, being thinner, are more susceptible to damage but as they are only used once, it is unlikely that such damage would occur on a single occasion.[2] The Pearl Index for condoms and diaphragms is 3–12 and is largely dependant upon the age of the woman and the experience of the user.[25]

Sterilization

Sterilization is a form of contraception that is considered to be permanent and irreversible. It is a voluntary act, with the request coming from the person who wishes to undergo the procedure. Between 30% and 35% of women over the age of 35 seek sterilization in the United Kingdom.

It is usual that a request for sterilization is made through the GP, although referrals may come from family planning clinics or be made at general gynaecology or antenatal outpatient clinics. According to the NHSLA database, failed sterilization claims represent 5.34% of all obstetric and gynaecology claims.[28]

Outpatient consultation/counselling

Counselling involves giving women non-directive and non-judgmental information, which is both comprehensive and intelligible. Such counselling should be backed up by information leaflets.[29–31]

The initial part of the interview should ascertain that the woman does not want – under *any* circumstances – to have (more) children. Other methods of contraception, both short-term and long-term should be discussed. These should relate particularly to IUCDs, which protect against pregnancy for up to eight years, progestogen-releasing devices, which last up to five years, and sub-dermal implants, which currently last up to three years. Some of these methods have failure rates comparable to female sterilization. In addition, it is important to discuss with the woman the possibility of a vasectomy for her partner.

Particular care must be taken when counselling women under the age of 25 or those without children. For women under the age of 25, even if they have two or three children, there is often regret at having undergone the procedure, and approximately 10% will request reversal at a later date. This is usually associated with forming a new partnership, particularly with a man who has no children.

The mental capacity of the person seeking sterilization must be taken into account. In September 1989, the Official Solicitor produced guidelines indicating that in virtually all cases where a mentally handicapped person was involved, prior sanction from a High Court judge would be necessary.[32]

In 1995, the Law Commission, in its report on mental incapacity, similarly advised that sterilization of mentally handicapped people for the purposes of contraception required the approval of a judicial forum.[33]

The outpatient consultation must include a full gynaecological and obstetric history, paying particular attention to previous abdominal surgery. Pelvic examination should be carried out to exclude any obvious gynaecological pathology.

A discussion should follow on the method of access to the Fallopian tubes and the method of occlusion. Access is normally by laparoscopy. It is important to explain to the patient that if this method fails, a further and different approach may be necessary (ie laparotomy). The most important aspects of the consultation are to explain to the patient the following:

1. Tubal occlusion, by whatever method, is associated with a failure rate and the lifetime risk is approximately 1 in 200,[34-39] although Peterson et al.[36] in the USA calculated a cumulative 10-year probability of pregnancy after clip sterilization of 16.6–18.5 per 1000 procedures. However, this study dealt with occlusive clips other than the Filshie clip, which is the clip generally used in the UK.
2. Should the procedure fail, the resulting pregnancy may be an ectopic pregnancy. If, following the procedure, the patient believes that she is pregnant, medical help must be sought as soon as possible.
3. The procedure is *not* associated with an increased risk of heavier periods or an increased incidence of other gynaecological problems.
4. The procedure is to be considered irreversible although, with occlusive methods involving the application of clips, successful reversal is possible, usually via an open procedure. Such procedures are not generally available on the NHS, however.

It is essential that these points are recorded in the notes and it is desirable that a précis of the consultation is made in the letter to the referring doctor.

It is important that the woman is told that she must continue to use whatever form of contraception she chooses *up to the time of the sterilization* and, in terms of the contraceptive pill, to the end of that current treatment cycle.

Admission to hospital

It is usual that the date of the last menstrual period is recorded and good practice dictates that a pregnancy test should be performed. The doctor or nurse admitting the patient should confirm the outpatient details, as described above, and again go over the main points regarding the irreversibility of the procedure and the failure rate. Ideally, consent for the procedure should be obtained by the operating surgeon himself. Most hospitals have special written forms of consent for sterilization detailing the appropriate risks. The consent form has to be signed by both the doctor and the patient. A signed form of consent to sterilization does not, in itself, provide absolute evidence that real consent has been obtained. Nevertheless documented evidence, as described above, detailing the counselling that the patient has received, does provide substantial evidence that informed consent has been obtained. There is no legal obligation to obtain the partner's written consent to the procedure, although the outpatient counselling should, preferably, involve participation of the partner.

Methods of sterilization

A number of methods of female sterilization are available; in the UK, the most popular is by laparoscopy with the application of an occlusive device. Laparoscopy is both quicker and less painful than other methods and is associated with a quicker return to normal activity. It is usually performed as a day-case procedure. It is essential that the surgeon is appropriately trained in laparoscopic techniques.

There are three techniques of laparoscopic tubal occlusion.

1. The application of clips

The Filshie clip replaced the original clip designed by Hulka and Clemens and has been available in the UK for more than 20 years. When using Filshie clips, it is essential that the clip applicator is assembled according to the manufacturer's instructions and that the machinery is maintained properly.[40] Failure to do so may lead to incomplete occlusion of the Fallopian tube. The clip applicator is inserted via a second portal under direct vision through the laparoscope. It is essential that the operator correctly identifies the Fallopian tube at the beginning of the procedure (usually by following its course to its distal end and observing the fimbriae) and checks at the end of the procedure that the clip is fully closed and completely across the tube. The clip should be placed over the isthmus of the uterine tube as this is the thinnest part – application elsewhere may not completely occlude the tube. The portion of tube contained within the clip becomes ischaemic and necrotic and it is not uncommon for the clip to fall off after a period of time leaving a proximal and distal portion of occluded tube. The patient should be informed that a subsequent X-ray on her abdomen or pelvis, which may be necessary for other reasons, might not demonstrate the clip to be in the area of her uterus. This does not mean that the sterilization has failed.

2. The Falope ring

This is a silastic band that is placed over a loop of Fallopian tube. The applicator is inserted through a second portal under direct vision. A loop of tube is drawn up into the lumen of the applicator and the band applied around the base of this loop. This leads to the loop becoming ischaemic and eventually necrotic. Failures have been reported because a fistulous connection can form between the proximal and distal parts of the tube.

3. Diathermy coagulation

This method has been superseded by the two methods described above, although it was popular in the 1970s. Its abandonment occurred because of the introduction of the occlusive clip and also because of the associated risks of damage to organs other than the uterine tubes. Chamberlain and Brown[41] estimated that the mortality rate was in the range of eight to ten per 100,000 operations. These accidents were the result of unipolar diathermy because this procedure generated high temperatures which spread to sites distant from the application of the forceps. Bipolar diathermy generates similar temperatures but there is little spread of the heat; however, the method is not generally used within the UK.

Laparotomy

This is the alternative route for sterilization and should be used when the surgeon is insufficiently skilled or experienced in laparoscopy, where the size of the patient precludes safe laparoscopy or where the patient has undergone previous extensive abdominal surgery making laparoscopy an inherently dangerous procedure. It is usually performed through a small transverse suprapubic incision. Once entry into the peritoneal cavity is achieved, an assistant should elevate the uterus so that the tubes are easily accessible and close to the abdominal incision. The most widely used method is the Pomeroy technique, which involves using absorbable sutures to tie the base of a loop of tube near to its mid portion and then removing the top of the loop. The suture material is rapidly absorbed and the two cut ends of the tube then separate. This procedure usually destroys 3–4 cm of the tube and makes reversal very difficult. It is a method commonly used at the time of Caesarean section.

Sterilization at the time of Caesarean section is not generally recommended and should never be carried out when consent has only been obtained shortly before the procedure. Should a woman seek sterilization during her pregnancy, the counselling procedures outlined above should be gone through and an interval laparoscopic procedure should be carried out about six weeks after the birth of the child. This allows the patient time to reconsider her decision and observe that her baby is healthy.

Sterilization at the time of a therapeutic termination of pregnancy is sometimes requested. Again, this is not an ideal time for the procedure to be carried out, partly because the woman may have felt pressurized into the decision because of her situation and partly because the Fallopian tubes are thicker than in the non-pregnant state, so that complete occlusion may be more difficult and the subsequent failure rate higher.

Failure of sterilization

Sterilization can fail for the following reasons:

▶ The patient was pregnant at the time of the procedure (luteal-phase sterilization).

▶ The wrong structure was occluded (eg the round ligament).

▶ The occluding device was incorrectly applied to the Fallopian tube.

▶ The applicator (particularly when using the Filshie clip) was faulty or incorrectly assembled.[40]

▶ The tube recanalizes or a fistula forms.

It is believed widely that any failure of sterilization is likely to occur within the first year of the operation. However, the risk persists for years after the procedure and varies with method of tubal occlusion and age.[42]

When a practitioner is faced with a failed sterilization that was his responsibility, he needs to consider if he is the best person to continue looking after the patient, whether she wishes to carry on with the pregnancy or seek a termination. It is probably best that he does not undertake the re-sterilization procedure should the woman decide upon this course of action.

Because of the nature of the sterilization procedure, the risk of an ectopic pregnancy is greatly increased. It follows that any patient who has been sterilized and who subsequently has a positive pregnancy test must be seen urgently and ultrasound examination undertaken in an attempt to visualize the site of the pregnancy. If it is extra-uterine, it should be dealt with speedily, either surgically by laparoscopy or laparotomy, or medically using methotrexate. In the event of a surgical procedure, it is essential that close attention is paid to the state of the Fallopian tubes and the relationship of the occluding device to them (*vide infra*).

Following a sterilization procedure, there is no need to check tubal patency unless it is felt that the procedure was technically difficult and occlusion may not have occurred. Usually it is best to apply another clip when in doubt, but if access or visualization is difficult, the patient must be told to continue to use contraception until such time that a tubal patency test can be performed (eg hystero-salpingography).

Resterilization

Once a decision has been made about the pregnancy, the question of resterilization may arise. In general it is advisable that this is carried out by another doctor, perhaps at a different hospital, so that an unbiased opinion as to the cause of the sterilization can be obtained. It is tempting to offer a further laparoscopy, as this will be least traumatic for the patient, although mini-laparotomy can be considered as a relatively minor procedure. Wherever possible, videophotography should be employed to demonstrate the position of the occluding device. Insufflation of blue dye at the time may demonstrate where tubal patency has occurred. Efforts should be made to remove both tubes in their entirety so that histological examination can take place. The histologist should be advised accordingly so that he might provide some supporting evidence of blockage or patency.[43]

Conclusion

Sterilization is an operation often used as a method of contraception. It has to be regarded as permanent but there is an associated failure rate. The woman undergoing sterilization must be properly informed of the associated problems and the gynaecologist must ensure that the operator is fully trained in the procedure, that proper skill is employed and that the equipment used is properly maintained and assembled. Should failure occur, he must take into account the circumstances that led to that failure, and the consequent needs of the individual woman.[44]

Litigation is common following failed sterilization and, in the case of a live birth, damages have been high, taking into account the costs of bringing up a child to adulthood. However, these have been somewhat moderated recently by a ruling that emphasized the joy gained from having a child, even when unplanned. The House of Lords ruled in *McFarlane v Tayside Health Board*[45] that there should be no damages recoverable for bringing up a *healthy* child – leaving open the question of whether damages would be recoverable in such cases for the cost, or any part of the costs, of the upbringing of a handicapped or sick child.

In cases involving termination of pregnancy or ectopic pregnancy, pain and suffering – both physical and emotional – are taken into account.

References

1   James C. Risk management in obstetrics and gynaecology. *Journal of the Medical Defence Union* 1991; 7: 36–38.
2   Bromham DR. Contraception. In: Clements RV (ed.) *Safe Practice in Obstetrics and Gynaecology: a Medico-Legal Handbook.* Edinburgh: Churchill Livingstone, 1994: 381–396.
3   Jones M. *Medical Negligence*, 2nd edition. London: Sweet and Maxwell, 1996 (paras 2-003–2-010).
4   Hannaford PC. Combined oral contraceptives: do we know all their effects? *Contraception* 1955; 51: 325–327.
5   Benagioni G. Venous thrombosis and the pill. *Human Reproduction* 1998; 13: 1115–1120.
6   *British National Formulary* 2000; 40: 371.
7   Guillebaud J. *Contraception – Your Questions Answered.* Edinburgh. Churchill Livingstone, 1993.
8   Bracken MB. Oral contraception and congenital malformations: a review and meta-analysis of the prospective studies. *Obstetrics and Gynaecology* 1990, 76: 552–557.
9   Fraser IS. A comprehensive review of injectable contraception with special emphasis on depot medroxyprogesterone acetate. *Medical Journal of Australia* 1981; 1(suppl 1): 1–20.
10 WHO Collaborative Study of Neoplasia and Steroid Contraceptives. Invasive cervical cancer and DMPA. *Bulletin of the WHO* 1985; 63(3): 505–511.
11 WHO. Steroid contraception and the risk of neoplasia. *World Health Organisation Technical Report Series* no. 619, 1978.
12 WHO Expanded Program of Research, Development and Research Training in Human Reproduction: Task Force on Long-Acting Systemic Agents for the Regulation of Fertility. Multinational comparative clinical evaluation of two long-acting injectable contraceptive steroids: norethisterone oenanthate and medroxyprogesterone acetate. *Contraception* 1978; 17: 395.
13 Cundy T, Evans M, Roberts H *et al.* Bone density in women receiving DMPA for contraception. *British Medical Journal* 1991; 303: 13–16.

14   Olsson SE, Odlind V, Johansson E. Clinical results with subcutaneous implants containing 3-keto desogestrel. *Contraception* 1990; 42: 1–11.

15   Mascarenhas L. Insertion and removal of Implanon. *Contraception* 1998; 58(Suppl 6): 79S–83S.

16   Burton R, Savage W, Reader F. The morning-after pill is the wrong name for it. *British Journal of Family Planning* 1990; 15: 119–121.

17   Faculty of Family Planning and Reproductive Health Care. *Recommendations for Clinical Practice: Emergency Contraception* (Interim Guidance), 1999.

18   Task Force on Postovulatory Methods of Fertility Regulation. Randomised controlled trial of levonorgestrel versus Yuzpe regimen of combined oral contraceptives for emergency contraception. *Lancet* 1998; 352: 428–433.

19   Ellison J, Thomson AJ, Greer I, Walker ID. Apparent interaction between warfarin and levonorgestrel used for emergency contraception. *British Medical Journal* 2000; 321: 1382.

20   Gillick v Wisbech and West Norfolk Area Health Authority [1985] 3 All ER 402 HL.

21   Section 2(4) of the Age of Legal Capacity (Scotland) Act 1991, as amended by the Children (Scotland) Act 1995.

22   Farley TM, Rosenberg MJ, Rowe PJ, Chan JH, Meirik O. Intrauterine devices and pelvic inflammatory disease: an international perspective. *Lancet* 1992; 339: 785–788.

23   Shelton JD. Risk of clinical pelvic inflammatory disease attributable to an intrauterine device. *Lancet* 2001; 357: 732.

24   Spillane H, Jackson R, Tang L, Newton J. A regional referral clinic for intrauterine removal problems. *British Journal of Family Planning* 1991; 16: 139–144.

25   Chamberlain GVP, Bowen-Simpkins P. *A Practice of Obstetrics and Gynaecology,* 3rd edn. Edinburgh: Churchill Livingstone, 2000: 214.

26   Barrington JW, Bowen-Simpkins P. The levonorgestrel intrauterine system in the management of menorrhagia. *British Journal of Obstetrics and Gynaecology* 1997; 104(5): 1014–1016.

27   Suhonen S, Holmstrom T, Lahteenmaki P. Three-year follow-up of a levonorgestrel-releasing intrauterine system in hormone replacement therapy. *Acta Obstetrica et Gynecologica Scandinavica* 1997; 76(2): 145–150.

28   Anderson C, NHS Litigation Authority. Personal communication, November 2000.

29   Edwards MH. Satisfying patients needs for surgical information. *British Journal of Surgery* 1990; 77: 463–465.

30   Hawkey GM, Hawkey CJ. Effects of information leaflets on knowledge of patients with gastro-intestinal diseases. *Gut* 1989; 30: 1641–1646.

31   Dixon M. Assertions about patient information are not supported. *British Medical Journal* 1995; 311: 946.

32   Practice note [1989] 2 FLR 447.

33   The Law Commission. *Mental Incapacity.* Law Commission No. 231. London: HMSO, 1995.

34   Bhiwandiwhala PP, Mumford SD, Feldblum PJ. A comparison of different laparoscopic sterilization occlusion techniques in 24,439 procedures. *American Journal of Obstetrics and Gynecology* 1982; 144: 319–331.

35   Chi IC, Potts M, Wilkens L. Rare events associated with tubal sterilizations: an international experience. *Obstetrical and Gynecological Survey* 1986, 4: 7–19.

36   Peterson HB, Xia Z, Hughes JM, Wilcox LS, Tylor LR, Trussell J. The risk of pregnancy after tubal sterilization: findings from the US Collaborative Review of Sterilization. *American Journal of Obstetrics and Gynecology* 1996; 174: 1161–1168.

37   Mumford SD, Bhiwandiwala PP. Tubal ring sterilization: experience with 10,086 cases. *Obstetrics and Gynecology* 1981; 57: 150–157.

38   Mumford SD, Bhiwandiwala PP, Chi IC. Laparoscopic and mini-laparotomy female sterilisation compared in 15,167 cases. *Lancet* 1980; 2: 1066–1070.

39   Vessey M, Huggins GR, Lawless M, McPherson K, Yeates D. Tubal sterilisation: findings in a large prospective study. *British Journal of Obstetrics and Gynaecology* 1983; 90: 203–209.

40   Femcare Ltd. Operating room instructions for Filshie clip laparoscopic equipment. Nottingham, 1995.

41   Chamberlain GVP, Brown JC (eds.) *Report of the Working Party on the Confidential Inquiry into Gynaecological Laparoscopy.* Royal College of Obstetricians and Gynaecologists. London, 1978.

42   Royal College of Obstetricians and Gynaecologists. *Evidence-Based Clinical Guidelines No 4. Male and Female Sterilisation.* London, 1995.

43   Chamberlain GVP. Sterilisation – clinical aspects. In: Orr CJB, Sharp F, Chamberlain GVP (eds.) *Litigation in Obstetrics and Gynaecology.* London: RCOG, 1985: 163–176.

44   Filshie GM. Sterilization. In: Clements RV (ed.) *Safe Practice in Obstetrics and Gynaecology: a Medico-legal Handbook.* Edinburgh: Churchill Livingstone, 1994: 337–344.

45   Watt J. McFarlane v Tayside Health Board. *Clinical Risk* 2001; 7: 20–22.

▶18

Induced Abortion

David Paintin

National guidelines

The Royal College of Obstetricians and Gynaecologists (RCOG) has recently produced evidence-based guidelines on the care of women requesting induced abortion.[1] These set national standards for audit and service accreditation in the National Health Service (NHS) and in the independent health sector. They are to be reviewed every three years. Other relevant guidelines have been published by the Royal College of Anaesthetists[2] and the Royal College of Nursing.[3] The Department of Health has made clear that independent sector providers of abortion will be licensed only if they adhere to such guidelines.[4] The RCOG guidelines includes the interpretation of the law on abortion, consent, the organization of services, the information required by women, and some aspects of clinical practice. It contains evidence-based 'recommendations' and 'good practice points' that express the experience of the RCOG Guideline Development Group. Future abortion practice in Great Britain will be assessed against these guidelines, and medical practitioners and service managers will have to be able to justify any deviation from the recommendations.

Providing an abortion service that is legal

Scope of the Abortion Act 1967

The primary law on abortion in England, Wales and Northern Ireland is the Offences Against the Person Act 1861. (Abortion is regulated by common law in Scotland.) The woman, or any other person, is prohibited from 'unlawfully... procuring a miscarriage' and, with the exception of the woman herself, the prohibition applies 'whether she be or be not with child'. The Abortion Act 1967 specifies when a medical practitioner may lawfully procure a miscarriage in Great Britain. The Abortion Act does not apply in Northern Ireland, where the legality of an abortion has to be interpreted through case law and, on cautious interpretation, is permitted only when continuing the pregnancy would have a grave adverse effect on the mental or physical health of the woman.

What is a legal abortion?

A miscarriage is not defined in the relevant statutes but can be interpreted as an intervention that ends a pregnancy without the production of a living child; the essential event is the death of the fetus. It follows that a lawful termination under the Abortion Act should not result in a live birth. The evacuation of the dead fetus is not necessarily an integral part of the abortion, as when the dead fetus remains *in utero* for many weeks following fetal reduction done to reduce the risk to the woman of continuing a high-multiple pregnancy. Conversely, the Abortion Act does not regulate obstetric interventions that end a pregnancy because of maternal complications or fetal distress, providing the intention is that the child should be born alive and, if possible, survive.

The Abortion Act 1967

The grounds under which a pregnancy may be terminated are defined in Section 2 of the Abortion Act 1967 (as amended in 1991). These are as follows:

1. That the pregnancy has not exceeded its 24th week and that the continuation of the pregnancy would involve risk – greater than if the pregnancy were terminated – of injury to the physical or mental health of the pregnant woman or any existing children of her family; or
2. That the termination is necessary to prevent grave permanent injury to the physical or mental health of the pregnant woman; or
3. That the continuance of the pregnancy would involve risk to the life of the pregnant woman, greater than if the pregnancy were terminated; or
4. That there is a substantial risk that if the child were born it would suffer from such physical or mental abnormalities as to be seriously handicapped.

Specific conditions for legal abortion

1. Two registered medical practitioners must decide 'in good faith'

All legal abortions, with the exception of those that are immediately necessary to save the life or to prevent grave permanent injury to health, require the opinion of two doctors. 'Good faith' implies that both have considered the effect that the pregnancy would have on the woman and both are of the personal opinion that abortion is both legal and in the woman's best interest. To meet the requirements of 'good faith', each should be sufficiently experienced to be able to form a valid judgement. They should not have a relationship in which the opinion of one would be dominated by the other, as might be if they were a consultant and a junior doctor undergoing specialist training.

The treatment for the termination of pregnancy must be carried out in a NHS hospital or a place approved for this purpose by the Secretary of State for Health. All NHS hospitals can provide legal abortion. The statutory Abortion Regulations specify that abortions *after the 24th week* must occur in a NHS hospital or in a hospital administered by a NHS Trust. Independent sector hospitals wishing to provide abortion must be registered by the local health authority under the Registered Homes Act 1984 and must be licensed by the Secretary of State for Health. Licence holders must comply with the required standard operating principles listed in *Procedures for the Approval of Independent Sector Places for the Termination of Pregnancy.*[4] The retention of the licence depends both on annual and on unannounced random inspections by the Department of Health.

Recently, the UK Department of Health has granted licences to independent-sector providers that permit day care for women who have had an early medical abortion or an abortion using vacuum aspiration under local anaesthesia in premises that are not within a private hospital and do not have an operating theatre equipped for general anaesthesia. This recognizes the published evidence for the safety and relative freedom from serious complications of these techniques. It is probable that NHS providers would obtain approval for day-care abortion in the first trimester in health centres that are not attached to a NHS hospital.

2. The pregnancy must not have exceeded the 24th week

The law does not indicate how the length of the pregnancy should be determined. This should be by the methods used in current gynaecological and obstetric practice (see below [The limitations of ultrasound scanning]).

3. Certification

The certificates specified in the Abortion Regulations must be completed. Before the abortion, the two doctors must both sign Certificate A (HSA 1 – the 'Blue form" in which they must state the legal grounds for the abortion. The doctor performing the abortion can, but need not necessarily be, one of the two doctors. The form asks each doctor whether they 'Have/have not*seen/and examined* the pregnant woman (*delete as appropriate)'. The need for the opinions to be in 'good faith' requires that at least one of the doctors should have both seen and examined the woman. A medical practitioner has been convicted of procuring a miscarriage under the Offences Against the Person Act 1861 because he did not enquire about the woman's medical history, make a physical examination, or obtain a second medical opinion.[5] The wording of Certificate A suggests that the second doctor could be considered to have acted within the law if he had not seen or examined the woman but had judged that he could rely on the information in the case records. This has not been tested in the courts and it is good practice for both doctors to have interviewed the woman independently. Certificate A must be preserved with the case records of the abortion for three years.

The Form of Notification (HSA4 – the 'Yellow form' must be completed by the doctor who performs the abortion, and must be sent within seven days to the Chief Medical Officer in either England or Wales, whichever is relevant. Related forms are used in Scotland and are sent to the Chief Medical Officer at the Scottish Office. Both the Form of Notification and a Stillbirth Certificate must be completed for abortions after the 24th week.

Interpreting the grounds for abortion

Threat to the life or physical health of the pregnant woman

Pathology sufficiently severe to justify abortion under these grounds is rare. It is desirable that one of the certifying doctors should be a specialist in relation to the disease in question.

Threat to the mental health of the pregnant woman

This is the ground for most abortions. 'Health' has not been defined in British law and the doctors can choose the definition that they consider appropriate. In 1948, the World Health Organization stated that health is '... a state of physical and mental well-being and not merely an absence of disease or infirmity'.[6] This broad definition is in tune with current medical attitudes to health which emphasize that disease and its management must be considered in the context of the life and environment of the sufferer and not, narrowly, as a disorder of human biology. The Abortion Act 1967 supports this wider view of mental health by stating 'Account may be taken of the pregnant woman's actual or foreseeable environment', and that abortion can be performed to 'prevent injury to the health of... existing children of her family'. The law does not require that the woman be mentally ill, but it *does* require that there should be factors in her life that are stressing her so that her mental health would be in danger if the pregnancy continued. There is usually no difficulty in identifying the stress factors that justify legal abortion. The case records should list these clearly so that the doctors could defend their decision if they were to be challenged. On the Form of Notification, in answer to the question 'State main medical diagnosis', it is acceptable to write 'Social factors threatening mental health'.

Abortions to prevent the birth of a seriously handicapped child

The two doctors have to decide what constitutes a substantial risk of serious handicap. The interpretation of 'substantial risk' poses no difficulties when antenatal investigation shows with certainty that the fetus has a specific abnormality, such as the wrong number of chromosomes or a defect such as spina bifida. But sometimes, as with maternal infection with rubella or toxoplasma, there is only a probability of fetal damage. The probability depends on known variables, such as the gestation at which the woman had active infection, and unknown variables, such as the virulence of the particular strain of infecting microorganism. A 50% probability of abnormality is clearly 'substantial' but the lower limit depends on the opinions of the doctors and the pregnant woman. A 2–3% probability of a significant fetal abnormality is clearly not 'substantial', as this is the level of risk associated with all pregnancies. However, the availability of high-quality ultrasound scanning means that many fetal abnormalities are diagnosed with a probability greater than 90%. Occasionally, a woman continues to insist on abortion when medical opinion is that the probability of a serious fetal abnormality is small. Such pregnancies can still be terminated legally if the woman's distress about the possibility of an abnormal fetus is considered sufficient to threaten her mental health. But this is possible only if gestation is less than 24 weeks. One of the more stringent criteria listed above under sections 2, 3 and 4 must be met for an abortion to be legal later in pregnancy.

Definition of 'serious handicap'

The RCOG has suggested that the decision could be based on the following criteria:[7]

 The probability of effective treatment, either *in utero* or after birth

The probable degree of self-awareness and of the child's ability to communicate with others

▶ The suffering that would be experienced by the child

▶ The extent to which actions essential to health that normal individuals perform unaided would have to be performed by others

▶ The probability of being able to live alone and to be self-supporting as an adult.

Advice from the British Medical Association[8] contains the first three of these criteria. It adds that consideration should be given to the suffering that would be experienced by the people caring for the child but does not include a consideration of the extent to which the child (or adult) would have to depend on the care of others. However, both Down syndrome and major open spina bifida have become accepted as resulting in serious handicap, and both are characterized by a need for considerable assistance in coping with adult life, by limitation of the quality of life and by a lack of methods of reasonably effective treatment. Whenever antenatal investigation detects an abnormal fetus, the doctors must provide the best available information about the expected outcome if the pregnancy is to continue. The decision about abortion has to be made in the context of the informed view of the pregnant woman – particularly her willingness to become the carer of a seriously disabled child. With unusual or debatably serious handicapping conditions, the obstetrician should arrange for the pregnant woman to consult, as appropriate, a medical geneticist, a developmental paediatrician or a paediatric surgeon. Such a medical specialist could be the second signatory on Certificate A.

'Reduction' of multiple pregnancy

The law allows the obstetrician to reduce the number of fetuses in a multiple pregnancy only when this is necessary within the grounds for abortion that are discussed above. Certification is straightforward if the fetus to be destroyed is severely abnormal. If not, the reduction is considered legal if continuing the multiple pregnancy would result in a greater risk to maternal health than a twin or single pregnancy or if there would be a risk to the mental health of the woman if all the fetuses were lost as a consequence of pre-term labour.

Termination of pregnancy after the 24th week

This is only permitted to preserve the life of the pregnant women, to protect her from grave permanent injury to her physical or mental health and, as described in the previous paragraph, when there is a substantial risk that the fetus has an abnormality that would result in serious handicap when born. In practice, almost all very late abortions are a consequence of the late diagnosis of serious fetal abnormality and very few are necessary because of grave risk to the physical health of the woman. A small number are done because a severe maternal complication of pregnancy gravely threatens the health of the woman and consequent severe chronic fetal distress has resulted in a substantial risk that a child would be severely handicapped.

The need to ensure fetal death *in utero* when the fetus is potentially viable

Legal opinion obtained by the RCOG has stated that the death of a baby as a result of immaturity but born alive as the result of a legal abortion would expose the registered medical practitioner who ended the pregnancy to a charge of murder. Case law suggests that a live birth is the birth of a baby that is capable of surviving by breathing air, even if respiration has to be assisted. On the basis of this definition, the RCOG advises that the fetal heart should be stopped *in utero* at the beginning of any abortion procedure at 21 weeks or more.[7] This can be achieved by an intervention such as the injection of potassium chloride solution into the fetal heart under ultrasound control, or by a procedure such as dilatation and evacuation.

Abortions that are immediately necessary to save the life or to protect the health of the woman from grave permanent injury

Such terminations can be performed at any gestational age without the agreement of a second doctor if there is no time for such consultation. A possible reason would be to facilitate urgent abdominal surgery. It is important that the case record should contain a detailed account of the reasons for the abortion. There were only two notifications under these grounds in England and Wales in 1998.

The 'conscience clause' in the Abortion Act

Section 4 of the Abortion Act 1967, states that '... no person shall be under any duty... to participate in any treatment authorised by the Act to which he has a conscientious objection'. The only exception is when the abortion is necessary to save the woman's life or to prevent grave permanent injury to her health. The doctor may subsequently have to establish his conscientious objection if this results in harm to the patient. Such doctors should make clear from the beginning of the consultation that the woman is entitled to further opinions from doctors who are willing to recommend and perform termination of pregnancy. An answer to a Parliamentary question stated that conscientious objection was intended to apply only to those who participate directly in the abortion treatment – doctors and nurses – but that hospital managers had been asked to apply the principle, at their discretion, to those ancillary staff who were involved in the handling of fetal tissue.[8] Case law has established that this section of the Act does not apply to support staff such as clinical secretaries.[9]

Status of the woman's partner in the abortion decision

Three legal cases have established that the man involved in the conception of the pregnancy cannot prevent the woman having an abortion when this is considered necessary by two medical practitioners acting in good faith within the grounds specified in the Abortion Act.[10]

Consent

Issues relating to consent by adults and children under 16 are discussed in Chapter 3. It is worth noting here several specific scenarios, however:

  High Court permission is *not* required when two doctors decide that a pregnant non-competent adult requires an abortion.

  The Gillick test of competence applies clearly to girls aged 14 and 15, but not necessarily to those aged 13 or less when parental consent and/or the initiation of local child protection procedures may be necessary.

▶ Only a person with parental responsibility can give consent for a non-competent minor

▶ The consent of the court is necessary for young women who are wards of court

(See BMA, *The Law and Ethics of Abortion*, 1997;[8] and MDU, *Consent to Treatment*, 1996.)

Characteristics of safe abortion practice

The abortion consultation

In most consultations with a doctor, the patient comes with an open mind and expects to be able to accept the advice she is offered. In contrast, in most consultations about abortion, the emphasis is on whether the doctor feels able to support the woman's own judgement of the situation. To assist her in making a final decision, she must be given impartial help to understand the methods and risks of abortion, and of continuing the pregnancy at her particular gestation, and to check that she has made a full and balanced assessment of her situation. The doctor is in a similar position when antenatal investigations have shown that the fetus is abnormal. It is only when serious maternal pathology gravely threatens a woman's life or health that the doctor may have to advise the termination of a wanted pregnancy. This is rare and accounted for only 1.6% of all the legal abortions notified in 1998 in England and Wales.[11]

Information required by the doctor

Existence of pregnancy

It is important to confirm that the woman is actually pregnant. Most women will have had a positive pregnancy test before the consultation. A further pregnancy test is not essential if the uterus is found to be appropriately enlarged on either abdominal or vaginal examination, or if a fetus is visualized by ultrasound scanning.

Gestational age

In women with regular 28-day cycles, gestation is calculated from the first day of the last menstrual period even though ovulation and closely associated conception do not occur until about 14 days later. It is usual to adjust the calculated gestation in women whose cycles are shorter or longer than 28 days to allow for the fact that ovulation takes place 14 days before the end of each menstrual cycle, whatever its length (ie deduct four days when the cycle is usually 32 days). The calculated gestation should always be confirmed by assessment of uterine size. In the first trimester, this is traditionally by vaginal examination but it is acceptable in an apparently healthy woman to rely on an ultrasound scan to check the normality of the pelvic organs and to measure the fetus.

Role of ultrasound scanning in estimating gestation

Many abortion services in Europe and North America scan all women requesting abortions but this is not current British practice. The RCOG recommends a pre-abortion scan in some circumstances, particularly when gestation is in doubt or where extra-uterine pregnancy is suspected.[1] Serious complications such as incomplete evacuation and uterine injury are more likely if abortion is attempted when the gestation is greater than anticipated, particularly if the operator has experience only of first-trimester abortions by vacuum aspiration. A scan is essential at gestations of more than 18–20 weeks to provide additional evidence that the gestation is within the statutory limit of 24 completed weeks.

Limitations of ultrasound scanning

Ultrasound scanning measures fetal size rather than fetal age and does not provide an exact determination of gestation. Crown–rump length is used in the first trimester and estimates gestation (to with 95% confidence limits) of about ±5 days,[12] but these limits increase progressively when biparietal diameter of the skull has to replace crown–rump length in the second trimester, and are ±12 days by 24 weeks.[13] The final estimate of gestation should be based on the menstrual and sexual history, clinical assessment, and ultrasound. Early extra-uterine pregnancies cannot be identified reliably using ultrasound but should be suspected if a woman has a positive pregnancy test and no gestation sac in the uterus.

The health of the pregnant woman

The woman must be asked to list any present or previous diseases or infections, any current treatment, previous surgery, and any sensitivity or abnormal reactions to medication or anaesthetic agents. Smoking, and the recreational use of alcohol and other drugs, has relevance if general anaesthesia is to be used. She must be asked about previous pregnancies and their outcome, particularly whether any surgical procedure has left a scar in her uterus. Assessment should include height, weight and blood pressure. Comprehensive physical examination need not be a routine but any current symptoms or a history of disease should lead to a clinical examination of the relevant organ system(s) and, when necessary, to appropriate diagnostic tests.

Laboratory investigations

The haemoglobin concentration is estimated routinely – further haematological investigation is necessary if this is lower than 10 g/dl. The ABO and rhesus blood groups should be determined and the serum screened for red cell antibodies (which should alert clinicians to the possibility of delay in identifying compatible blood should transfusion become necessary). All women should have a serum sample saved by the laboratory until after the abortion. Routine cross-matching of blood for transfusion is not necessary.

All Afro-Caribbean women should be screened for haemoglobinopathy. Women homozygous for sickle cell disease (or thalassaemia) are not suitable for day care. Carriers – heterozygotes – can be managed as day cases but with special attention to oxygenation during and after general anaesthesia.

Women at special risk of having hepatitis B/C or the human immunodeficiency virus (HIV) should have the option of screening (with appropriate counselling). Women with acquired immune deficiency syndrome (AIDS) have an increased risk of post-abortion infection from a variety of microorganisms. Screening for HIV or hepatitis should not be made a pre-condition for the termination, however. Abortion providers must regard blood from both high- and low-risk women as potentially infectious and ensure that protocols are in place to minimize any risk to staff.

Information required by the woman

Most women are poorly informed about the methods and risks of abortion. Providers must appreciate that information given orally during a consultation is often remembered incompletely, or inaccurately, and that women should take home an explanatory leaflet or an audiotape in a language that they can understand. Women claiming negligent treatment often state that they were not told what was to be done to them or that there was a risk of the complication in question.

Women need to know:

 The details of methods of abortion available to her at the gestation of her pregnancy.

 The approximate risk of immediate complications for the method(s) that could be used (the probabilities shown below are approximate and are for first-trimester abortion using vacuum aspiration by experienced staff):

> haemorrhage requiring blood transfusion (1 in 1000);

> uterine injury that might require immediate abdominal surgery (1 in 1000, but more likely in women who have had a Caesarean section);

> anaesthetic complications (1 in 1000).

 The approximate risk of complications in the early weeks following abortion, particularly of:

> incomplete abortion requiring re-evacuation (1 in 100);

> continuing pregnancy (1 in 1000);

 pelvic infection requiring hospital admission (1 in 50 to 1 in 100 if prophylactic antibiotics are used).

 There is no convincing evidence that abortion is followed in the long term by:

339

infertility (providing there was no serious pelvic infection, or a uterine injury requiring immediate repair);

 psychiatric illness (but women with a history of psychiatric illness continue to be at risk);

breast cancer.

'Counselling'

The RCOG guidelines read: 'Clinicians caring for women requesting abortion should try to identify those patients who require more support in decision making than can be provided in the routine clinic setting. Facilities for additional support, including access to social services, should be available'.[1] Most women have made their decision to have an abortion before they see a doctor, but some are ambivalent, and up to10% decide to continue the pregnancy because of the additional information obtained during the assessment process. Few need the help of a professional counsellor; but most welcome time with a specially trained support worker who, in private, unhurried and comfortable surroundings, can help them to check their reasons for requesting a termination, their understanding of the abortion process, and go over any other options they might be considering.

Arranging the abortion

Women who have shown any uncertainty should not have their abortion until they have had time for reflection. Three to five days is a suitable interval. Formal consent should be obtained on the day on which the abortion is to be performed.

Day care

Surgical methods of abortion – vacuum aspiration and dilatation and evacuation – are provided routinely for healthy women though day care up to about 18 weeks. Medical abortion is a day-care procedure up to nine weeks, and in a recent report from Scotland, about two-thirds of women having a medical method at 13–18 weeks were able to return home the same day.[14] The RCOG suggests that up to 10% of women will require day care – the proportion relating directly to gestational age.[1] Reasons include women with a variety of potentially serious medical conditions that require special management before, during or after general anaesthesia (including severe obesity); social problems, such as a lack of an adult companion at home; geographic reasons; and unplanned admission because of complications. Criteria for suitability for day care should be agreed locally between the anaesthetists and the medical staff of the abortion service. All day care services should have a telephone helpline through which women can obtain emergency medical assessment and, when necessary, immediate hospital admission.

Contraception

An enquiry into previous experience with contraception should be integral to pre-abortion assessment. It must be understood that contraception is necessary as soon as intercourse is resumed and that ovulation occurs within a month of first trimester abortion in over 90% of women. Many women will already have decided on a future method and should be supported by immediate post-abortion provision. The primary purpose of a follow-up examination is to encourage effective contraception in the future. This should be about two weeks after an uncomplicated abortion and should be with a health professional to whom the woman feels able to return for further contraceptive support – her GP or regular family planning doctor, for example, rather than with the abortion provider.

The insertion of an intra-uterine contraceptive device immediately following abortion

Randomized controlled trials have shown that an intra-uterine contraceptive device can be inserted safely immediately after a first-trimester abortion.[15] There is anecdotal evidence that the expulsion rate is increased when insertion immediately follows second trimester procedures.

Sterilization

Tubal occlusion to prevent future conception can be provided at the same time as first-trimester termination of pregnancy but has a higher failure rate and is more often followed by regret.[16] There have been no recent studies of sterilization with second-trimester termination. The Medico-Legal Committee of the RCOG has questioned whether abortion and sterilization should ever be combined;[17] however, this can be acceptable if the woman has sound reasons for being sterilized, particularly if she had been considering tubal ligation before the conception of the unwanted pregnancy, and providing she understands and accepts the increased risks of failure and regret.

Measures to minimize post-abortion complications

Prevention of isoimmunization to a blood-group antigen

Feto-maternal haemorrhage occurs in about 7% of first-trimester suction terminations and about 20% of second-trimester abortions by intra-amniotic injection. In women who are rhesus negative, this results in isoimmunization in about 4% in the first trimester (and presumably in a higher proportion in the second trimester).[18] All women who are rhesus negative should receive an intramuscular injection of anti-D immunoglobulin (250 iU) after abortions performed up to the 20th week. After the 20th week, 500 iu should be the routine dose but a Kleihauer test or its equivalent should be performed and a larger amount given if feto-maternal haemorrhage has exceeded 4 ml of fetal red cells (National Blood Transfusion Service, 1991). The injection is protective up to 72 hours after the feto-maternal haemorrhage but is best given before the woman returns home after the abortion. When medical abortion is induced in the first trimester using mifepristone and prostaglandin, the anti-D immunoglobulin is given on the same occasion as the mifepristone. A significant level of anti-D will remain in circulation for 10–14 days and will protect from the effects of repeated feto-maternal haemorrhage during that period.

Anti-D immunoglobulin will not protect the woman against other blood-group antigens. Consequently, a very small number of women will develop antibodies to rhesus factors other than D, or to the Kell or Duffy antigens. Currently, this is unavoidable.

Screening for sexually transmitted infections and the prophylaxis of post-abortion infection

The RCOG recommends that there should be '...a strategy for minimising the risk of post abortion infection, and that this includes antibiotic prophylaxis, or screening for lower genital-tract organisms, with treatment of positive cases.[1] (See below [Infection].)

Methods of abortion: first-trimester methods

Early medical abortion

The drug regimens

The manufacturer's data sheet specifies that amenorrhoea should be less than 63 days, and that mifepristone (600 mg by mouth) should be followed 36–48 hours later by the prostaglandin analogue gemeprost (1 mg vaginally). Since the British licence was granted in 1991, randomized controlled trials have shown that 200 mg of mifepristone is as effective as 600 mg; and the prostaglandin analogue misoprostol (400 µg by mouth up to 49 days, and 800 µg vaginally up to 63 days of amenorrhoea) is as effective as gemeprost (1 mg vaginally).[1] Anecdotal evidence suggests that most early medical abortions in Great Britain are now provided by the unlicensed regimen of mifepristone 200 mg followed 36–48 hours later by misoprostol (800 µg vaginally).

What happens

The woman attends the providing unit three times: to take the mifepristone, to be given a prostaglandin analogue, and for follow-up. About 50% of women begin to bleed, and up to 2% abort, in the 48 hours following the administration of mifepristone. The women are asked to return to a day-care unit two days after taking the mifepristone and, if abortion has not occurred, are given a prostaglandin analogue either orally or vaginally. This induces uterine contractions that expel the pregnancy. Up to 1% of women have bleeding that is heavy enough for the abortion to have to be completed by vacuum aspiration on the day the prostaglandin is given. Women return home when pain and bleeding have diminished to an acceptable level – usually after three to six hours – even if there is uncertainty whether the pregnancy has been expelled (see below [Incomplete abortion]). Complete abortion occurs ultimately in about 95% of women. Up to 5% have a vacuum aspiration in the ensuing week or so because of persistent bleeding due to incomplete abortion. The method fails and the pregnancy continues in about 0.5% of women – abortion should then be completed by vacuum aspiration (see below [Continuing pregnancy: Early medical abortion]). It is mainly to identify continuing pregnancy that all women are asked to return for a follow-up assessment 10–14 days after administration of the prostaglandin.

Vacuum aspiration at 7–14 weeks

This method is used for most terminations in the first trimester and may be preceded by cervical preparation (see below [Reducing the risk of cervical injury]). The cervix is dilated to a diameter that does not exceed and may be up to 2 to 3 mm less than the gestation expressed in weeks. A suction cannula of the same diameter is passed through the cervical canal into the uterine cavity and the pregnancy aspirated through a flexible tube into a suction bottle. The cannula is usually made of translucent plastic and the operator can monitor the passage of the pregnancy tissues. Fetal tissue may block the eye of the cannula when the gestation is of 10 weeks or more. Narrow forceps (polyp forceps) are then used to remove the bulk of the residual material from the uterus before the cannula is reinserted to complete the evacuation (see below [Incomplete abortion: Routine inspection of the material evacuated from the uterus...]).

Vacuum aspiration at less than seven weeks

The RCOG recommends that vacuum aspiration should be provided at less than seven weeks only if a strict protocol is in use.[1] This is because the fetus and gestation sac are very small and are difficult to recognize in the relatively large volume of decidual tissue which the uterus contains at this stage of pregnancy. It is also because the uterus contains decidua even when the implantation is extra-uterine – as when in the uterine tube. Failure can occur in up to 3% of pregnancies; a minority of these being unrecognized extra-uterine implantations that ultimately will rupture with danger to the woman's life. A protocol has been published that resulted in the early recognition of all continuing pregnancies, and the identification of symptom-less extra-uterine pregnancies in nine of 1530 (0.6%) women with less than six weeks amenorrhoea.[19] All women had an ultrasound scan prior to the abortion; the aspirate was carefully inspected with a hand lens in the operating room – if no chorionic villi or fetal parts were seen, serum chorionic gonadotrophin (β-hCG) was measured twice, with a further scan taken three days later.

Second-trimester methods of abortion

Medical abortion: drug regimens at 13–20 weeks

Mifepristone followed by a prostaglandin analogue has become the standard medical method in the second trimester. The licensed regimen between 13 and 20 weeks is mifepristone (600 mg orally) followed 36–48 hours later by gemeprost (1 mg vaginally every three hours up to a maximum of five doses). A randomized controlled trial[20] had shown that this regimen, when compared with repeated doses of gemeprost alone, reduced the length of the abortion labour by about 50% and lessened the risk of serious complications such as haemorrhage and unexpected reactions to abortifacient drugs. This is also true for older methods of second-trimester abortion using extra- or intra-amniotic prostaglandins E_2 or $F_{2\alpha}$. Since the licence was granted, randomized controlled trials have shown that 200 mg of mifepristone is as effective as 600 mg, and that misoprostol is as effective as gemeprost. A comprehensive review is provided in the RCOG guidelines.[1] As a result of this research, there is widespread unlicensed use: an established regimen is 200 mg mifepristone followed 36–48 hours later by misoprostol 800 μg vaginally and then 400 μg orally every three hours. Further doses of misoprostol are given if abortion has not occurred in the first 24 hours.

After 20 weeks

The original studies on which the licence was based were of abortions from 13 to 20 weeks, but a randomized controlled trial[21] has shown that mifepristone (200 mg), followed by prostaglandin, will induce abortion later in pregnancy and can be used safely to induce labour in the third trimester in wanted pregnancies. However, when used for abortion at 21 or more weeks, the fetus may be expelled alive and the fetal heart should be stopped *in utero* before the prostaglandin is given (see above [The need to ensure fetal death *in utero* . . .]). Fetal death *in utero* is probable but not certain when second-trimester abortion is induced with an intra-amniotic injection of prostaglandin E_2 and hypertonic urea. This older method is still used by some gynaecologists because they lack the skill or the equipment necessary to make ultrasonically guided intra-uterine injections into the fetal heart.

What happens

As with early medical abortion, the woman attends the providing unit, where she is observed while she takes mifepristone by mouth. She returns 36–48 hours later for the prostaglandin. She needs a bed and must have visual and acoustic privacy. The abortion process lasts a median time of 6.5 hours and about 97% occur within15 hours of the first dose of prostaglandin. A small number take more than 24 hours. A midwife or a specially trained nurse should provide care and support. About 10% of women have an incomplete abortion and require uterine evacuation under general anaesthesia. There is convincing evidence that routine surgical exploration of the uterus is unnecessary.[1]

Dilatation and evacuation

The fetal parts become too large to be aspirated through a suction cannula after about 13 weeks, and dilatation and evacuation provides an important alternative to medical abortion. In Britain, the method is used much more frequently in the independent sector than in the NHS. Dilatation and evacuation requires special skills – the gynaecologist must have been trained in the method and appropriate instruments must be used. The RCOG guidelines recommend routine pre-abortion preparation of the cervix, but some independent sector operators do not do this and have developed the skill to evacuate the uterus through a relatively narrow cervical canal.

Appropriate anaesthesia is critical in minimizing blood loss (see below [Haemorrhage]). In Britain, many operators supplement light general anaesthesia (intravenous propofol, or methohexitone, with fentanyl and nitrous oxide/oxygen) with a para- or intra-cervical block of about 20 ml of adrenaline (1 in 200,000) in 0.5% or 1.0% lignocaine. This may reduce blood loss and is believed by some to make the cervix more easily dilatable. At 14–15 weeks, a pregnancy can be evacuated through a cervix that has been dilated to 12 mm; at 15–18 weeks, 14–16 mm; and at 19–24 weeks, 18–21 mm. Robust but narrow evacuation forceps of the Sopher or Bierer type are passed through the dilated cervical canal and are used to crush, fragment and remove the fetus and placenta. The parts of the fetus should be identified as they are obtained to ensure that the abortion is complete. It has been recommended that real-time ultrasound is used routinely during all second-trimester evacuations.[22] This has not become standard practice in Britain. But real-time ultrasound is very helpful when problems occur during cervical dilatation or evacuation of the fetus, and it is desirable that the equipment should be available for use in the operating room.

Two-stage dilatation and evacuation

This technique has been used for abortions after about 18 weeks in the independent sector in Britain since the 1970s. A general anaesthetic is given for each stage. On the first occasion, the cervix is dilated sufficiently to allow the membranes to be ruptured and a pair of narrow sponge forceps (or a suction cannula) to be used to pull down and sever the umbilical cord. Hygroscopic tents of laminaria or Dilapan may be left in the cervix to dilate the canal. The emphasis in the first stage is to intervene sufficiently only to ensure the death of the fetus. This, with or without cervical preparation, makes further dilatation of the cervix and the evacuation of the uterus much easier under a second anaesthetic the following day.

Hysterotomy

An abdominal incision is made and pregnancy removed through either a longitudinal or, preferably, a low transverse incision in the uterus. Only 23 abortions were carried out using this method in 1998. It is associated with much greater morbidity and mortality than any of the surgical or medical vaginal methods. It is necessary only when abortion cannot be safely achieved through the vagina (eg when serious uterine injury occurs during an attempt at vaginal abortion, when severe fibrosis and stenosis of the cervix from previous surgery prevents cervical dilatation, when congenital malformation of the uterus makes the pregnancy inaccessible), or when a pregnancy must be ended promptly under general anaesthesia because of an acute medical condition and a vaginal method is considered impracticable or unsafe.

Hysterectomy

This is necessary very occasionally – for example, as an emergency when severe accidental uterine injury or haemorrhage during a vaginal abortion cannot be controlled by other means. It has the highest morbidity and mortality of all abortion methods. Eleven terminations in England and Wales were by hysterectomy in 1998.[11] It is used occasionally to terminate a pregnancy electively when a woman is found to have malignant disease of the reproductive tract – usually carcinoma of the cervix.

Selective termination – the 'reduction' of multiple pregnancies

This procedure is so uncommon that it should be provided only by obstetricians who specialize in feto-maternal medicine, who have been trained in the technique, and have a sufficient case load to maintain their skills. Sixty-five cases of selective reduction of the number of fetuses in multiple pregnancies were notified in England and Wales in 1998. Discussion of the clinical reasons for selective reduction and of the details of technique is outside the scope of this chapter.

Litigation and induced abortion

Communication with the patient

The risk of litigation is minimized if a woman is kept well informed about the occurrence of any complication. The operator should tell her of any unexpected outcome as soon as possible. An account of the interview should be recorded in the case record and a copy offered to the woman. She should be given the opportunity of a second interview at which she can choose to have the support of her partner, family member or friend. With the consent of the woman, a summary should be sent promptly to the general practitioner (and to any referring doctor). All women who have serious complications should be offered a follow-up consultation either with the operator in person or the most senior member of the surgical team.

Complications with abortions in which licensed drugs have been used in an unlicensed way

Regimens for medical abortion currently in use in Britain involve the use of licensed pharmaceuticals in an unlicensed way. Such use is supported by randomized controlled trials and the evidence is presented in the RCOG guidelines.[1] The Medicines Act 1968 (section 9) allows medical practitioners to prescribe licensed medicines outside the officially authorized recommendations listed in the manufacturers' data sheets, but they do this on their personal professional responsibility.[23] Medicines prescribed in this way can be dispensed by pharmacists and administered by nurses. Such prescribing should:

▶ be a practice endorsed by a responsible body of professional opinion;

▶ be carried out only with the valid consent of the patient who must:

  ▶ know that the medicine is unlicensed for this purpose;

  ▶ have been given written information on the benefits and risks of its use;

  ▶ have signed a specifically designed consent form (that must be preserved in the case records).

These requirements have special importance for medical abortion because of the reluctance of the manufacturers of abortifacient drugs to risk commercially adverse publicity by applying for a licence (misoprostol) or for a modification of a licence (mifepristone).

Apparent failure to obtain fetal tissue

Apparent failure to obtain fetal or placental tissue is an occasional problem with vacuum aspiration and may be associated with the following:

failure during pre-abortion assessment to identify:

> secondary amenorrhoea

> gestational age less than suggested by the duration of amenorrhoea

 extra-uterine pregnancy

miscarriage since abortion was agreed

acute ante- or retroflexion of the uterus with failure to dilate the internal os and so to enter the uterine cavity

congenital malformation of the uterus with failure of the cannula to enter the part of the uterus containing the pregnancy

failure to enter the uterine cavity because of the formation of a false passage in the cervix or a perforation of the uterine body.

Management

Investigation must begin before the woman is allowed to recover from anaesthesia.

Any tissue that has been obtained from the uterine cavity must be examined for unexpectedly small fetal parts and chorionic villi. This can be done in the operating room if the tissue is suspended in saline and examined with a hand lens against a lighted background.[24] The tissue should be put into fixative and sent for histological examination (unless the examination shows a fetus and chorionic material has been removed).

If no pregnancy tissues are found, there should be:

> a careful bimanual examination to check the size and position of the uterus and any adnexal masses;

> a gentle exploration of the cervical canal and the uterine cavity with a blunt sound;

> a pregnancy test (using a catheter specimen of urine). A negative result identifies the woman who is not actually pregnant. A positive result suggests an ongoing pregnancy or a recent miscarriage;

> an immediate ultrasound scan (if the equipment is available in the operating theatre). This will show any pregnancy within the uterus. An empty uterus suggests either a recent miscarriage or an extra-uterine implantation;

> if ultrasound is not immediately available and the uterus does not feel to be pregnant, the anaesthetic should be discontinued and a scan arranged as soon as possible.

An extra-uterine pregnancy is a possibility if the pregnancy test is positive and a bimanual examination, with or without ultrasound, suggests that the uterus is empty. Early extra-uterine pregnancies are difficult to visualize with ultrasound and may not distend the uterine tube enough for an adnexal mass to be felt. If there is no suggestion of a tubal mass and the woman shows no signs of significant internal blood loss, she may be allowed to recover consciousness but must be observed closely. She must be informed of the possibility and potentially serious consequences of an extra-uterine pregnancy and must be advised to become an inpatient immediately until this diagnosis has been excluded.

▶ If the uterus contains a pregnancy and no false passage or perforation has been detected, it is usually possible to identify the internal os with a probe and then to evacuate the pregnancy by suction after further carefully directed dilatation. With either a septate or a double uterus, the pregnant half of the uterus flops to one side so that the instruments tend to enter the empty half.[25] If the uterus contains a pregnancy and there is a false passage, the same procedure can be followed, but it may be better to allow the woman to recover from the anaesthetic and to attempt vaginal termination about a week later after cervical preparation with misoprostol.

▶ If the uterus contains a pregnancy and there is any suggestion that the uterus has been perforated, the procedure described in the section on uterine injury (below) should be followed.

▶ Follow-up is essential if extra-uterine pregnancy has been excluded and there remains uncertainty regarding whether an intra-uterine pregnancy continues. Protocols include an ultrasound scan after about seven days, an immediate measurement of plasma β-hCG, with a repeat measurement after three to seven days (β-hCG levels fall by about 50% every 36–48 hours if a pregnancy has ended but rise if it is continuing[26]). Repeated urinary pregnancy tests are of no value as β-hCG is removed from the blood stream quite slowly and, after a successful first-trimester abortion, a test sensitive to 20 mU/ml β-hCG can remains positive for 30 or more days.[27]

Continuing pregnancy

After early medical abortion

Continuing pregnancy is reported after about 0.5–1.0% of early medical abortions with mifepristone-prostaglandin. Misoprostol (400 μg orally) is as effective as vaginal gemeprost (1 mg when the gestation is 49 days or less. Gemeprost (1 mg) and misoprostol (800 μg vaginally) are probably equally effective at 50–63 days but a randomized comparison has not been published. Women choosing early medical abortion must understand that the method can fail and that vacuum aspiration would then be appropriate. They must also be aware that all abortifacient drugs are potentially teratogenic. The importance of the follow-up examination 10–14 days after treatment with the prostaglandin must be emphasized both orally and in an information leaflet. There is no clear evidence that mifepristone causes fetal abnormality in pregnancies that continue and in which prostaglandin was not used;

but a Brazilian case-control study has suggested an association between misoprostol used for attempted clandestine abortion and neonatal abnormalities.[28]

Continuing pregnancy is most effectively detected at the follow-up consultation by ultrasound scan – vaginal examination is frequently inconclusive. Reliance should not be placed on a urinary pregnancy test as this may remain positive for at least 21 days even when the abortion has been successful.

After vacuum aspiration at less than seven weeks
This has been discussed above in the section on surgical abortion methods.

After vacuum aspiration at seven weeks or more
No large British study has been published but a review of 37,235 first-trimester abortions in the US reported 26 pregnancies that continued, an overall rate of 0.7 per 1000, and with rates at eight and at nine or more weeks of 0.47 and 0.38 per 1000, respectively.[29] To prevent this complication, the operator must always be certain that an appropriate volume of placental and fetal tissue has been removed from the uterine cavity (see above [Apparent failure to obtain fetal tissue]; and below [Routine inspection of the material evacuated from the uterus immediately after the abortion]).

Continuing pregnancy due to multiple pregnancy
A rare cause of pregnancy continuing after an apparently successful abortion is a twin conception when the suction cannula has removed one gestation sac but not the other. The frequency of such continuing pregnancies is unknown; however, I have unintentionally aspirated a known triplet pregnancy incompletely at nine weeks so that the amniotic sac and placentation of one fetus remained intact. The pregnancy was allowed to continue but miscarriage and early neonatal death from immaturity occurred at 23 weeks. It is easy to assume that an abortion is complete when the aspirate is voluminous and contains multiple fetal parts, and relatively difficult to assess by bimanual examination of the uterus after the aspiration that there is a remaining pregnancy.

Twin pregnancy but with separate implantations in the compartments of a congenitally abnormal uterus is another reason for pregnancy continuing after an apparently successful vacuum aspiration. A case report has been published in which this occurred following the termination of four separate twin pregnancies in a woman who proved to have a bicornuate uterus.[30]

Cervical injury
Incidence
Minor injury to the cervix occurs relatively frequently during mechanical dilatation. This ranges from a trivial tear in the anterior lip due to the vulsellum pulling off during dilatation, to a split in the side of the cervix that extends to or beyond the internal os. In the first trimester, vulsellum tears occur in at least 1/100 and tears needing suturing in about 1/1000 abortions.[1] The risk increases with gestation, and is at least twice as great with dilatation and evacuation in the second trimester.[31]

The consequences of cervical injury

Most injuries of the external cervical os are relatively trivial: they may predispose slightly to post-abortion infection but have no long-term significance. Injuries to the internal os can result in haemorrhage that can be difficult to control, and a high cervical tear may extend through the wall of the uterus to become a perforation. Injury to the internal os can result in cervical incompetence that predisposes to second-trimester miscarriage or pre-term labour in future wanted pregnancies. Early, uncontrolled studies[32,33] suggested that cervical incompetence was a relatively frequent consequence of first-trimester abortion; but larger, more sophisticated, research reported that the relative risk of a subsequent pregnancy ending unsuccessfully was negligible in parous women, and from 1.6 to 1.9 in those who were nulliparous at the time of their abortion.[34]

Reducing the risk of cervical injury

Cervical preparation has been shown to be effective in reducing the risk of cervical injury and is recommended by the RCOG[1] when the gestation is ten or more weeks or the woman is under the age of 18 – misoprostol (400 µg vaginally) given three hours before the abortion has been shown to be effective.[1] There is evidence from the US that cervical injury is much less likely if the an osmotic dilator (laminaria) had been used to prepare the cervix, if local rather than general anaesthesia was used, and if the operator was a senior member of staff rather than a trainee.[35] Further American research has shown that tapered Hawkins–Ambler dilators require less force to achieve cervical dilatation than the parallel-sided Hegar dilators that are used in many NHS units in the UK.[36,37]

Management of cervical injury

Vulsellum tears in the external os should be sutured if bleeding continues or if they are more than superficial. Deep tears should be probed to check that they are not associated with a perforation of the cervical canal and then closed using interrupted sutures. The control of severe haemorrhage from a high tear of the cervix can be difficult and require the urgent assistance of a specialist gynaecologist. Vaginal access may be possible by dissecting between the front of the cervix and the bladder but laparotomy may be necessary to allow ligation of the uterine artery on the affected side or, at the last resort, hysterectomy. Techniques under development may lessen the need for open surgery; these include the hysteroscopic use of electro-cautery or clips, embolism of the uterine artery under radiological control, and the laparoscopic application of clips to uterine blood vessels.

Uterine injury (perforation or rupture)

Incidence

All gynaecologists occasionally perforate the uterus during surgical abortion. The RCOG guideline suggests an average incidence of perforation of about 1.3 per 1000 abortions, with a range of 0.3–3.6 per 1000.[1] Many perforations may not be recognized clinically – in a study of 706 women having a first-trimester abortion followed immediately by a laparoscopic sterilization, two perforations were recognized during the abortion process and a further 12 were discovered during the subsequent laparoscopy, an overall incidence of 19.8/1000.[38] Rupture of the uterus as a result of drug-induced uterine contractions during second-trimester medical abortion is less frequent than perforation during surgical methods. It may occur in no more than 0.1 per 1000 abortions in women who have had no previous uterine surgery[11] but in up to 2% of those who have had a Caesarean section.[39] There is no information available so far on the risk of uterine rupture with the recently introduced mifepristone/prostaglandin method but this is likely to be less than with the older medical regimens.

How perforations happen

A relatively thin wall of soft uterine muscle surrounds a normally sited pregnancy. In the early stages of an abortion, the uterus is relaxed and the walls of the cavity are difficult to feel with the instruments. The uterine walls contract and become thicker and firmer as the pregnancy is removed. The force necessary to perforate the body of the uterus is small – so small that the operator is usually unaware that it has happened – the injury is detected when the next instrument meets little or no resistance and reaches an unexpected depth. In contrast to the uterus, the cervix consists of fibrous tissue and tends to resist dilatation. The internal os is the most vulnerable point and may split if too much force is applied during dilatation or if too great a degree of dilatation is attempted. Such a split may become a perforation if a further dilatation is attempted or, when the cervical canal is distended as fetal tissue is removed with evacuating forceps. It is also possible for the tip of an instrument, usually a small dilator, to make a false passage in the wall of the cervical canal if the internal os resists dilatation, or if the instrument is inadvertently directed not at the internal os itself but towards the wall of the cervical canal. The introduction of further instruments may then enlarge the false passage and lead to perforation.

The site and severity of the injuries

Many perforations are in the body of the uterus and are often small. These tend to cause relatively little haemorrhage unless they involve the major blood vessels on the lateral aspects of the uterus. Perforations of internal cervical os and the lower part of the uterus are more serious. Such injuries are often lateral and can involve the branches of the uterine artery and vein, with haematoma formation in the broad ligament or serious haemorrhage into the peritoneal cavity. There is a danger with all perforations that instruments may have passed through the perforation and damaged an abdominal organ such as intestine, ureter, urinary bladder or a major blood vessel. Injury to the intestine has been reported in from 3%[40] to 7.5%[41] of women with clinically significant perforations.

Risk factors for perforation

The experience of the operator

Trainees are more likely to perforate the uterus than experienced operators. The increase was fivefold in a large prospective study of surgical abortions from the US[40] and, in a large retrospective review of first-trimester abortions in Singapore, 82% of perforations were by junior medical staff.[41] Experience results not only in fewer perforations but also in early recognition of uterine injury so that there is less risk of the dangerous use of a suction cannula or grasping forceps in the woman's abdominal cavity.

Gestational age

Clinical studies from the US and Australia, and national notification data from England and Wales[11] show that perforation during surgical abortion increases with gestation and is about twice as frequent in the second as in the first trimester. There is a greater risk of haemorrhage and of injury to abdominal organs as gestation advances.

Previous Caesarean section or other uterine surgery

An American study of second-trimester medical abortion reported uterine rupture in 3.6% of women who had had a Caesarean section compared to 0.2% in those with an unscarred uterus.[42]

Position and attitude of the uterus

The perforation is more likely if the uterus is retroverted (angled backwards in relation to the long axis of the vagina), or if it is acutely anteflexed or retroflexed (referring to the angle between the long axes of the cervical canal and the body of the uterus). The uterus is usually anteverted and anteflexed and instruments such as uterine sounds and cervical dilators are made with a curve to assist in negotiating the vagino-uterine angle. All surgical abortions should begin with a bimanual examination to check the position of the uterus and then the gentle exploratory insertion of a uterine sound or a narrow dilator to detect anteflexion or retroflexion.

Managing serious uterine injury

The possibility of a perforation should be investigated as soon as the gynaecologist becomes aware that an instrument may have passed through the wall of the uterus.

Investigation

The perforation is confirmed by gentle exploration with a uterine sound. The anaesthetist should monitor pulse rate and blood pressure to detect any severe intra-abdominal haemorrhage. A urinary catheter should be passed to exclude damage to the bladder wall and to ensure it is empty. Operators with little personal experience of managing uterine injury should seek the immediate assistance of a senior colleague with the appropriate skill. It is safe practice to assess the severity of the injury using a laparoscope to view the abdominal aspect of the pelvic organs. It is important to appreciate that an apparently normal laparoscopic appearance does not necessarily mean that the bowel has not been injured – a probability of serious bowel injury should be investigated by laparotomy.

Management

Small perforations with little associated bleeding do not require repair. In such cases, an assistant can monitor the perforation through the laparoscope while the most experienced operator available completes the abortion by the vaginal route. This ensures that the evacuating instruments remain in the uterine cavity and cause no further damage. The woman can be allowed to recover from the anaesthetic without further action, providing there is no persistent haemorrhage and the perforating instruments were not used in a way that could have caused serious bowel injury. A stable pulse rate and normal temperature, blood pressure and bowel sounds during the next 24 hours are reassuring, but signs of bowel injury – abdominal pain, distension and vomiting, for example – can be delayed for several days. In a woman who is apparently recovering normally, it is reasonable for her to return home after 24 hours but with instructions to call for medical assessment if she develops symptoms. Some experienced gynaecologists manage perforations in the body of the uterus caused by a narrow blunt instrument, such as a uterine dilator or suction cannula, by observation alone and do not pass a laparoscope routinely – they complete the abortion cautiously, taking care that the instruments do not pass into the woman's uterine cavity. This benefits the majority of women who recover without needing abdominal surgery (laparoscopy has some risks), but the down-side is that the small number of women who prove to require laparotomy are likely to have increased morbidity because of the delay.

When is laparotomy necessary?

Laparotomy is necessary if laparoscopy shows continuing haemorrhage or an enlarging broad ligament haematoma, if the uterine perforation is large enough to require suturing, if it is probable that bowel has been damaged, or if the urinary tract requires repair. Only a gynaecologist with appropriate experience should undertake this. This means that women with a major injury who were having their abortion in a day unit or a small independent sector hospital should be assessed, resuscitated if necessary, and transferred for specialist care rather than have a laparotomy on site. All such units should have an arrangement that provides for immediate consultant advice and transfer to hospital when such emergencies occur. Experienced gynaecologists can usually repair the uterus but occasionally the damage is so great that hysterectomy is necessary. Hysterectomy is more likely if the surgeon was inexperienced, and if there was delay in opening the abdomen. This is because traumatized tissues rapidly become oedematous, dissection is impeded by extensive haematoma and the condition of the patient may have deteriorated because of inadequate blood volume replacement. In the report from the US referred to above,[40] 9% of women who had a clinically recognized perforation had a hysterectomy – a rate of seven per 100,000 abortions.

Long-term consequences of a uterine perforation

Reliable information is lacking because serious uterine injury is so uncommon and long-term follow-up is difficult to achieve. Case reports show there is a small risk of uterine rupture in future wanted pregnancies. The risk after a small perforation is probably less than after lower-section Caesarean section – perhaps 1% – but could be greater if the uterine injury was extensive and repair difficult. Women should be warned of the possibility of uterine rupture in a future pregnancy and told to tell their obstetrician that the uterus was injured during an abortion. Knowledge of the scar in the uterus will make an obstetrician more likely to recommend a Caesarean section if a future labour proves to be slower than average. Midwives and obstetricians should be alert for signs and symptoms of uterine rupture in such women, both in the second half of pregnancy and in labour. Apart from the risk of uterine rupture, there is a possibility that fertility might be reduced by any adhesions forming around the uterine tubes and ovaries.

Haemorrhage

Incidence

Haemorrhage – defined either as a need for blood transfusion or as a loss exceeding 500 ml – complicates about one in 1000 abortions in the first trimester. The incidence increases with gestation and is about eight per 1000 at 20 or more weeks.[1] Haemorrhage is more likely with medical methods than with surgical methods.

Causes of excessive blood loss

Failure of the uterus to contract

This occurs occasionally without any apparent cause but usually is associated with general anaesthesia, particularly with inhalational agents that relax the uterus, such as halothane,[43] enflurane[44] and trilene. A randomized controlled trial has shown that total blood loss is reduced and clinically significant haemorrhage is less frequent when local anaesthesia is used.[45]

Uterine injury

Brisk bright haemorrhage when the uterus is found to be firm and contracted suggests damage to the internal os or lower lateral uterine wall. A probe should be used to search for a perforation but further action is not necessary providing the rate of loss becomes acceptable in the course of a few minutes. Otherwise, the management is as described above for uterine injury.

Incomplete abortion

Haemorrhage may persist because the abortion is incomplete but this is uncommon – the uterus will usually contract around the remaining products and the rate of blood loss will then appear within normal limits.

Abnormalities of placentation

A small clinical study has shown that placenta praevia is associated with a small increase in mean blood loss during second-trimester abortion by dilatation and evacuation but with no rise in the need for blood transfusion.[46] In contrast, placenta accreta results in severe haemorrhage that may be controllable only by expert abdominal surgery.[47] Placenta accreta is very rare except in association with placenta praevia and previous Caesarean section. A clinical study of women with placenta praevia at term reported that 5% had placenta accreta but that this increased to 27% or more in women who had had one or more previous Caesarean sections.[48] This suggests that women who have had a Caesarean section should have an ultrasound scan before a second-trimester abortion. This has not become standard practice because of the difficulties of the ultrasound diagnosis of placenta praevia in the second trimester and the expertise necessary to recognize placenta accreta. Nevertheless, there is a need to warn women who have had a Caesarean section that there is an increased risk of haemorrhage and of emergency abdominal surgery.

Disseminated intravascular coagulopathy

This is a rare cause of life-threatening haemorrhage that complicates about one in 12,500 first-trimester and 1 in 500 second-trimester abortions.[49] Disseminated intravascular coagulopathy (DIC) should be suspected if there is persistent excessive bleeding from the uterus, the blood fails to clot, and venipuncture points ooze and are surrounded by subcutaneous bruising. DIC was particularly associated with second trimester medical abortion by methods such as the intra-amniotic injection of hypertonic urea and prostaglandin but can also be a consequence of continued severe blood loss from other causes. The risk with mifepristone/vaginal prostaglandin methods has not been established; but no cases have occurred in the published reports, and it is probable that the efficiency of the abortion process, and the absence of any invasion of the uterine cavity reduces the risk considerably. DIC is an uncommon complication of second-trimester abortion by dilatation and evacuation but may be rather more frequent when the two-stage method is used at 20 or more weeks. The cause of DIC is uncertain. Hypothetically, amniotic fluid, trophoblast or fetal tissue may have been forced into an open maternal vein in the uterine wall. The risk of DIC may be higher if the fetus is dead at the time of the abortion.

Management of excessive blood loss

Haemorrhage from the uterus can usually be controlled by inducing a contraction by bimanual massage of the uterus, and by the intravenous injection of oxytocin (5–10 U). Any inappropriate anaesthetic agent should be withdrawn. The uterine contraction can be maintained by Syntometrine® (Alliance; oxytocin 5 U: ergometrine 0.5 mg), or ergometrine 0.5 mg, by intramuscular injection. If blood loss continues in spite of these measures, an intravenous infusion of normal saline should be used to maintain circulating volume and compatible blood for transfusion arranged urgently. Occasionally, uncross-matched antibody-screened group O rhesus negative blood has to be given until compatible blood is available. Monitoring should always include pulse rate and blood pressure and central venous pressure should be included if significant blood loss continues. The possibility of unsuspected uterine injury should be considered (see above [Uterine injury]). If uterine injury is unlikely, other treatments that increases uterine tone should be tried, such as the insertion of 800 μg of misoprostol into the uterine cavity or the upper vagina; carboprost (250 μg) by deep intramuscular injection repeated at intervals of 15 minutes or more for a maximum of eight doses; the injection into the cervical tissue of oxytocin (10 U); the intravenous infusion of oxytocin 50 mU/min. An intra-uterine pack can be helpful but should be removed after about four hours – recurrent bleeding is not likely and there is a risk of infection if it is left in place. DIC is an emergency that requires the immediate advice of a consultant haematologist. Early transfer to an intensive care unit should be arranged if dangerous blood loss persists, or if abdominal surgery is likely to be necessary because of uterine injury.

Reducing the risk of clinically significant haemorrhage
Delay in providing the abortion

Clinically significant haemorrhage, although uncommon, becomes more frequent as gestation increases.

Method of anaesthesia
General anaesthesia should be administered by an anaesthetist with experience of the special requirements of abortion surgery. The regimen should be chosen to minimize relaxation of the uterus – typically, this would be an intravenous agent such as propofol or methohexitone, supplemented with intravenous fentanyl and inhaled nitrous oxide and oxygen. This is particularly important for dilatation and evacuation in the second trimester. Local anaesthesia should be available as an option in the first trimester – many women find this acceptable but there is always discomfort and some women have quite severe pain.

Use of oxytocic agents
The routine administration of oxytocin (10 U intravenously) at the beginning of an abortion by vacuum aspiration significantly reduces blood loss[50] but the mean reduction is small and clinically insignificant. Practice varies – many operators do not inject oxytocin routinely, particularly when local anaesthesia is used. None of the published studies is large enough to show if routine oxytocin reduces the occurrence of clinically significant haemorrhage. Oxytocin for intravenous injection, and ergometrine or Syntometrine® for intramuscular injection, should be always be immediately available for the treatment of excessive haemorrhage. Ergometrine (and ergometrine-containing mixtures) are no longer licensed for intravenous use because of an association with vasospasm, causing a rise in blood pressure and, rarely, coronary occlusion or cerebral haemorrhage.

Incomplete abortion

How an abortion is judged to be complete
It is never possible to be completely certain that an abortion by vacuum aspiration is complete. The instruments are passed through a cervical opening 6–12 mm wide into a relatively large cavity that is surrounded by a soft vulnerable wall of uterine muscle. The uterine muscle contracts and the cavity becomes smaller as the pregnancy is evacuated. The abortion is judged to be complete from the amount of material that has been seen passing though the semi-translucent cannula and the feeling that the cannula is now contained in a small space with a firm granular surface. Some operators use a small curette or a narrow pair of evacuating (polyp) forceps to check that no further fragments of membrane or fetal tissue can be removed. A bimanual examination is now made to confirm that the uterus is firm and much reduced in size. But a minor degree of incomplete evacuation is still possible. This is not detectable either from the size of the uterus or from an inspection of the fragments of fetus and trophoblast in the suction bottle. Complete removal of the fetus is easier to determine during second-trimester abortions by dilatation and evacuation – the fetal parts are large and easy to recognize, but there may still be some uncertainty whether the entire placenta has been obtained.

Routine inspection of the material evacuated from the uterus immediately after the abortion
The introduction of policies to safeguard staff from infection with the HIV and hepatitis viruses has resulted in the development of closed disposable systems for vacuum

aspiration of the uterus, and has discouraged routine immediate examination of the sieved and washed contents of the suction bottle. Until the past few years, such examination was considered mandatory – to confirm that there had been a pregnancy, that the abortion was reasonably complete, and to diagnose relatively rare abnormalities such as hydatidiform change in the trophoblast. Some experienced operators now consider that routine examination of the material removed is unnecessary. But, inspection remains essential if the volume of material removed seems too small, or when the tissue appears to be abnormal. Under these circumstances, the contents of the suction bottle must be inspected immediately and safe facilities for this must be available within the operating suite. Routine histological examination of the tissues obtained at abortion has little clinical value.[51] But tissue must be sent for histological examination when placental pathology, such as hydatidiform change, is suspected or if an apparent absence of products of conception suggests an extra-uterine pregnancy.

Early medical abortion

Many clinicians do not check the material passed by women having early medical abortion. The pregnancy tissues are mixed with blood clot and the small fetus is difficult to find. In practice, complete abortion results in a marked reduction in bleeding and pain, and persistence of bleeding and pain indicate that the abortion has not happened or is incomplete. It has proved to be safe to allow women to return home once the acute reaction to the prostaglandin is over – most will have aborted by then but some will expel the pregnancy at home and some will be readmitted because of persistent symptoms. An early medical abortion service must have a help line that can arrange assessment and surgical evacuation if necessary. Completeness of the abortion is assessed at the follow-up clinic from the absence of pain, the slow reduction in blood loss and the finding of a small firm uterus. Any uncertainty is resolved by an ultrasound scan.

Second-trimester medical abortion

With medical abortion in the second trimester, the fetus is large and intact, and it is usually easy to judge whether the placenta has been completely expelled.

Incidence of incomplete abortion

Vacuum aspiration

A review of nine clinical studies of 500 or more first-trimester abortions by vacuum aspiration reported re-evacuation in from 0.35–2.9%.[1] The rates below 1% were obtained from specialist abortion-providing organizations with experienced gynaecologists that had a large caseload and serve a large area (but probably have incomplete follow-up data). The higher rates were associated with hospital-based gynaecological services in which some operators were trainees, with a relatively low caseload, and in which complications were managed within the providing service. On balance, it can be assumed that a re-evacuation rate of about 1% is associated with an acceptable standard of care.

Dilatation and evacuation

There are no large British studies of re-evacuation after dilatation and evacuation in the second trimester. An American study of 9527 abortions at 13–16 weeks reported a rate of 0.7%.[52]

Second-trimester medical abortion

Recent clinical experience with second-trimester medical methods suggests that no more than 10% of women will have enough retained products to require a uterine evacuation before they return home.[14]

Infection

Infection is the most important cause of post-abortion morbidity and may result in infertility and dispose to extra-uterine pregnancy. Without the screening or prophylaxis with antibiotics recommended by the RCOG,[1] up to 4% of women develop clinically significant pelvic infection in the month after the abortion (a temperature of 38^0C, abdominal pain. and uterine tenderness). Infection is more frequent in women under 20, and in those with multiple partners, clinical cervicitis/vaginitis or with previous pelvic infection. Prompt treatment of acute pelvic infection often results in complete recovery with normal fertility, However, research in Sweden has shown that one attack of laparoscopically proved acute salpingitis was followed by tubal infertility in 13% of patients and that the risk of extra-uterine pregnancy was considerably increased.[53]

Most infections are due to sexually transmitted organisms that were being carried in the lower genital tract, the most frequent of which is *Chlamydia trachomatis*. Some are due to the chance carriage in the vagina of the group B streptococcus, or to the various anaerobes that are normally found in the rectum and peri-anal areas. Pre-abortion screening for chlamydia is practicable but the limited nature of the screening possible in an abortion clinic, and the reluctance of women to attend elsewhere for full investigation,[54] means that all women, whatever their chlamydia status, should be offered prophylactic antibiotics. Unfortunately, the routine use of an antibiotic by unscreened women does no more than halve the rate of post-abortion infection.[55] All women found to carry a sexually transmitted microorganism or who develop an infection must be encouraged to persuade their sexual partners to attend a genito-urinary medicine clinic for investigation and treatment.

Psychological effects of abortion

Immediately after abortion, some women are almost euphoric with relief that a traumatic experience is over but others react with distress and may weep. This reflects the ambivalence that women feel; the abortion was necessary but the need is regretted. In the following weeks, up to 50% have some depression but this usually resolves without professional help. There have been no formal studies of the value of pre-abortion counselling. There is no evidence for an incapacitating post-abortion syndrome.[56] The published reports of the long-term psychological effects of abortion, and of women who had to continue unwanted pregnancies, were comprehensively reviewed by Dagg.[57] He wrote, 'Adverse sequelae occur in a minority of women, and when such symptoms occur, they usually seem to be the continuation of symptoms that appeared before the abortion, and are on the wane immediately after the abortion. Many women denied abortion show ongoing resentment that may last for years, while children born when the abortion is denied have numerous broadly based difficulties in social, interpersonal and occupational functions that last at least into early adulthood'. A large British prospective controlled study has shown that in previously healthy women psychiatric illness was no more likely after induced abortion than after giving birth at term.[58] Professional advice and support-counselling should be available for women with distress after abortion; however, few women take up offers of such help when it is made routinely at the time of the termination.

References

1   Royal College of Obstetricians and Gynaecologists (RCOG). *The Care of Women Requesting Induced Abortion.* London, 2000.
2   Royal College of Anaesthetists and The Association of Anaesthetists of Great Britain and Northern Ireland. *Good Practice – A Guide for Departments of Anaesthesia.* London, 1998.
3   Royal College of Nursing. *Guidelines on the Termination of Pregnancy.* London, 1997.
4   Department of Health. *Procedures for the Approval of Independent Sector Places for the Termination of Pregnancy.* London: HMSO, 1999.
5   R v Smith [1974] 1 All ER 376.
6   World Health Organization. *Constitution (1946).* London, 1985.
7   RCOG. *Termination of Pregnancy for Fetal Abnormality in England and Wales.* London, 1996.
8   Medical Ethics Department: British Medical Association. *The Law and Ethics of Abortion.* London, 1997.
9   Janaway v Salford HA [1988] All ER 1051 HL.
10 Paton v BPAS [1978] 2 All ER 987.
11 Office for National Statistics. *Abortion Statistics 1998 Series AB No. 25.* London: The Stationery Office, 1999.
12 Pedersen JF. Fetal crown–rump length measurement by ultrasound in normal pregnancy. *British Journal of Obstetrics & Gynaecology* 1982; 89: 926–930.
13 Chitty LS, Altman DG, Henderson A, Campbell S. Charts of fetal size: 2. Head measurements. *British Journal of Obstetrics and Gynaecology* 1994; 101: 35–43.
14 Ashok PW, Templeton AT. Nonsurgical mid-trimester termination of pregnancy: a review of 500 consecutive cases. *British Journal of Obstetrics & Gynaecology* 1999; 106: 706–710.
15 Bitsch M, Jakobsen AB, Prien-Larsen JC, Frølund C, Sederberg-Olsen J. IUD (Nova T) insertion following induced abortion. *Contraception* 1990; 42: 315–322.
16 RCOG. *Male and Female Sterilisation.* London, 1999.
17 Medico-Legal Committee: RCOG. *How to Avoid Medico-Legal Problems.* London, 1992.
18 Queenan JT, Kubarych SF, Shah S, Holland B. Role of induced abortion in rhesus immunisation. *Lancet* 1971; i: 815–817.
19 Creinin MD, Edwards J. Early abortion: surgical and medical options. *Current Problems in Obstetrics Gynecology & Fertility* 1997; 20(1): 1–32.
20 Rodger MW, Baird DT. Treatment with mifepristone (RU486) reduces the interval between prostaglandin administration and expulsion in second-trimester abortion. *British Journal of Obstetrics and Gynaecology* 1990; 97: 41–45.
21 Lelaidier C, Baton C, Benifla JL, Fernandez H, Bourquet P, Frydman R. Mifepristone for labour induction after previous Caesarean section. *British Journal of Obstetrics & Gynaecology* 1994; 101: 501–503.
22 Darney P, Sweet R. Routine intraoperative ultrasonography for second trimester abortion reduces incidence of uterine perforation. *Journal of Ultrasound Medicine* 1989; 8: 71–75.
23 Mann RD. Unlicensed medicines and the use of drugs in unlicensed indications. In Goldberg A, Smith I (eds.) *Pharmaceutical Medicine & the Law.* London: Royal College of Physicians, 1991: 103–110.
24 Munsick RA. Clinical test for placenta in 300 consecutive menstrual aspirations. *Obstetrics & Gynecology* 1982; 60: 738–741.
25 Valle RF, Sabbagha RE. Management of first trimester pregnancy termination failures. *Obstetrics & Gynecology* 1980; 55: 625–629.
26 Edwards J, Carson SA. New technologies permit safe abortion at less than six weeks' gestation and provide timely detection of ectopic gestation. *American Journal of Obstetrics & Gynecology* 1997; 176: 1101–1106.
27 Thyssen HH, Christensen H, Schebye O *et al.* Elimination of human chorionic gonadotropin in serum and urine after uncomplicated induced abortion during the first trimester (English translation). *Ugeskrift for Laeger* 1992; 154: 2071–2072.
28 Gonzalez CH, Marques-Dias MJ, Kim CA *et al.* Congenital abnormalities in Brazilian children associated with Misoprostol misuse in first trimester pregnancy. *Lancet* 1998; 351: 1624–1627.
29 Fielding WL, Lee S-Y, Borten M, Friedman EA. Continued pregnancy after failed first trimester abortion. *Obstetrics & Gynecology* 1984; 63: 421–424.

30   Mukhopadhyay M, Killick SR, Guthrie K, Speck E. A bizarre history in a woman requesting repeat termination of pregnancy. *Journal of Obstetrics & Gynaecology* 2000; 20(2): 200.

31   Peterson WF, Berry FN, Grace MR, Gulbranson CL. Second trimester abortion by dilatation and evacuation: an analysis of 11,747 cases. *Obstetrics & Gynecology* 1983; 62: 185–189.

32   Wright CS, Campbell S, Beazley J. Second-trimester abortion after vaginal termination of pregnancy. *Lancet* 1972; 1: 1278–1279.

33   Richardson JA, Dixon G. Effects of legal termination on subsequent pregnancy. *BMJ* 1976; 1: 1303–1304.

34   Harlap S, Shiono PH, Ramcharan S, Berendes H, Pellegrin F. A prospective study of spontaneous fetal losses after induced abortions. *New England Journal of Medicine* 1979; 301(13): 677–681.

35   Schulz KF, Grimes DA, Cates W Jr. Measures to prevent cervical injury during suction curettage abortion. *Lancet* 1983; i: 1182–1185.

36   Hulka JF. Pratt dilators: resistance at 9 mm is an instrumentation artifact. *American Journal of Obstetrics & Gynecology* 1988; 159: 166–174.

37   Hulka JF, Lefler HT Jr., Anglone A, Lachenbruch PA. A new electronic force monitor to measure factors influencing cervical dilation for vacuum curettage. *American Journal of Obstetrics & Gynecology* 1974; 120: 166–173.

38   Kaali SG, Szigetvari IA, Bartfai GS. The frequency and management of uterine perforations during first trimester abortions. *American Journal of Obstetrics & Gynecology.* 1989; 161: 406–408.

39   Atienza MF, Burkman RT, King TM. Midtrimester abortion induced by hyperosmolar urea and prostaglandin F2a in patients with previous Cesarean section: clinical course and potential for uterine rupture. *American Journal of Obstetrics & Gynecology* 1980; 138: 55–59.

40   Grimes DA, Schulz KF, Cates WJ Jr. Prevention of uterine perforation during curettage abortion. *Journal of the American Medical Association* 1984; 251: 2108–2111.

41   Chen LH, Lai SF, Lee WH, Leong NK. Uterine perforation during elective first trimester abortions: a 13-year review. *Singapore Medical Journal* 1995; 36: 63–67.

42   Chapman SJ, Crispens M, Owen J, Savage K. Complications of mid-trimester pregnancy termination: the effect of prior Cesarean delivery. *American Journal of Obstetrics & Gynecology* 1996; 177(4): 889–892.

43   Cullen B, Margolis A, Eger EI II. The effects of anesthesia and pulmonary ventilation on blood loss during elective therapeutic abortion. *Anesthesiology* 1970; 32: 108–113.

44   Hall J, Ng W, Smith S. Blood loss during first trimester termination of pregnancy: comparison of two anaesthetic techniques. *British Journal of Anaesthesia* 1997; 78: 172–174.

45   Andolsek L, Cheng M, Hren M *et al.* The safety of local anesthesia and outpatient treatment: a controlled study of induced abortion by vacuum aspiration. *Studies in Family Planning* 1977; 8: 118–124.

46   Thomas AG, Alvarez M, Friedman F Jr., Brodman ML, Kim J, Lockwood C. The effect of placenta previa on blood loss in second-trimester pregnancy termination. *Obstetrics & Gynecology* 1994; 84: 58–60.

47   Rashbaum W, Gates E, Jones J, Goldman B, Morris A, Lyman WD. Placenta accreta encountered during dilatation and evacuation in the second trimester. *Obstetrics & Gynecology* 1995; 85: 701–703.

48   Clark SL, Koonings PP, Phelan JP. Placenta previa/accreta and prior Cesarean section. *Obstetrics & Gynecology* 1985; 66(1): 89–92.

49   Kafrissen ME, Barke MW, Workman P, Shultz KF, Grimes DA. Coagulopathy and induced abortion methods: rates and relative risks. *American Journal of Obstetrics & Gynecology* 1983; 147: 344–345.

50   Ali PB, Smith G. The effect of syntocinon on blood loss during first trimester suction curettage. *Anaesthesia* 1996; 51: 483–485.

51   Heath V, Chadwick V, Cooke I, Manek S, MacKenzie IZ. Should tissue from pregnancy termination and uterine evacuation routinely be examined histologically? *British Journal of Obstetrics & Gynaecology* 2000; 107: 727–730.

52   Kafrissen ME, Schulz KF, Grimes DA, Cates W Jr. Mid-trimester abortion: intra-amniotic instillation or hyperosmolar urea and prostaglandin $F_{2\alpha}$ v dilatation and evacuation. *Journal of the American Medical Association* 1984; 251: 916–919.

53   Lim BH, Lees DAR, Bjornsson S *et al.* Normal development after exposure to Mifepristone in early pregnancy. *Lancet* 1990; 336: 257–258.

54   Penney GC, Thomson M, Norman J *et al.* A randomised comparison of strategies for reducing infective complications of induced abortion. *British Journal of Obstetrics & Gynaecology* 1998; 105: 599–604.

55   Sawaya GF, Grady D, Kerlikowske K, Grimes DA. Antibiotics at the time of induced abortion: the case of universal prophylaxis based on a meta-analysis. *Obstetrics and Gynaecology* 1996; 87: 884–890.

56   Stotland NL. The myth of the abortion trauma syndrome. *Journal of the American Medical Association* 1992; 268: 2078–2079.

57   Dagg PKB. The psychological sequelae of therapeutic abortion – denied and completed. *American Journal of Psychiatry* 1991; 148: 578–585.

58   Gilchrist AC, Hannaford PC, Frank P, Kay CR. Termination of pregnancy and psychiatric morbidity. *British Journal of Psychiatry* 1995; 167: 243–248.

►19

Fertility and Assisted Conception

Gillian M Lockwood and David H Barlow

The epidemic of infertility

In most branches of gynaecology, a great source of anxiety for the clinician stems from unwanted or inadvertently preserved fertility. However, about one in six couples seek specialist help because of difficulty or delay in conceiving a first or subsequent child. Hence, the problem of infertility and the preservation of fertility will continue to play a significant and increasing role in the consultation load.

There are several reasons for the current apparent 'epidemic of infertility'. The human species is relatively inefficient at reproducing itself and there is a fairly narrow window of opportunity in a woman's life in which she is reasonably fecund. Although about half of couples having regular unprotected intercourse will have conceived within three months of discontinuing contraception and approaching 90% will have conceived within a year, the rapid, age-related decline in natural fertility in women is increasingly apparent. Current demographic trends towards delayed child-bearing due to career or financial pressures, in conjunction with a high rate of divorce, which results in many women seeking to conceive in a new partnership and at an older age, contribute to this picture. In the UK, 12% of live births are to women aged 35 years or older and *first* live births to women 35 years old or older now account for 7% of all births. Moreover, the option of adoption, especially of a *baby*, is no longer available, except to a tiny minority of childless couples. This situation is due, in part, to the wide availability of effective contraception and the provision of legal termination for unwanted pregnancy. With wider social acceptance of single motherhood, there is less pressure on unsupported women to give up their babies for adoption.

The main predictive factors for successful pregnancy in infertile couples undertaking assisted conception are the female partner's age, the duration of infertility, previous reproductive history and sperm quality. The media attention given to the conspicuous success of 'state-of-the-art' fertility treatments has also encouraged many couples, who in former years would quietly have tolerated their childlessness or claimed it was voluntary, to request access to investigation and treatment.

The prime role of counselling in infertility

Fundamental to the treatment of infertility, whether or not 'high tech' solutions eventually need to be adopted, is the role played by counselling of the infertile couple.

It may appear, during the course of investigations, that one or other partner is primarily 'responsible' for their problem of infertility. However, it is vital that the couple's state of childlessness is seen as a 'shared' problem and the attribution of sole responsibility should be avoided in all but the most overt cases. This position is supported by recognition of the fact that in at least one-third of all cases of infertility, there are mutifactorial causes predisposing to a fertility problem.

Considered overall, and given ready access to available techniques and resources, it is likely that modern fertility practice can achieve successful pregnancies for about two-thirds of all couples referred for treatment. But provision of fertility services within the NHS has reflected a view, held by both the general public and the medical profession, that scarce resources should be directed preferentially at life-saving and disability-relieving indications, and this has resulted in significant under funding of fertility provision.

Compared with other European countries, where techniques such as *in vitro* fertilization (IVF) are generally provided to most eligible couples at little, or no, cost as part of a national or insurance-based healthcare package, NHS provision in the UK is funded at a low level. Less than 10% of IVF cycles are publicly funded and there is wide regional variation in the level of provision. This situation has led to the proliferation of private provision of fertility care, and private ART (artificial reproductive technology) centres have often been at the forefront of scientific developments in the field of infertility research. Nowadays, the vast majority of patients undergoing treatments such as IVF are fee-paying consumers rather than NHS recipients of medical services.

The recent referral of the tertiary Royal College of Gynaecologists (RCOG) guidelines (which recommend that ART should be available on the NHS for specific clinical indications) to NICE (National Institute of Clinical Excellence) may indicate that wider provision of fertility treatments on the NHS is being considered.

This trend has rightly focused on the need for audit of fertility care provision in both the public and private sectors. Clinicians involved in the provision of fertility services must be ever conscious of the need to strike a balance between offering hope to childless couples and not raising unrealistic expectations in a potentially highly vulnerable social group. One of the most important undertakings of the HFEA (Human Fertility and Embryology Authority) is to provide information (including individual clinic's 'success rates') for all the licensed IVF clinics in the UK, to facilitate patient choice.

Patient autonomy and infertility

Patients seeking help with a fertility problem are quite unusual in that the treatment they seek is elective, optional and voluntary. They are not 'ill' by any usual definition of illness (although their infertility may have an underlying pathological cause), and yet a medical solution to their 'problem' is likely to have a greater impact on their lives than almost any other medical intervention. Fertility patients need a high level of information about options for investigation and treatment and are often extremely well informed about their diagnosis and about the therapies that could help them. Fertility patients also differ from 'normal' patients in that their expectations about any course of treatment are likely to be unrealistically high. Achieving successful pregnancy is an 'all or none' event and so 'failure' in any given cycle of treatment (which, even with very successful treatments such as IVF, occurs in 75% of cycles) results in devastating disappointment. It is simply not possible to have infertility 'symptoms' improved by anything other than a baby, whereas in other conditions a less than totally successful operation may nevertheless provide palliation or improved quality of life. In addition, fertility patients are particularly sensitive to any implication that they are in some sense responsible for their childlessness; that aspects of their lifestyle – such as deliberate delay in embarking on a pregnancy or previous termination of unplanned or ill-timed pregnancies – might be involved in their failure to conceive. They are usually suffering anyway from feelings of guilt or remorse, and treating this morbidity with appropriate counselling and sympathy is often just as important as the ability to diagnose and treat their fertility problem.

Normal fertility and assisted conception

The graphs below (Figures 19.1–19.4) show the basic parameters of fertility, within which all fertility treatments, including IVF, must operate

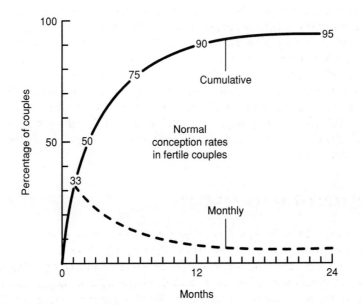

Fig. 19.1. Graph of highest conception rates in a normal population of proven fertility during the first two years of trying.

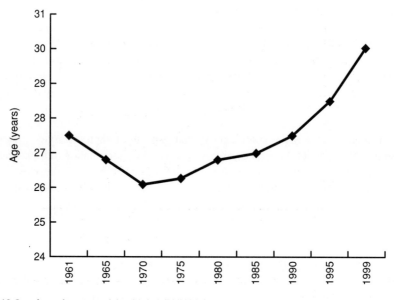

Fig. 19.2. Age of women giving birth (all UK births).

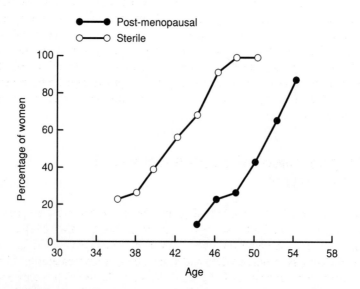

Fig.19.3. Proportion of British women with 'biological infertility' and menopause. Biological infertility commences ten years before menopause.

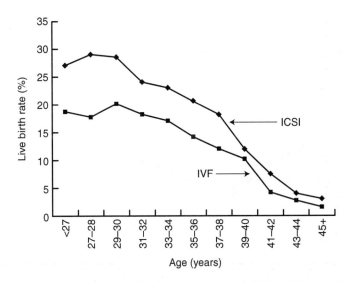

Fig. 19.4. IVF live birth rates by female age (using own eggs): IVF and intracytoplasmic sperm injection (ICSI) (HFEA UK data).

Confidentiality and the investigation of infertility

During history taking and routine investigation, factors related to one partner's medical or reproductive history may emerge that are not known by the other partner. For example, eliciting a history of previous undisclosed paternity, termination of pregnancy, sexually transmitted disease (STD) or even sterilization may involve a breach of confidence between couples. Early on in the course of infertility consultations, it is therefore vital that an opportunity is made for the partners to be seen separately; and where significant features emerge, patients should be asked if their partners are aware of these facts. In order to provide optimal care, both partners should be encouraged to register with the same GP so that any such issues may be resolved and investigations coordinated.

Infertility treatment when pregnancy itself presents dangers

There are many medical conditions that may be exacerbated by pregnancy – for example: diabetes, multiple sclerosis, hypertension, renal disease, myotonic dystrophy, cardiac dysfunction, post-transplant immunosuppression, acquired immunodeficiency syndrome (AIDS) and systemic lupus erythematosus (SLE). In all circumstances, the clinician is obliged to consider the possible consequences of achieving pregnancy for his patient, especially where complex techniques involving superovulation and IVF are required. Even for women enjoying good health, pregnancy may present predictable hazards and the latest Confidential Enquiry has highlighted the marked excess maternal mortality rate amongst mothers over the age of 40. The technique of ovum donation, which permits technically post-menopausal women to become pregnant via IVF, may be contra-indicated on general medical grounds. Where complex fertility treatments are not required, clinicians may be reluctant to counsel young patients with chronic diseases about the wisdom of embarking on a pregnancy that may significantly worsen their prognosis. Where women with such conditions require treatments such as IVF or egg donation to achieve pregnancy, the health consequences for the woman and the prospect that she may not survive to see her child reach independence should be discussed before treatment is undertaken. Advice of an ethics committee and/or the support of counselling also should be sought.

Role of genetic counselling

Fundamental to these more general issues is the role of genetic considerations. Historically, most conditions associated with very poor health outlook, such as cystic fibrosis, Duchenne muscular dystropy, renal failure, haemophilia and Kartegener's Syndrome, were incompatible with reproductive success. However, improved medical care now offers these individuals the chance of living beyond their teens and the new reproductive technologies (especially intracytoplasmic sperm injection [ICSI]–IVF) offer the chance of biological parenthood to individuals with significant inheritable health problems. ICSI is a method of fertilizing eggs *in vitro* by the injection of a single sperm into the cytoplasm of each egg. Therefore, men with extremely poor sperm parameters, whose sperm could never have achieved fertilization even with conventional IVF, or azoospermic men, from whom sperm may be surgically recovered directly from the testis, may be able to father pregnancies via IVF. Where severe sperm dysfunction or azoospermia is associated with a genetic defect such as in the oligospermia found in men with a gene deletion on the Y chromosome, or congenital bilateral absence of the vas deferens (CBAVD), as seen in some cystic fibrosis carriers, there is a significant risk that any male offspring could inherit a similar or more severe genetic problem. Patients with sex-chromosome abnormalities, such as Turner's Syndrome (XO) in women or Klinefelter's Syndrome (XXY) in men, can be helped to achieve pregnancy via IVF with donated eggs and ICSI–IVF, respectively. There has been some concern regarding the apparent small excess of sex chromosome and gonadal abnormalities in babies born following the ICSI procedure. However the vast majority of couples would rather accept these risks for the chance of achieving a pregnancy that was genetically entirely their own, than resort to using donated gametes.

Modern techniques of prenatal diagnosis (eg chorionic villus sampling [CVS], maternal serum screening, amniocentesis, cordocentesis and anomaly scanning) can now be augmented by pre-implantation genetic diagnosis (PGD) in which a single blastomere from an early fertilized embryo can be analysed for its chromosomal structure (using fluorescent *in situ* hybridization [FISH]) or for specific gene defects (using the polymerase chain reaction [PCR]). Only embryos with a normal genetic composition then would be transferred to the womb and the couple would be confident that if implantation and pregnancy *were* achieved that prenatal diagnosis leading to therapeutic termination would not be necessary.

Fertility treatment as a 'ladder of assistance'

Contemporary fertility treatment is best regarded as a 'ladder of assistance', in which the lowest rungs are perhaps the most important, not least because they offer significant opportunities for early and successful intervention. The ladder shown below (Table 19.1) illustrates the hierarchy of therapies available to the

Table 19.1. The 'ladder of assistance'.

Indication	Therapy	
Premature ovarian failure (POF) Menopause	'Extraordinary procedures'	Ovum donation
Uterine anomaly or absence	Host surrogacy	IVF
Very severe male factor	Micromanipulation IVF	ICSI
Azoospermia	Surgical sperm retrieval	PESA, TESA
	Donor insemination (DI)	
Blocked tubes Cervical hostility Endometriosis Idiopathic infertility	Extracorporeal fertilization	IVF–ET*
Oglio/asthenozoospermia Anti-sperm antibodies	Extracorporeal gamete enhancement	GIFT, ZIFT, IUI
Anovulation Oligo-ovulation PCOS	Superovulation Ovulation induction Secondary investigation	Anti-oestrogens Gonadotrophins Laparoscopy Hysteroscopy HSG, PCT
	Primary investigation	Day 21 progesterone Hormone profile Semen analysis
	Counselling and general health advice	

PESA = percutaneous sperm aspiration; TESA = testicular sperm aspiration; ICSI = intracytoplasmic sperm injection; IVF–ET = *in vitro* fertilization and embryo transfer; GIFT = gamete intrafallopian transfer; ZIFT = zygote intrafallopian transfer; IUI = intrauterine insemination; HSG = hysterosal pinogram; PCT = postcoital test.

infertile couple, although it must be recognised that treatment has to be guided both by the clinical findings on examination and investigation, and by the couple's own wishes.

The graph below (Figure 19.5) shows the cumulative conception rates resulting from conventional management of couples with a single cause of infertility, compared with conception rates for the normally fertile. It is clear that the ovulatory disorders and idiopathic/unexplained infertility have the best chance of responding to relatively simple procedures such as ovulation induction and IUI (intrauterine insemination). However, great progress has been made in IVF in the past ten years, particularly since the introduction of the micromanipulation techniques such as ICSI. Now, even patients with irremediably blocked fallopian tubes or severe sperm disorders can be offered a chance of pregnancy that is as high as that in each cycle of treatment, as a normally fertile couple trying to conceive

In infertility, as in other non-acute specialities, time is a great healer; and in many specialist referral centres that operate a 'waiting list' system of appointments post-referral, up to 20% of potential fertility patients never attend their first appointment because pregnancy has intervened or the couple have achieved a spontaneous pregnancy during initial investigations. However, fertility specialists are well-advised to consider the speed at which intervention should be suggested and offered. Age, cause and duration of infertility taken together with female follicular phase follicle-stimulating hormone (FSH) levels and female gynaecological and family reproductive history all should be taken into account. Since women in their late thirties and early forties have such a significantly lower success rate, not only in

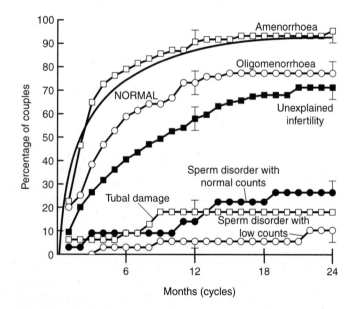

Fig. 19.5. Cumulative conception rates resulting from conventional management of couples with a single cause of fertility.

achieving pregnancy, but also in successful pregnancy outcome, expeditious referral for specialist opinion and treatment after even a relatively short period of perceived infertility is usually necessary.

Time is a particularly significant factor where the diagnosis is one of idiopathic or 'unexplained' infertility. As the graph below shows (Figure 19.6), the chance of pregnancy occurring after more than three years have elapsed if the diagnosis is one of 'unexplained' infertility is sufficiently low that intervention with either stimulated IUI or IVF is justified at this point, even though there is objectively 'nothing wrong'.

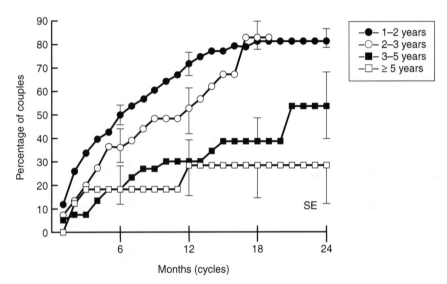

Fig. 19.6. Cumulative conception rates in couples with 'unexplained' infertility, related to duration of infertility at time of referral. SE, standard error.

The need to safeguard fertility

The expectation of successful fecundity is so great nowadays that it cannot be stressed too strongly the need to safeguard future fertility considerations in even apparently unrelated medical conditions. One in a thousand children in the UK will become adult survivors of serious malignant diseases such as leukaemia and Hodgkin's lymphoma. Many life-saving therapies such as chemotherapy, radiotherapy and total body irradiation (TBI) prior to bone marrow transplant may have profound consequences for the individual's future fertility.

Women who have a partner with whom they may wish to have a child in the future may be offered IVF with cryopreservation of embryos before starting their cancer treatment. Some women without a partner at the time of their diagnosis may elect to undergo an IVF cycle and have embryos created from their eggs with donor sperm. For very young women, the technique of cryopreservation of mature eggs generated in an ovarian hyperstimulation cycle is still at the experimental stage, and although some 20 healthy babies have been born worldwide following IVF of cryopreserved eggs, clinicians should be guarded in their optimism about this technique. Psychologically, however, it can be very valuable for the young patient about to undergo cancer treatment (and her parents) to know that there is, at least, a chance that she may be able to bear her own genetic children one day. Cryopreservation of ovarian tissue, with the hope that *in vitro* maturation of primordial follicles to produce oocytes suitable for IVF is another option that can be offered to young women about to undergo potentially sterilizing cancer therapy. Storage of mature gametes can only take place in HFEA-licensed centres, and at present, oocytes derived from cryopreserved ovarian tissue cannot be used for fertility treatment.

Post-pubertal men who are going to undergo chemotherapy, radiotherapy or orchidectomy should be offered the opportunity to 'bank' sperm with a view to future use in artificial insemination by husband (AIH), IUI or IVF cycles. Spermatozoa are usually obtained from the ejaculate but when this is impossible, it is feasible to obtain sperm directly by testicular needle biopsy (TESA) or aspiration of the epididymis (PESA) for cryopreservation and subsequent use in ICSI–IVF cycles. It should be recognised that sperm parameters often deteriorate very rapidly at an early stage in severe malignant illness and discussion about the possibility of sperm banking should not be delayed.

For pre-pubertal boys sperm storage is not an option. Spermarche occurs at a median age of 13.4 (range: 11.7–15.3) years and, with ICSI, normal fertilization can be achieved with immature sperm (round and elongated spermatids) although this is not currently an HFEA-licensed procedure in the UK. Storage of testicular material from a boy who has reached Tanner stage 2 is a licensable activity under the HFEA. Thus, consent to storage of testicular tissue cannot be given on behalf of any boy who has reached Tanner stage 2. If a boy is pre-pubertal (Tanner stage 1), his testicular tissue can be stored on unlicensed premises since it does not contain gametes within the meaning of the Human Fertilization and Embryology Act. If such material were subsequently to be developed *in vitro* to create gametes, effective consent and a licence would be required.

In women, relatively minor surgical interventions, such as laparotomy for appendicitis and salpingectomy for ectopic pregnancy, may have devastating consequences for future fertility, and it is vital that minimally invasive and/or conservative surgery is undertaken wherever future fertility may be an issue. These issues are equally relevant when treating young children and adolescents as – for example – failure to recognize and treat undescended testes in young boys (ideally orchidopexy should be performed before the age of three) or failing adequately to treat possible pelvic sepsis in young women; both of which may have disastrous consequences for future fertility. Delayed diagnosis and inadequate treatment of pelvic infection continues to be a common cause of avoidable tubal factor infertility and too many cystic or endometriotic ovaries are removed when more limited, if technically more difficult, surgery would have been preferable in the interests of fertility conservation. A young woman who is to undergo bilateral oophorectomy for ovarian teratoma should have her uterus preserved (and cyclical hormone replacement therapy prescribed) since she could achieve pregnancy in future by means of ovum donation and IVF.

Risks associated with fertility treatment

Approximately 25% of female factor infertility is due to disorders of ovulation, of which the numerically most significant is that characterized by hormone imbalance as in polycystic ovarian syndrome (PCOS). Twenty percent of all women have polycystic ovaries on ultrasound scan, but only a minority will have significant fertility problems due to hyperandrogenism and irregular ovulation. The underlying pathogenesis of PCOS, however, involves a fundamental disorder of metabolism including increased insulin resistance, and these women are at increased risk of obesity, endometrial hyperplasia, hypertension and type-II diabetes. In anovular women with PCOS, standard therapy involves increasing endogenous FSH levels by giving anti-oestrogens such as clomiphene citrate. This treatment proves effective at inducing regular ovulation in approximately 50% of women so treated and the majority of those will conceive. The side effects are generally minimal, the incidence of twin pregnancies is significantly increased over the background rate (10%), but with ultrasound monitoring, greater degrees of multiple pregnancy are rare.

Patients who fail to respond to oral therapy may be treated with injected gonadotrophins (either human menopausal gonadotrophin [HMG] or purified/recombinant FSH). This treatment is most likely to achieve superovulation (the production of multiple, mature ovarian follicles) and is associated with two significant risks which are sufficiently serious that gonadotrophin therapy should only be undertaken in centres equipped with facilities for ovarian scanning and rapid oestradiol assessment.

Ovarian hyperstimulation syndrome

The most significant risk associated with superovulation is that of ovarian hyperstimulation syndrome (OHSS), which occurs in approximately 2% of ovulation induction or IVF cycles. The rapid enlargement of the ovaries, due to the presence of multiple maturing follicles which secrete large amounts of oestradiol, may result in abdominal distension with bloating, pain, ascites, nausea and vomiting. Severe haemoconcentration is marked by oligouria and renal shut-down and abnormalities of coagulation leading to stroke, thrombosis and adult respiratory distress syndrome (ARDS) can prove fatal. The syndrome is explained by a sudden increase in capillary permeability, induced by prostaglandin synthesis, stimulated in part by excess oestrogens. There follows intravascular haemoconcentration and a hypoproteinaemic state, with hepatic and renal dysfunction. The accumulation of ascites may be associated with pleural effusions, and the patient requires urgent hospitalization and may need high-dependency care. If human chorionic gonadotrophin (hCG) has been given to trigger ovulation, or if pregnancy occurs, the time course and severity of OHSS is extended; thus, hCG should be withheld (or embryo transfer cancelled and all embryos cryopreserved in an IVF cycle) if the clinician judges the woman to be at significant risk of OHSS.

High multiple pregnancies

The risk of multiple pregnancy is present in all fertility treatments involving superovulation, such as ovulation induction, stimulated IUI, GIFT (gamete intrafallopian transfer) and IVF–ET (embryonic transfer). Half of all triplet pregnancies conceived in the UK are the result of IVF treatment and many of the others result from ovulatory therapies such as clomiphene citrate or gonadotrophins. Around 25% of all conception cycles following IVF, GIFT or stimulated IUI will result in multiple pregnancies (twins or higher order) compared with <1% in spontaneous conceptions. A twin pregnancy is often welcomed, or even actively sought, by couples with longstanding infertility problems, but all multiple pregnancies have significant consequences that need to be assessed at several levels. There are risks to the mother and her babies and costs to the community resulting from the distortion these pregnancies produce in the provision of obstetric and neonatal care. There are also less tangible, but nevertheless significant, risks associated with even successful multiple pregnancies. 'Instant' families produced by the arrival of triplets or even higher order multiple births are subject to great psychological, emotional and financial stress.

Multiple births are associated with a significant risk of prematurity: twins typically being delivered before 36 weeks gestation and triplets before 34 weeks. Modern neonatal intensive care offers a reasonable chance of intact survival for babies born even as early as 26 weeks gestation, but multiples at 26 weeks are likely to be of lower birth weight and have a generally poorer prognosis. Just two sets of premature triplets delivering simultaneously can effectively overwhelm a Special Care Baby Unit for many weeks, since their neonatal needs, involving assisted ventilation, parenteral nutrition and intensive care nursing, impose a great strain both on healthcare resources *and* their parents.

Premature babies have a significantly higher neonatal death rate than do full-term infants, and multiple pregnancy is the most common cause of prematurity. Triplets are about six times (twins, three times) more likely to be stillborn and twelve times (twins, five times) more likely to die than singletons in the first year of their life. Babies born very prematurely are also more likely to have complications that can lead to long-term morbidity and handicap. Triplet pregnancies produce a child with cerebral palsy 47 times more often than a singleton pregnancy. The rate for cerebral palsy in twins is 7.4 per thousand births and for triplets 26.7, compared with 1.6 for singletons.

The current recommendation of the RCOG is that two, rather than the maximum allowable (ie three), embryos should be transferred in most embryo transfers following IVF–ET and especially in the case of young women and women with previous IVF pregnancies.

Recent legal cases – both in the UK and the United States – have highlighted the need for clinicians working in the field of assisted reproduction to provide evidence to demonstrate that couples at risk of multiple pregnancy (ie those couples requesting more than two embryos to be transferred at ET following IVF) were appropriately counselled about the risks of multiple pregnancy and gave full, written informed consent.

High-order multiple pregnancies can be detected by ultrasound scan as early as three weeks post-ovulation and the technique of selective fetal reduction (which is covered by the revised Abortion Act 1967 (amended 1990), may be used to reduce the pregnancy to twins or a singleton. This technique, which involves passing a fine needle under ultrasound guidance into some of the supernumery gestational sacs (ideally before 12 weeks gestation), thus preventing any further embryonic development, is associated with a 10% risk of losing the entire pregnancy and a similar risk of provoking a significantly premature delivery. These risks must be balanced against the statistically greater risk that a high multiple pregnancy will end in a spontaneous miscarriage or the premature delivery of non-viable infants if the reduction is not attempted. It has been estimated that for any triplet pregnancy, selective reduction to twins at 12 weeks gestation or earlier would significantly increase the chance of at least one healthy baby being born. The technique of selective fetal reduction must not, however, be regarded as a 'safety net' to relieve clinicians of the responsibility for producing high-order births, and strenuous efforts should be made to avoid multiple conceptions, even if this does mean accepting a lower overall pregnancy rate.

Other risks associated with GIFT and IVF–ET

Both IVF and GIFT also involve hazards associated with egg collection. Laparoscopic egg collection and gamete transfer require a general anaesthetic and an extended conventional laparoscopy. IVF is usually performed under ultrasound guidance with the patient sedated with intravenous sedo-analgesia. In both techniques, there is a small but non-negligible risk of bleeding, perforation of other pelvic organs, infection and abscess formation. Many infertile women undergoing IVF may have had extensive pelvic surgery for tubal disease, ectopic pregnancy or endometriosis and are clearly at higher risk during apparently routine laparoscopic or ultrasonic egg retrieval.

Ovarian cancer and assisted conception

Several series of cases of ovarian cancer occurring in women treated with fertility drugs have been published. However, interpretation of the data has often been masked by methodological flaws, as well as difficulties separating known risk factors, such as low parity and infertility, from any effect of controlled ovarian stimulation. Ovarian cancer is the most common cause of death from gynaecological malignancy, but it presents at a late stage and the peak incidence is during the mid-sixties. Ovarian cancer decreases significantly with increased parity by a mechanism probably similar to that demonstrated for the contraceptive pill in that the overall number of ovulations are reduced. Since infertility itself is a significant risk factor for gynaecological malignancy, the current available data do not lead to a firm link between fertility drugs and ovarian cancer. The current recommendation of the Committee of Safety of Medicines, however, is that anovulatory women should be restricted to a lifetime maximum of six to 12 cycles of ovulation induction with clomiphene citrate.

Pregnancy outcome after IVF

Recorded rates of spontaneous abortion in IVF pregnancies are higher than those following spontaneous conception. Early reports gave figures of >20% spontaneous abortion and 2–4% ectopic pregnancy. The 'vanishing twin' syndrome, in which a multiple pregnancy undergoes spontaneous reduction leading to a live birth of a singleton or twins from an original triplet or twin pregnancy, is a relatively common occurrence. Although most of the increased incidence of miscarriage after IVF may be attributed to the number of multiple pregnancies and advanced maternal age, there is an excess rate in IVF singleton pregnancies. However, recent studies that restrict comparisons to singleton data have shown that there are no significant excess risks of prematurity, low birthweight or pregnancy morbidity over pregnancies resulting from ovulation induction without ART.

The incidence of maternal complications in pregnancy is generally reassuringly low for singletons. Major complication such as placenta praevia (1.6%), placental abruption (2%) and gestational diabetes (2%) are no more common than in spontaneous conceptions. The exception is the high incidence of pregnancy-associated hypertension (9.6%), which, at about twice the expected figure, may represent a problem of early placentation and early development secondary to IVF and ET.

During the early years of IVF, most IVF pregnancies – singletons *and* multiples – were delivered by Caesarean section. Now, at least for singleton pregnancies, the elective Caesarean rate is comparable to that of an age-matched population. However, the complex obstetric and gynaecological histories of IVF patients, and the high level of anxiety surrounding an IVF delivery, means that there is earlier and more frequent resort to instrumental or operative deliveries *intra partum*.

Future trends in assisted conception

The new technologies of ICSI and testicular sperm extraction (TESE), allied with cryopreservation of oocytes and embryos, have revolutionized the way in which society looks at reproductive behaviour and relationships. Now that it is possible to separate – both temporally and spatially – the acts of gamete production or extraction from those of fertilization or conception, society and the clinician working in the field of assisted conception are faced with new ethical dilemmas.

Although the success rate in establishing pregnancies from cryopreserved oocytes (as opposed to embryos) is low, the existence of this technology does theoretically allow women to put their reproductive options 'on hold'. Similarly contentious is the use of cryopreserved sperm from a deceased partner to impregnate or otherwise achieve a pregnancy in the surviving spouse. The Warnock Report, which gave rise to the Human Fertilisation and Embryology Act (1990), considered the issue of the posthumous use of gametes and expressed grave misgivings because of the presumed profound psychological problems these pregnancies could cause for mother and child. The Act did not prohibit the retrieval, storage and use of such gametes, but required the written consent of the gamete donor before retrieval.

Whatever the legal status of gametes or even embryos cryopreserved after or beyond the death of their 'genetic origin', the sheer speed of research-based developments in this field is such that clinicians may encounter scenarios not envisaged when legislation was framed. Of particular relevance is the responsibility of the clinicians and scientists involved in the handling and storage of gametes and embryos to ensure that they are identified accurately and adequately safeguarded against accidental damage, contamination or destruction.

Bibliography

Barlow DH. Short- and long-term risks for women having IVF – what is the evidence? *Human Fertility* 1999; 2: 102–106.

Botting B, MacFarlane AJ, Price FV (eds.) *Three, Four or More: a Study of Triplet and Higher Order Births.* London: HMSO, 1990.

Hull MGR. Indication for assisted conception. *British Medical Bulletin* 1990; 46: 358B.

Lockwood GM. Ethical dilemmas arising from the cryopreservation of gametes. *Human Fertility* 1999; 2: 115–117.

Quasim SM, Karacan M, Kemmanne E. An eight-year review of hospitalisation for ovarian hyperstimulation syndrome. *Clinical Experiments in Obstetrics and Gynaecology* 1997; 24: 45–52.

RCOG Working Party. *Storage of Ovarian and Prepubertal Testicular Tissue.* London, 2000.

RCOG. *Guidelines on the Provision of Tertiary Level Fertility Treatment.* London, 2000.

Report of the Committee of Inquiry into Human Fertilisation and Embryology. DHSS Cmnd 9314. London: HMSO, 1984.

Rossing MA, Daling JR, Weiss NS *et al.* Ovarian tumours in a cohort of infertile women. *New England Journal of Medicine* 1994; 331: 771–776.

Serour GI, Aboulgar M, Mansour R *et al.* Complications of medically assisted conception in 3500 cycles. *Fertility and Sterility* 1998; 70: 638–642.

Templeton A, Morris JK. Reducing the risks of multiple births by the transfer of two embryos after *in vitro* fertilization. *New England Journal of Medicine* 1998; 339: 573–577.

Tucker MJ, Wright G, Morton PC, Massey JB. Birth after cryopreservation of immature oocytes with subsequent *in vitro* maturation. *Fertility and Sterility* 1998; 70: 578–579.

►20

Urogynaecology

Gerry Jarvis

Introduction

The term 'urogynaecology' relates to the management of a specific group of benign pelvic disorders in women. Traditionally, the soft tissues which lie within the maternal pelvis have been divided artificially into three compartments: the anterior compartment relating to the bladder and urethra; a middle compartment relating to the ovaries, fallopian tubes, uterus and vagina; and a posterior compartment related to the rectum and anus. Such a division may be useful in defining anatomical landmarks but it is of limited value in managing patients. All three compartments require physical support to avoid prolapse and it is the same tissues that support all of these structures – namely, the pelvic floor divided into its muscular component – the lavator ani – and fascial component – the endopelvic fascia. Similarly, common pathological processes affect all of these tissues, including the effects of childbirth and ageing. Not surprisingly, pathological conditions overlap such that a woman with, say, urinary incontinence is more likely to have ano-rectal incontinence than a woman in the general population.

This chapter will discuss three major areas within urogynaecology:

1. The effect of childbirth upon urinary continence.
2. Urological damage associated with gynaecological surgery.
3. The assessment and treatment of genuine stress incontinence.

Effect of childbirth upon urinary continence

Childbirth is arguably one of the most eagerly anticipated events in the life of any woman, and for most people childbirth and its consequences are highly pleasurable experiences. However, for a significant minority of women, the complications of childbirth are a source of misery.

The complications of vaginal childbirth do not necessary need to have a high incidence for there to be a significant population problem. There are approximately 600,000 vaginal deliveries in England and Wales every year and it requires only a low incidence of complication to produce a large number of significant clinical problems which may or may not be associated with an allegation of negligence. That negligence may not simply relate to the management of particular problems; it may also include an increasing risk of litigation related to informed choice. All obstetricians currently are aware that not only is the Caesarean section rate within the UK rising, but there is an increasing request from healthy pregnant women to be allowed elective Caesarean section as a prophylaxis against some of the potential problems of vaginal childbirth. This appears to have been embraced by some female obstetricians – in a recent survey, 31% said they would prefer elective Caesarean section to vaginal delivery and 80% of those who would choose Caesarean section do so because of fear of perineal damage.[1]

Urinary incontinence

Urinary incontinence is defined as involuntary loss of urine that is a social or hygienic problem and is objectively demonstrable. The most common cause of urinary incontinence in women of reproductive age is genuine stress incontinence, but other causes, including detrusor instability and a vesico-vaginal fistula, must be excluded.

Whilst the management of this condition will be discussed later in the chapter, the association between genuine stress incontinence and pregnancy and childbirth is important.

Urinary incontinence occurring for the first time during pregnancy is different from that which occurs for the first time following delivery. Pregnancy is associated with a large increase in circulating levels of progesterone, which relaxes smooth muscle and predisposes to urinary incontinence. Similarly, the greatly increased intra abdominal pressure related to the weight of a fetus, liquor and increased uterine muscle mass may also predispose towards transient genuine stress incontinence. It is the genuine stress incontinence that occurs for the first time following delivery that is of greater importance, since that which occurs for the first time during pregnancy generally regresses spontaneously following delivery.

Vaginal delivery predisposes to genuine stress incontinence in a number of ways, including the following:

1. Mechanical strain upon the pelvic floor, both lavator ani muscle and endopelvic fascia, during pregnancy augmented by the potential for tears of the pelvic floor during labour and childbirth.
2. Damage, particularly during the second stage of labour, to the pudendal nerve, which runs through the pelvis, crossing the ischial spines, and supplies striated muscle within the wall of the urethra – the so-called distal urethral sphincter. (The pudendal nerve also supplies the external anal sphincter.)

Caesarean section may protect against genuine stress incontinence, which relates to the effect of labour and delivery but cannot protect against the less severe and more transient incontinence related to pregnancy itself. In a large study from New Zealand,[2] it was demonstrated that 8% of all women in their first pregnancy had noted some degree of urinary stress incontinence before pregnancy, 27.2% noted incontinence arising for the first time during pregnancy, whilst 7.6% complained of genuine stress incontinence occurring for the first time following delivery. As a generalization, it was incontinence that arose for the first time following delivery which was the most disruptive for the patient.[2]

When the New Zealand data is analysed in greater detail, it may be found that 24.5% of all women had some evidence of urinary incontinence following their first vaginal delivery compared with only 5.2% who delivered their first child by Caesarean section. The New Zealand data found no association between the risk of incontinence and such factors as the length of labour, the length of the second stage, the type of vaginal delivery, or the birthweight of the baby. The only factor which seemed to predict incontinence following vaginal delivery in this study was increased pre-pregnancy weight.

The Berkshire Episiotomy Trial[3] found a significant persistence of urinary incontinence following vaginal delivery. Some 4% of women had urinary incontinence three years after vaginal delivery regardless of whether they were in the restricted episiotomy or liberal episiotomy group.

Whilst it may be difficult to separate mechanical tearing of pelvic tissues from pudendal nerve injury as aetiological factors, the evidence does suggest that denervation is the more important factor. Neurophysiological studies[4-6] have demonstrated a reduced rate of conduction of nerve impulses in the pudendal nerve in women with genuine stress incontinence compared with women without pelvic pathology. Single-fibre electromyography (EMG) studies of the pubococcygeus muscle have suggested changes compatible with both denervation and re-innervation of this muscle, whilst histological and histochemical studies of biopsy samples have shown evidence compatible with a denervation injury.

Urological damage associated with gynaecological surgery

It is not uncommon in clinical practice that women who have previously undergone a hysterectomy for benign gynaecological disease date any subsequent symptoms of bowel dysfunction to the previous hysterectomy. There is, in fact, conflicting scientific information as to whether or not such an association is causal. The bladder is in close proximity to the uterus and hysterectomy involves the dislocation of the posterior wall of the bladder from the anterior wall of the uterus and at least in theory allows for a mechanism by which bladder function could be altered, either to the benefit or detriment of the patient. Theoretically, such an alteration in terms of detriment could be reflected in terms of a urinary voiding disorder or the onset of genuine stress incontinence.

There is evidence – both in terms of symptoms and in terms of neurophysiological studies – that abdominal hysterectomy for benign disease may cause an increase in lower urinary tract symptoms. Parys et al.[7] demonstrated that there was an increase in lower urinary tract symptoms from 58% in women before hysterectomy to 75% following, of which the major increase was in relation to urinary frequency and incomplete bladder emptying. Moreover, neurophysiological studies demonstrated an increase in pudendal nerve latency following hysterectomy.

Prospective series have not always confirmed such an increase. In a series comparing the effects of hysterectomy with the effects of dilatation and curettage, which obviously cannot disrupt bladder function, there were no significant differences.[8] Others have demonstrated a similar finding comparing symptoms before and after abdominal hysterectomy with symptoms before and after endometrial ablation, which similarly would not be expected to disrupt bladder function.[9] However, it may be that there is an incidence of disturbance of bladder function following hysterectomy, especially a voiding disorder, but that the incidence of such a complication is so small that the studies have not been powerful enough to identify it.

If the chance of bladder dysfunction following hysterectomy is real, albeit small, then it ought to occur less frequently with subtotal hysterectomy than with total abdominal hysterectomy, since in the former less dislocation of the bladder is required. There is early evidence that following subtotal hysterectomy, voiding disorder is less common. In a series of 105 women undergoing total abdominal hysterectomy, 28.6% of patients reported pre-operative incomplete bladder emptying compared with 22.1% postoperatively.[10] In a series of 107 women undergoing subtotal hysterectomy, 35.5% reported incomplete bladder emptying pre-operatively but only 10.3% postoperatively.[10] Further studies are needed, and indeed are in progress, but it would seem that many patients undergoing hysterectomy have symptoms of lower urinary tract dysfunction prior to surgery, that surgery may not increase such symptoms, but that there is frequently an inadequate recording of such symptoms in pre-operative clerking.

Of more serious risk to the patient is the chance of bladder injury or ureteric injury at the time of gynaecological surgery in general and hysterectomy in particular. The close proximity of the bladder to the uterus has already been noted and the ureters run along the pelvic side wall, being crossed by the uterine artery and vein and lying some 1–2 cm lateral to the supra-vaginal cervix. From this point, both ureters then curve medially towards the bladder and hence even closer to the uterus.

Good surgical technique will reduce the likelihood of injury to bladder or ureter. The ureter is at particular risk when clamps are placed or sutures inserted. Appropriate surgical practice is to be aware of the anatomy of the ureter and never to clamp or ligate until the ureter has been excluded from the operative field either by visual identification or by attempting to roll the ureter between finger and thumb. However, there are occasions when the ureter is difficult to identify, perhaps because of the pathology for which the hysterectomy is to be performed.

It is during operations for cancer, endometriosis and pelvic inflammatory disease that the anatomy of the ureter, including its blood supply, is most likely to be disturbed. In such difficult cases, it should be possible to identify the ureter as it crosses the pelvic brim at the bifurcation of the common iliac vessels and trace the ureter down into the operation site, but the presence of fibrosis may make it virtually impossible to identify (and therefore to protect) the ureter with absolute certainty when there is significant pathology present.

The bladder is at greatest risk of injury whilst opening the peritoneum and whilst separating the bladder from the uterus. By emptying the bladder pre-operatively and by the use of transillumination, the risk of injury to the bladder whilst opening should not occur. When separating the bladder from the uterus there is, in the absence of previous surgery, a satisfactory plane of cleavage and the two structures should be identifiable and the bladder uninjured. However, in the presence of previous surgery, especially previous Caesarean section, this plane of cleavage may be lost; there may be only a thin layer of scar tissue separating the bladder from the uterus and however careful the surgeon, the bladder might be inadvertently opened at this point.

A major complication of bladder or ureteric injury is the creation of a fistula. As can be seen from Table 20.1, vesico-vaginal fistula complicates one total abdominal hysterectomy per 1000, only 0.2 vaginal hysterectomies per 1000, and is rare after subtotal hysterectomy. Uretero-vaginal fistula is more common after total abdominal hysterectomy than subtotal (0.4 compared with 0.3 per 1000) and occurs in 0.2 per 1000 vaginal hysterectomies. Both types of fistula are more common after laparoscopically assisted vaginal hysterectomy than after open surgery.[11]

Table 20.1.

Operation	UVF per 1000	VVF per 1000
Laparoscopically assisted vaginal hysterectomy	13.9	2.2
Total abdominal hysterectomy	0.4	1.0
Subtotal	0.3	0
Vaginal hysterectomy	0.2	0.2

UVF, uretero-vaginal fistula; VVF, vesico-vaginal fistula.

If there is recognition at the time of surgery that either the bladder has been opened or the ureter injured, immediate repair is indicated. Closure of the bladder should be within the capability of all gynaecological surgeons and most surgeons would close the bladder in two layers, drain the bladder with a catheter for a variable period of time postoperatively (views seem to vary between seven and ten days) and ideally a cystogram should be performed in the X-ray department in order to check the integrity of the bladder before the catheter is removed. Ureteric injury may require splinting, re-anastomosis or re-implantation into the bladder and whilst this may be within the expertise of a small number of gynaecologists, most would require the assistance of a urological surgeon to complete repair.

A vesico-vaginal fistula occurs postoperatively for one of several reasons. There may have been a cystotomy unrecognized at the time of operation; therefore, there would be haematuria in the immediate postoperative period. If there was a cystotomy and it was recognized, then almost always the bladder would heal without complication.

In other circumstances, the bladder is intact at the end of the procedure but leaks subsequently because of avascular necrosis. Classically, such a fistula becomes manifest between seven and ten days postoperatively. There are numerous causes for avascular necrosis, including previous gynaecological surgery, partial thickness injury of the bladder wall with an instrument, or the insertion of a suture inadvertently through the bladder. A haematoma between the bladder wall and vagina may discharge into both creating a fistula.

If a fistula is suspected, it may be confirmed by a variety of methods, including the finding of a pool of urine in the vagina on speculum examination, the leakage of blue fluid after the insertion of methylene blue into the bladder, cystoscopy, or micturating cystogram. A vesico-vaginal fistula may heal spontaneously after a period of catheter drainage; but if catheter drainage fails, surgical intervention is required. Depending upon the clinical circumstances and the experience of the surgeon, such surgery may be transabdominal or transvaginal and with or without the interposition of a piece of tissue (omentum or Martius fat pad) between the closed bladder defect and the closed vaginal defect. Regardless of the approach taken, primary repair of an uncomplicated fistula is associated with a success rate in excess of 80%.[12]

The presentation of a uretero-vaginal fistula depends to some degree upon the site of the fistula and its cause. The ureter may become obstructed either by encirclement of a suture or by kinking related to a suture placed near the ureter but not through or around the ureter. There may be a diathermy injury. All three of these mechanisms will result in avascular necrosis, with the fistula becoming apparent in the postoperative period – usually beyond the 4th or 5th day and in almost any timecourse thereafter. Indeed, silent obstruction of a ureter is well recognized. If the mechanism is division of the ureter intra-operatively then the fistula will be apparent within a very short period of time postoperatively. If a uretero-vaginal fistula is suspected, either an intravenous urogram or an ultrasound scan should be performed. In ureteric obstruction, a temporary percutaneous nephrostomy may be required to salvage renal function.

Once a fistula is confirmed, the two most important principles of management relate to making the patient continent and to the preservation of renal function on the affected side. Repair generally will involve a urological colleague and, depending upon the circumstances, will involve either retrograde stenting of the ureter or ureteric re-implantation with or without a Boari flap or psoas hitch.

Assessment and treatment of genuine stress incontinence

Genuine stress is the commonest cause of urinary incontinence in adult women. Possible aetiological factors have already been described above. Treatment may be conservative, involving some form of pelvic floor exercise regime, or surgical. The choice between these major modalities will depend upon a number of factors, including the severity of the incontinence, the presence or absence of previous intervention, and the wish of the patient.

The single most important issue before embarking upon surgery for genuine stress incontinence is to ensure that the diagnosis is correct and that co-existing pathology is not present, which, if recognized, may influence the choice of therapy.

It has long been acknowledged that the symptom of stress incontinence is not pathognomonic of the condition of genuine stress incontinence. History will undoubtedly assess the severity of the incontinence but not necessarily the diagnosis. The most important symptoms to assess are the presence or absence of stress incontinence, urgency and urge incontinence. If the only symptom present is stress incontinence, it would be reasonable to progress to surgical intervention without confirming the diagnosis on a filling cystometrogram, since the chance of there being detrusor instability is small. If the patient should admit to urgency but no urge incontinence as well as the symptom of stress incontinence, however, there is a 10% chance of detrusor instability. Should she admit to urgency, urge incontinence and stress incontinence, there is a 41% chance of detrusor instability. Under such circumstances, it is inappropriate to offer surgery for genuine stress incontinence without confirming the diagnosis with a urodynamic assessment.[13]

An equally important co-existing pathology to exclude is a voiding disorder. Virtually all operations for genuine stress incontinence are to some degree obstructive and the most successful operations are potentially the most obstructive. Some degree of voiding disorder will be found, for instance, in 12.5% of patients following colposuspension and in 10.4% of patients after a pubo-vaginal sling.[14] If a voiding disorder is already present pre-operatively, there is a risk that the patient may ultimately require intermittent clean self-catheterization for life following surgical intervention. It is therefore important to exclude a pre-existing voiding disorder.

The classical symptoms of a voiding disorder – namely hesitancy, poor stream and incomplete bladder emptying – are frequently unrecognized in women and only 40% of those women with a urodynamically demonstrated voiding disorder will complain of such symptoms.[15] A voiding disorder can only therefore be excluded by a pre-operative urodynamic voiding study. If there is no evidence of a voiding disorder, the surgeon can choose the procedure that would appear to be the most appropriate for the patient; but if there *is* a voiding disorder, the choice lies between a less obstructive procedure – even though that will mean a lesser chance of urinary incontinence – or a procedure with a greater chance of restoring continence but with a risk of the need for clean intermittent self-catheterization.

None of the surgical procedures described for the treatment of genuine stress incontinence are associated with a 100% cure rate. Depending upon the procedure chosen, the patient can expect a cure rate of between 45% and 94%.[14] Guidance on the choice of procedure has been provided recently by both the American Urological Association and the World Health Organization.[16,17] Both have come, not surprisingly, to similar conclusions. To quote the advice of the American Urological Association, 'Surgical treatment of female stress urinary incontinence is effective, offering a long-term cure in a significant percentage of women. The evidence supports surgery as initial therapy or in the secondary form of therapy after failure of other treatments for stress urinary incontinence. Retropubic colposuspension and slings are the most efficacious procedures for long-term success based on pure-dry rates'.[16] In specific circumstances, however, the patient and surgeon might opt for less efficacious forms of treatment, including the anterior repair and bladder buttress, long needle suspensions, or the injection of materials such as collagen into the wall of the proximal urethra.[14,17]

References

1 Al-Mufti A, McCarthy A, Fisk NM. Obstetricians' personal choice and mode of delivery. *Lancet* 1996; 347: 544.
2 Wilson PD, Herbison GP. Obstetric practice and the prevalence of urinary incontinence 3 months after delivery. *British Journal of Obstetrics and Gynaecology* 1996; 103: 154–161.
3 Sleep J, Grant A. West Berkshire Perineal Management Trial. *British Medical Journal* 1987; 295: 749–781.

4   Smith ARB, Hosker GL, Warrell DW. The role of pudendal nerve damage in the aetiology of genuine stress incontinence. *British Journal of Obstetrics and Gynaecology* 1989; 96: 29–32.

5   Varma JS, Fides A, McInnes A *et al*. Neurophysiological abnormalities in genuine female stress incontinence. *British Journal of Obstetrics and Gynaecology* 1988; 95: 705–710.

6   Gilpin SA, Gosling JA, Smith ARB *et al*. The pathogenesis of genito-urinary prolapse and stress incontinence of urine. *British Journal of Obstetrics and Gynaecology* 1989; 96: 15–23.

7   Parys BT, Haylen BT, Hutton JL *et al*. The effects of simple hysterectomy on the vesico-urethral function. *British Journal of Urology* 1989; 64: 594–599.

8   Griffiths-Jones MD, Jarvis GJ, McNamara YHM. Adverse urinary symptoms after total hysterectomy. *British Journal of Urology* 1991; 67: 295–297.

9   Bhattacharya S, Mollison J, Pinion S *et al*. A comparison of bladder and ovarian function following hysterectomy or endometrial ablation. *British Journal of Obstetrics and Gynaecology* 1996; 103: 898–903.

10   Kikku P. Supravaginal uterine amputation versus hysterectomy with reference to bladder symptoms and incontinence. *Acta Obstetrica et Gynaecological Scandinavica* 1995; 64: 375–379.

11   Harrki-Siren P, Sjoberg J, Tiitinen A. Urinary tract injuries after hysterectomy. *Obstetrics and Gynecology* 1998; 92: 113–118.

12   Stanton SL, Shah J. Recognition and management of urological complications of gynaecological surgery. *Clinical Risk* 2000; 6: 94–101.

13   Jarvis GJ, Hall S, Stamp S *et al*. An assessment of urodynamic examination in incontinent women. *British Journal of Obstetrics and Gynaecology* 1988; 87: 893–896.

14   Jarvis GJ. Surgery for genuine stress incontinence. *British Journal of Obstetrics and Gynaecology* 1994; 101: 371–374.

15   Jarvis GJ. *The Management of Urinary Incontinence in Obstetrics and Gynaecology.* Oxford: Oxford University Press. 1994, 260–299.

16   Leach GE, Dmochowski RR, Appell RA *et al*. Female stress urinary incontinence clinical guidelines. *Journal of Urology* 1997; 158: 875–880.

17   Jarvis GJ, on behalf of WHO Subcommittee. The surgery of urinary incontinence in women. In: Abrams and Khoury (eds.) *Incontinence.* London: World Health Organization. 1999, 637–668.

Index

Note: page numbers in *italics* refer to figures and tables

Also available from RSM Press

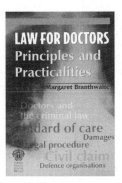

Law for Doctors
Principles and Practicalities
Margaret Branthwaite

'an excellent introduction ... concise, informative and lucid ... this book stands out from the rest.'
Medical Litigation

'This is an excellent book. I think that Dr Branthwaite has explained everything which is explicable. Every doctor would benefit from reading it.'
British Journal of Anaesthesia

This book provides a clear, concise and non-technical guide to medical law and has been written for doctors who often do not have the time or legal background to read detailed books on medical law written for lawyers. *Law for Doctors: Principles and Practicalities* focuses on aspects of English law that are particularly relevant to medical practice such as civil claims, legal procedure, funding, complaints, whistle-blowing, disciplinary proceedings, coroner's courts and criminal law.

Read a sample chapter online at www.rsm.ac.uk/pub/bkbranth.htm
£7.50 paperback, 1-85315-465-2, August 2000

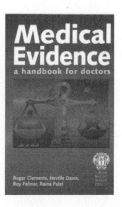

Medical Evidence
A handbook for doctors
Roger Clements, Neville Davis, Roy Palmer and Raina Patel

Every doctor will at some stage in their career need to give evidence, either as defendants, witnesses or medical experts. This book is a comprehensive guide to giving evidence in a range of different contexts, including civil, criminal and coroner's courts, as well as employment, mental-health and other tribunals.

The authors, all experienced in different areas of medico-legal practice, highlight the pitfalls of giving evidence and provide practical, reassuring advice. Recommended to all doctors and healthcare professionals involved in giving evidence, including police surgeons, staff in accident and emergency departments, occupational physicians and lawyers specializing in medico-legal practice.

£17.50 paperback, 1-85315-387-7, April 2000

Ordering information
Marston Book Services
PO Box 269, Abingdon, Oxon OX14 4YN
Tel +44 (0)1235 465550   Fax +44 (0)1235 465555
Cheques made payable to 'Marston Book Services'

Browse our book and journal catalogue & order online at www.rsmpress.co.uk

Also available from RSM Press

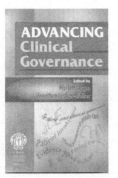

Advancing Clinical Governance
Edited by Myriam Lugon, Jonathan Secker-Walker

' ... this book is a most helpful review of current trends ... and will be of help to every clinician.'
Hospital Doctor'

'We all have to get a grip on quality control ... A good start would be to read this book. Read this and you won't be caught out in this brave new world.'
Bandolier

This long awaited follow-up to *Clinical Governance — Making it Happen* considers the implications of clinical governance for a wide range of health care professionals, including nurses, medical directors and chief executives. *Advancing Clinical Governance* will enable health professionals to implement clinical governance effectively and with confidence. This book is recommended to clinicians and managers at all levels within trusts, health care purchasers and academics.
£18.50, 1-85315-471-7, paperback, February 2001

Ordering information
Marston Book Services
PO Box 269, Abingdon, Oxon OX14 4YN
Tel +44 (0)1235 465550   Fax +44 (0)1235 465555
Cheques made payable to 'Marston Book Services'

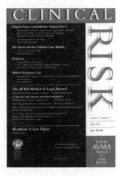

Clinical Risk
Edited by Roger V Clements

This leading journal provides best practice guidelines for doctors and risk managers and is the only journal dealing exclusively with medical negligence cases. *Clinical Risk* gives both the medical and legal professions an indispensable analysis of key medicolegal issues through authoritative articles, reviews and news on the prevention and management of clinical risk.

FREE ONLINE ACCESS FOR SUBSCRIBERS
Annual subscription **Volume 7, 2001** (6 issues starting in January), 1356-2622
Europe **£142.00**, USA **US$253.00**, Rest of the world **£146.00**

Ordering information for Clinical Risk
Publications Subscription Department
The Royal Society of Medicine Press
1 Wimpole Street, London W1G 0AE
Tel: +44 (0)20 7290 2928   Fax: +44 (0)20 7290 2929
E-mail: rsmjournals@rsm.ac.uk

Browse our book and journal catalogue & order online at www.rsmpress.co.uk